Voice Science

About the Author

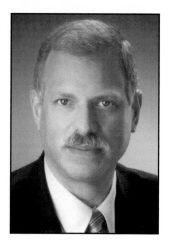

Robert Thayer Sataloff, MD, DMA, who has organized this volume especially for speech-language pathology students and clinicians who are new to the field of voice care, is Chairman of the Department of Otolaryngology-Head and Neck Surgery at the Graduate Hospital in Philadelphia and Professor of Otolaryngology-Head and Neck Surgery at Jefferson Medical College, Thomas Jefferson University. He is President-Elect of the American Laryngeal Associa-tion; Chairman of the Speech, Voice and Swallowing Committee of the American Academy of Otolaryngology-Head and Neck Surgery; and Chairman of Board of Directors of the Voice Foundation and the American Institute for Voice and Ear Research. A prolific author, Dr. Sataloff has contributed to more than 500 publications, including 23 textbooks. Dr. Sataloff is also Editor-in-Chief of the *Journal of Voice* and the *Ear, Nose and Throat Journal*.

Voice Science

Robert Thayer Sataloff, MD, DMA

Plural Publishing, Inc.

SAN DIEGO   OXFORD

PLURAL PUBLISHING
5521 Ruffin Road
San Diego, CA 92123

e-mail: info@pluralpublishing.com
Web site: http://www.pluralpublishing.com

49 Bath Street
Abingdon, Oxfordshire OX14 1EA
United Kingdom

Voice Science is one of three student editions prepared for speech-language pathology students and clinicians who are new to the field of voice care from selected chapters of the third edition of *Professional Voice: The Science and Art of Clinical Care* to provide relevant information in an affordable format.

© Plural Publishing, Inc.

Typeset in 10/12 Palatino by So Cal Graphics

For permission to use material from this text, contact us by
Telephone: (866) 758-7251
Fax: (888) 758-7255
e-mail: permissions@pluralpublishing.com

Care has been taken to confirm the accuracy of the information presented in this book and to describe generally accepted practices. However, the authors, editors, and publisher are not responsible for errors or omissions or for any consequences from application of the information in this book and make no warranty, expressed or implied, with respect to the currency, completeness, or accuracy of the contents of the publication. Application of this information in a particular situation remains the professional responsibility of the practitioner

ISBN 1-59756-038-3
Library of Congress Control Number: 2005905961

Contents

Foreword

In our time, knowledge expands at a rate that probably has never been achieved before. Some years ago, it was claimed that the number of active scientists equaled the total number of scientists who have ever been active throughout history. Thus, much effort is spent today on understanding better various aspects of the world in which we live.

This interest in scientific research is not difficult to understand. Many bad things that have happened, and that keep happening, reflect lack of understanding, lack of knowledge, and lack of competence. Often we have reasons to say: "Had I only known, I would not have made that mistake" or "Had I only known how that thing works, I could have fixed it much more efficiently."

An explosion of new knowledge has occurred in our time also in the field of voice. The reason is not merely society's thirst for new knowledge. Another important reason is that the voice is one of the most frequently used communication tools. This is true in spite of the huge amount of communication transported in digital form today. That, in turn, might be related to the fact that we tend to hover in large cities. This implies that we have contact and interaction with a great number of people. In addition to that we have the telephone, the conventional as well as its cellular cousin. Also important is that the voice is one of the most common working tools in our time. Therefore, voice disorders have a large impact on daily life for a great number of people who cannot work when their voices do not function properly; and sick-leave is quite expensive for society.

Doing research is one thing; ensuring that all the people for whom the results are relevant get to know about them is quite another. One of a researcher's nightmares is to work in vain, to write in water. This risk is not negligible. For example, it is quite difficult for a voice physician, therapist, or teacher to follow all the journals in which results of relevance to their daily work appear. If they fail, they are likely to pursue methods less efficient than the state of the art.

The solution to this problem is textbooks that compile the present state of knowledge within a specific field. Exactly this is the aim of this new and substantially expanded edition of Robert Sataloff's *Professional Voice: The Science and Art of Clinical Care*. It gives a broad overview of the many scientific aspects of voice that have been developed up to present. It is a valuable up-to-date overview of the field, and it will certainly be useful as an extensive source of knowledge for those interested in various scientific aspects of voice. The book is an impressive monument of the voice as we know it today. The portions of that book contained in this student edition entitled *Voice Science* make this important information available and affordable for those without access to the entire book. *Voice Science* should be a valuable asset for teachers and students in the communication sciences.

Johan Sundberg
KTH, June 2005

Preface

Voice Science is part of a 5-book student edition of selected chapters from the third edition of *Professional Voice: The Science and Art of Clinical Care*. That compendium fills approximately 2000 pages including 160 chapters and numerous appendices, and it is not practical for routine use by students. However, *Professional Voice: The Science and Art of Clinical Care*, Third Edition, was intended to be valuable to not only laryngologists but also to speech-language pathologists, voice teachers, performers, students, and anyone else interested in the human voice. *Voice Science* and other volumes of the student edition have been prepared to make relevant information available to students in a convenient and affordable form, suitable for classroom use as well as for reference.

Chapter 1 provides introductory information about the physics of sound and helps students understand concepts and terms such as decibels and hertz. *Chapter 2* is an exceptionally interesting chapter on Music and the Brain. It reviews much of what is known currently about central development and processing of musical information; and this science should be extremely valuable in expanding the vision of voice researchers. *Chapter 3* reviews much of what is known about genetics of the voice from a clinical perspective. *Chapter 4* offers extraordinary insight into the complex topics of genomics and proteomics as they relate to the larynx. *Chapter 5* is a classic exposition of laryngeal embryology. *Chapter 6* provides an extensive and comprehensive chapter on the clinical anatomy and physiology of the voice. It contains a great deal of information about laryngeal anatomy, neuroanatomy, respiratory function, and other topics that have not been synthesized in similar detail in a single source elsewhere. *Chapter 7* on arytenoid cartilage movement is similarly unique. In *chapter 8*, Susan Thibeault and Steven Gray summarize their extraordinary insights into the structural response to vocal fold injury. This information is essential in understanding vocal fold scar. In *chapter 9*, Leslie Malmgrem crystalizes current knowledge regarding cellular and molecular mechanics of vocal fold aging.

Chapter 10 is speculative and introductory to the voice literature. So far, little is known about the effects of nutrition on vocal aging, healing, and health in general. This chapter reviews information about one good candidate (glutathione) for clinical and basic research into the effects of nutraceutical manipulation. *Chapter 11*, Baken's overview of laryngeal function, presents the complex topic with remarkable clarity. In *chapter 12*, Ronald Scherer expands on Baken's information from chapter 11 and provides insights into more complex aspects of laryngeal function. Johan Sundberg has synthesized and summarized his many contributions to our understanding of vocal tract resonance in *chapter 13*. *Chapter 14*, Chaos and the Voice, contains basic information on chaos theory and new ideas on application of nonlinear dynamics to voice care and research. In *chapter 15*, Baken expands extensively on applications of chaos theory to understanding and caring for the human voice. *Chapter 16* by Harry Hollien capsulizes his extraordinary insights into the voice and forensic voice science and its potential for future application to clinical voice assessment.

Every effort has been made to maintain style and continuity throughout the book. Although the interdisciplinary expertise of numerous authors has been invaluable in the preparation of this text, contributions have been edited carefully where necessary to maintain consistency of linguistic style and complexity. I have written or coauthored 6 of the 16 chapters and made every effort to preserve the concept and continuity of a single-author text with generous input from colleagues, rather than an edited text with numerous authors each writing independently. This paradigm was used in a conscious effort to minimize repetition and provide consistent reading from cover to cover. All of us who have been involved in the preparation of this book hope that readers will find it not only informative but also enjoyable to read.

Robert T. Sataloff, MD, DMA

Contributors

Ronald J. Baken, PhD
Professor and Director of Laryngology Research
Department of Otolaryngology
New York Eye and Ear Infirmary
New York, New York

Rajeev Bhatia, BSEE, MS, PhD
Assistant Professor, Computer Science and
Information Science
Temple University
Narberth, Pennsylvania

Gustavo Bounous, MD, FRCS(C)
Director of Research and Development
Immunotec Research Ltd
Quebec, Canada

Mary J. Hawkshaw, RN, BSN, CORLN
Otolaryngologic Nurse Clinician
Executive Director
American Institute for Voice and Ear Research
Philadelphia, Pennsylvania

David H. Henick, MD
Clinical Assistant Professor
Department of Otolaryngology
Albert Einstein College of Medicine
New York, New York

Kelly Gilrain, MA
Psychology Intern
Department of Psychiatry
Pennsylvania Hospital
Philadelphia, Pennsylvania

Steven D. Gray, MD (deceased)
Formerly Professor and Hetzel Presidential Chair
Division of Otolaryngology–Head and Neck Surgery
Department of Surgery
University of Utah
Salt Lake City, Utah

Harry F. Hollien, PhD
Courtesy Professor
Department of Communiation Sciences and
Disorders
University of Florida
Gainesville, Florida

Thomas A. Kwyer, MD
Otolaryngologist
Private Practice
Toledo Ohio

James A. Letson, Jr., MD
Associate Clinical Professor
Michigan State University
Adjunct Faculty Member
Central Michigan University
Valley ENT Associates
Saginaw, Michigan

Leslie T. Malmgren, PhD
Professor
Department of Otolaryngology and Communication
Sciences
SUNY Upstate Medical Center
Syracuse, New York

Elisabeth Mandel, BA
Philadelphia, Pennsylvania

Steven Mandel, MD
Clinical Professor of Neurology
Thomas Jefferson University
Philadelphia, Pennsylvania

Robert Thayer Sataloff, MD, DMA
Professor
Department of Otolaryngology–Head and Neck
Surgery
Thomas Jefferson University
Adjunct Professor of Otolaryngology
Georgetown University
Chairman, Department of Otolaryngology–Head
and Neck Surgery
The Graduate Hospital
Chairman, Board of Directors
The Voice Foundation
Faculty, Academy of Vocal Arts
Faculty, The Curtis Institute of Music
Chairman, American Institute for Voice and Ear
Research
Philadelphia, Pennsylvania

Ronald C. Scherer, PhD
Professor, Department of Communication Disorders
Bowling Green State University
Bowling Green, Ohio

Johan Sundberg, PhD
Professor, Department of Speech Communication
and Music Acoustics
Royal Institute of Technology
Stockholm, Sweden

Thomas Swirsky-Sacchetti, PhD
Clinical Associate Professor Neurology and Psychiatry
Jefferson Medical College
Thomas Jefferson University
Philadelphia, Pennsylvania

Renny Tatchell, PhD
Chairman, Department of Communication
Disorders
Central Michigan University
Saginaw, Michigan

Susan L. Thibeault, PhD, CCC-SLP
Assistant Professor
Speech Language Pathology
Research Director
University of Utah School of Medicine
Division of Otolaryngology–Head and Neck Surgery
University of Utah, Primary Children's Hospital
Salt Lake City, Utah

Joseph Tracy, PhD
Associate Professor of Neurology and Radiology
Director, Neuropsychology Division
Jefferson Medical College
Thomas Jefferson University
Philadelphia, Pennsylvania

Riitta Ylitalo, MD
Associate Professor
Karolinska Institute
Department of Logopedics and Phoniatrics
Huddinge University Hospital
Stockholm, SwedenI am indebted to the many

Acknowledgments

distinguished colleagues who collaborated in writing this book. Their friendship and wisdom are appreciated greatly. I also remain indebted to the many friends and colleagues who have helped develop the field of voice over the last few decades, particularly the late Wilbur James Gould.

As always, I cannot express sufficient thanks to Mary J. Hawkshaw, RN, BSN for her tireless editorial assistance, proofreading, and scholarly contributions. Without her help, many of my books would still be unfinished. I am also indebted to Helen Caputo and Beth V. Luby for their tireless, painstaking preparation of the manuscript and for the many errors they found and corrected and to my associates Joseph Sataloff, MD, DSc, Karen M. Lyons, MD, and Yolanda D. Heman-Ackah, MD. Without their collaboration, excellent patient care, and tolerance of my many academic distractions and absences, writing would be much more difficult. In addition, I am indebted to Sandy Doyle from Plural Publishing Company, Inc. who has done a truly superb job editing this book and preparing it for publication.

My greatest gratitude goes to my wife Dahlia M. Sataloff, MD, and sons Ben and John who patiently allow me to spend so many of my evenings, weekends, and vacations writing.

Dedication

To my wife Dahlia Sataloff, MD, my sons Benjamin Harmon Sataloff and Johnathan Brandon Sataloff,
my parents Joseph Sataloff, MD and Ruth Sataloff, and my friend and editorial assistant
Mary J. Hawkshaw RN, BSN, for their unfailing patience and support
and
To Wilbur James Gould, MD, friend, scholar, educator, and founder of the Voice Foundation,
who devoted his life to improving, understanding, and caring for the human voice.

and

To Howell S. Zulick, my voice teacher for twenty-nine years and an inspiration for life.

and

To Walter P. Work, Charles J. Krause, and Malcolm D. Graham, the professors who trained me and
cultivated the love for academic medicine inspired by my father and for which he wisely sent me to Ann Arbor.

1

The Physics of Sound

Robert Thayer Sataloff

Fortunately, one need not be a physicist in order to function well in professions involved with hearing, sound, and music. However, a fundamental understanding of the nature of sound and terms used to describe it is essential to comprehend the language of otolaryngologists, audiologists, music acousticians, and engineers. Moreover, studying the basic physics of sound helps one recognize complexities and potential pitfalls in measuring and describing sound. These concepts are important to musicians interested in understanding concert hall acoustics, evaluating studies of risk from musical noise exposure, understanding the effects of vocal efficiency (like going from pressed to flow phonation), and other situations surrounding the professions above.

Sound

Sound is a form of motion. Consequently, the laws of physics that govern actions of all moving bodies apply to sound. Because sound and all acoustic conditions consistently behave as described by the laws of physics, we are able to predict and analyze the nature of a sound and its interactions. Sound measurement is not particularly simple. The study of physics helps us understand many practical aspects of our daily encounters with sound. For example, why does an audiologist or otologist use a different baseline for decibels in his office from that used by an engineer or industrial physician who measures noise in a factory? Why is it that when hearing at high frequencies is tested, a patient may hear nothing and then suddenly hear a loud tone when all the examiner did was move the earphone a fraction of an inch? Why is it when two machines are placed close together, each making 60 dB of noise, the total noise is not 120 dB?

Sound Waves

Sound is the propagation of pressure waves radiating from a vibrating body through an elastic medium. A vibrating body is essential to cause particle displacement in the propagating medium. An elastic medium is any substance or particles returned to their point of origin as soon as possible after they have been displaced. Propagation occurs because displaced particles in the medium displace neighboring particles. Therefore, sound travels over linear distance. Pressure waves are composed of areas of slightly greater than ambient air pressure compression and slightly less than ambient air pressure (rarefaction). These are associated with the bunching together or spreading apart of the particles in the propagating medium. The pressure wave makes receiving structures such as the eardrum move back and forth with the alternating pressure. For example, when a sound wave is generated by striking a tuning fork, by vocalizing, or by other means, the vibrating object moves molecules in air, causing them to be alternately compressed and rarefied in a rhythmical pattern. This sets up a chain reaction with adjacent air molecules and spreads at a rate of approximately 1100 ft/sec (the speed of sound). This is propagation of the pressure waves.

Sound requires energy. Energy is used to set a body into motion. The energy is imparted to particles in the propagating medium and is then distributed over the surface of the receiver (eardrum or microphone) in the form of sound pressure. Energy is equal to the square of pressure ($E = P^2$). However, we are unable to directly measure sound energy. Only the pressure exerted on the surface of a microphone can be quantified by sound-measuring equipment.

Characteristics of Sound Waves

Sound waves travel in straight lines in all directions from the source, decreasing in intensity at a rate inversely proportional to the square of the distance from their source. This is called the inverse-square law. This means that if a person shortens his distance from the source of a sound and moves from a position 4 feet away to only 2 feet from the source, the sound will be four times as intense rather than merely twice as intense. In practical application, this inverse-square law applies only in instances in which there are no walls or ceiling. It is not strictly valid in a room where sound waves encounter obstruction or reflection, and increasing the distance of a whisper or a ticking watch from the subject can rarely be truly accurate or reliable.

Sound waves travel through air more rapidly than through water. They are conducted through solids also at different speeds. An ear placed close to the iron rail of a train track will detect the approach of a train before the airborne sounds can reach the observer. Thus, sounds travel through different media at different speeds; the speed also varies when the medium is not uniform. However, sound waves are not transmitted through a vacuum. This can be demonstrated by the classic experiment of placing a ringing alarm clock inside a bell jar and then exhausting the air through an outlet. The ringing will no longer be heard when the air is exhausted, but it will be heard again immediately when air is readmitted. This experiment emphasizes the importance of the medium through which sound waves travel.

The bones of the head also conduct sounds, but ordinarily the ear is much more sensitive to sounds that are airborne. Under certain abnormal conditions, as in cases of conductive hearing loss, a patient may hear better by bone conduction than by air conduction. Such an individual can hear the vibrations of a tuning fork much better when it is held directly touching the skull than when it is held next to the ear but without touching the head.

Distortion of sound waves by wind is common. The effect also varies according to whether the wind blows faster near the ground or above it. When sound travels through the air and encounters an obstruction such as a wall, the sound waves can bend around the obstacle almost like water passing around a rock in a stream. The behavior of sound waves striking an object depends upon several factors, including wavelength. Sound waves may pass through an object unaffected, be reflected off the object, or may be partially reflected and partially passed through or around the object (shadow effect). Low-frequency sounds of long wavelength tend to bend (diffraction) when encountering objects, while diffraction is less prominent with sounds above 2000 Hz. The behavior of sound waves encountering an object also depends upon the nature of the object. The resistance of an object or system to the transmission of sound is called impedance. This depends upon a variety of factors such as mass reactants, stiffness reactants, and friction. The ability of an object to allow transmission of sound is called its admittance, which may be thought of as the opposite of impedance.

Components of Sound

A simple type of sound wave, called a pure tone, is pictured in Figure 1–1. This is a graphic representation of one and one-half complete vibrations, or cycles, or periods, with the area of compression represented by the top curve and the area of rarefaction by the bottom curve. Although pure tones do not occur in nature, the more complicated sounds that we actually encounter are composed of combinations of pure tones. Understanding the makeup of this relatively simple sound helps us analyze more complex sounds. Fourier analysis is used to separate complex signals into their simple tonal components.

A pure tone has several important characteristics: One complete vibration consists of one compression and one rarefaction (Fig 1–2). The number of times

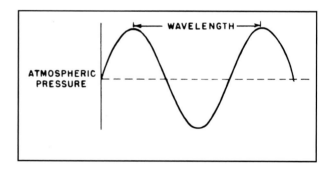

Fig 1–1. Diagram of a pure tone (sine wave).

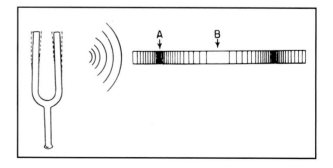

Fig 1–2. Areas of compression (A) and rarefaction (B) produced by a vibrating tuning fork.

such a cycle occurs in a given period of time (usually 1 second) is called frequency. Frequency is usually recorded in cycles per sound, or hertz. The perceptual correlate of frequency is pitch. In general, the greater the frequency, the higher the pitch, and the greater the intensity, the louder the sound. However, there is a difference between actual physical phenomena (such as frequency or intensity) and peoples' perceptions of them (pitch and loudness). A tuning fork is constructed so that it vibrates at a fixed frequency no matter how hard it is struck. However, although it will vibrate the same number of times per second, the prongs of the tuning fork will cover a greater distance when the fork is struck hard than when it is softly struck. We perceive this increased intensity as increased loudness. In the sine wave diagram of a pure tone, a more intense sound will have a higher peak and lower valley than a softer sound. Greater intensity also means that the particles in the propagating medium are more compressed. The height or depth of the sine wave is called its amplitude. Amplitude is measured in decibels (dB). It reflects the amount of pressure (or energy) existing in the sound wave.

Wavelength is the linear distance between any point in one cycle and the same point on the next cycle (peak to peak, for example). It may be calculated as the speed of sound divided by the frequency. This is also one period. Wavelength is symbolized by the Greek letter lambda (λ) and is inversely proportional to frequency (Fig 1–3). This is easy to understand. If it is recalled that sound waves travel at about 1100 ft/sec, simple divi-

sion tells us that a 1000-Hz frequency will have a wavelength of 1.1 ft/cycle. A 2000-Hz tone has a wavelength of about 6.5 inches. A 100-Hz tone has a wavelength of about 11 feet. The wavelength of a frequency of 8000 Hz would be 1100 divided by 8000, or 0.013 feet (about 1 inch). Wavelength has a great deal to do with sound penetration. For example, if someone is playing a stereo too loudly several rooms away, the bass notes will be clearly heard, but the high notes of violins or trumpets will be attenuated by intervening walls. Low-frequency sounds (long wavelengths) are extremely difficult to attenuate or absorb, and they require very different acoustic treatment from high-frequency sounds of short wavelengths. Fortunately, they are also less damaging to hearing.

Any point along the cycle of the wave is its phase. Because a sine wave is a cyclical event, it can be described in degrees like a circle. The halfway point of the sine wave is the 180-degree phase point. The first peak occurs at 90 degrees, etc. The interaction of two pure tones depends on their phase relationship. For example, if the two sound sources are identical and are perfectly in phase, the resulting sound will be considerably more intense than either one alone (constructive inference). If they are 180 degrees out of phase, they will theoretically nullify each other and no sound will be heard (destructive interference) (Fig 1–4). This is the principle behind the concept of anti-sound, which is a sound generated to silence an unwanted sound that is equally loud but of opposite phase (180° phase). Interaction of sound forces also depends upon other com-

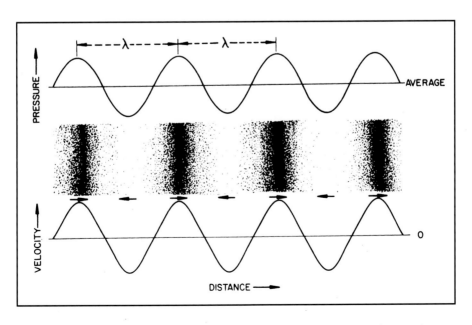

Fig 1–3. Diagram showing wavelength in relation to other components of a sound wave. (Adapted from Van Bergeijk.[1])

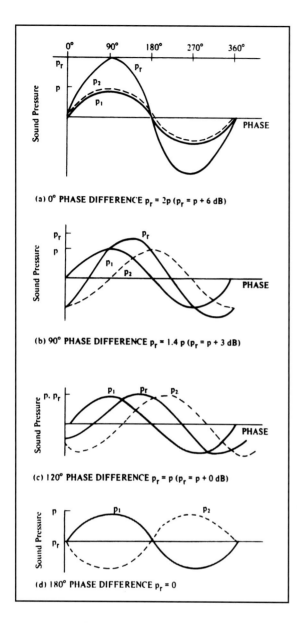

Fig 1–4. Combination of two pure tone noises (p_1 and p_2) with various phase differences.

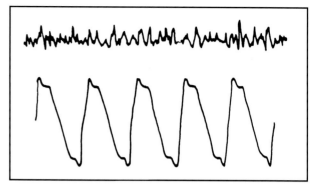

Fig 1–5. Upper graph, typical street noise. Lower graph, C on a piano.

plicated factors such as resonance, which is affected by the environment and the characteristics of the receiver (such as the ear canal and ear).

Speech, music, and noise are complex sounds rather than pure tones. Most sounds are very complex with many different wave forms superimposed on each other. Musical tones are usually related to one another and show a regular pattern (complex periodic sound), whereas street noise shows a random pattern (complex aperiodic sound) (Fig 1–5).

It is somewhat difficult to accurately define noise, because so much of its meaning depends on its effect at any specific time and place, rather than on its physical characteristics. Sound in one instance or by one individual may be considered as very annoying noise, whereas on another occasion or to another observer the same sound may seem pleasant and undeserving of being designated "noise." For the purpose of this book, the term "noise" is used broadly to designate any unwanted sound.

An interesting aspect of sound waves is a phenomenon called the standing wave. Under certain circumstances, two wave trains of equal amplitude and frequency traveling in opposite directions can cancel out at certain points called "nodes." Figure 1–6 is a diagram of such a situation. It will be noted that when a violin string is plucked in a certain manner, at point "n" (node) there is no displacement. If this point falls at the eardrum, the listener will not be aware of any sound because the point has no amplitude and cannot excite the ear. This phenomenon occasionally occurs in hearing tests, particularly in testing at 8000 Hz and above. These higher frequencies are likely to be involved, because the ear canal is about 2.5 cm long and the wavelength of sound at such high frequencies is of the same order of magnitude. The point of maximum displacement is called the antinode.

Furthermore, when sound waves are produced within small enclosures, as when an earphone is placed over the ear, the sound waves encounter many reflections and much of the sound at high frequencies is likely to be in the form of standing waves. Such waves often do not serve as exciting stimuli to the inner ear and no sensation of hearing is produced because of the absence of transmission of sound energy.

Sometimes, by simply holding the earphone a little more tightly or loosely to the ear in testing the higher frequencies, suddenly no sound may be produced at all when it should be loud, or a loud sound may be heard when a moment before there seemed to be no sound. This phenomenon occurs because of the presence of standing waves. During hearing testing, one often uses modulated or "warbled" tones to help eliminate standing wave problems that might result in misleading test results. Analogous but more complex problems may occur in acoustical environments such as concert halls.

In addition, resonant characteristics of the ear canal play a role in audition. Just like organ pipes and soda bottles, the ear may be thought of as a pipe. It is closed at one end and has a length of about 2.5 cm. Its calculated resonant frequency is approximately 3400 Hz (actually 3430 Hz if the length is exactly 2.5 cm and if the ear were really a straight pipe). At such a resonant frequency, a node occurs at the external auditory meatus (opening to the ear canal), and an antinode is present at the tympanic membrane, resulting in sound pressure amplification at the closed end of the pipe (ear drum). This phenomenon may cause sound amplification of up to 20 dB between 2000 and 5000 Hz. The res-

onance characteristics of the ear canal change if the open end is occluded, such as with an ear insert or muff used for hearing testing; and such factors must be taken into account during equipment design and calibration and when interpreting hearing tests.

The form of a complex sound is determined by the interaction of each of its pure tones at a particular time. This aspect of a sound is called a complexity and the psychological counterpart is timbre. This is the quality of sound that allows us to distinguish between a piano, oboe, violin, or voice all producing a middle "C" (256 Hz). These sound sources differently combine frequencies and consequently have different qualities.

Measuring Sound

The principal components of sound that we need to measure are frequency and intensity. Both are measured with a technique called scaling. The frequency scale is generally familiar because it is based on the musical scale, or octave. This is a logarithmic scale with a base of 2. This means that each octave increase corresponds to a doubling of frequency (Fig 1–7). Linear increases (octaves) correspond with progressively increasing frequency units. For example, the octave between 4000 and 8000 Hz contains 4000 frequency units, but the same octave space between 125 and 250 Hz contains only 125 frequency units. This makes it much easier to deal with progressively larger numbers and helps show relationships that might not be obvious if absolute numbers were used (Fig 1–8).

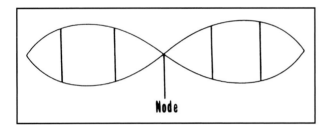

Fig 1–6. Diagram of a standing wave, showing the nodal point at which there is no amplitude.

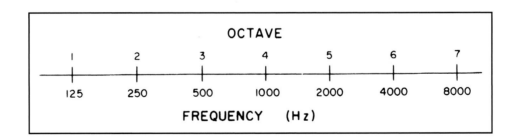

Fig 1–7. Scaling for octave notation of frequency levels.

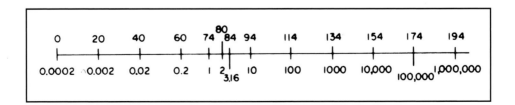

Fig 1–8. Decibel scaling (SPL). (After Lipscomb.[2])

Another reason for using an octave scaling was pointed out in the 19th century by psychophysicist Gustav Fechner. He noted that sensation increases as the log of the stimulus. This means that ever-increasing amounts of sound pressure are needed to produce equal increments in sensation. For example, loudness is measured in units called sones. Other psychoacoustic measures include the PHON scale of loudness level, and the MEL scale for pitch. The sone scale was developed by asking trained listeners to judge when a sound level had doubled in loudness relative to a 1000-Hz reference at 40 dB. Each doubling was called one sone. This is similar to doubling in pitch being referred to as one octave. One-sone increments correspond to approximately 10-dB increases in sound pressure, or about a 10-fold energy increase. So, in addition to being arithmetically convenient, logarithmic scaling helps describe sound more as we hear it.

In the kind of noise measurement done in industry, the chief concern is with very intense noise. In the testing of hearing, the primary concern is with very weak sounds, because the purpose is to determine the individual's thresholds of hearing. Accurate intensity measurement and a scale that covers a very large range are necessary to measure and compare the many intensities with which we have to work.

The weakest sound pressure that the keen, young human ear can detect under very quiet conditions is about 0.0002 μbar, and this very small amount of pressure is used as the basis or the reference level for noise measurements. This basis usually is determined by using a 1000-Hz tone (a frequency in the range of the maximum sensitivity of the ear) and reducing the pressure to the weakest measurable sound pressure to which the young ear will respond. In some instances, the keen ear under ideal conditions will respond to a pressure even weaker than 0.0002 μbar, but it is the 0.0002-μbar pressure that is used as a base.

Of course, sound pressures can be tremendously increased above the weakest tone. The usual range of audible sound pressures extends upward to about 2000 μbar, a point at which the pressure causes discomfort and pain in the ears. Higher pressures can damage or even destroy the inner ear. Because this range (0.0002 μbar) is so great, the use of the microbar as a measurement of sound is too cumbersome.

Intensity

Measuring intensity or amplitude is considerably more complex than measuring frequency. Intensity is also measured on a logarithmic ratio scale. All such scales require an arbitrarily established zero point and a statement of the phenomenon being measured.

Sound is usually measured in decibels. However, many other phenomena (such as heat and light) are also measured in decibels.

Decibels

The term "decibel" has been borrowed from the field of communication engineering, and it is the term most generally used to describe sound intensity. The detailed manner in which this unit was derived and the manner in which it is converted to other units is somewhat complicated and not within the scope of this book. However, a very clear understanding of the nature of the decibel and the proper use of the term is most valuable in understanding how hearing is tested and noise is measured.

A Unit of Comparison

The decibel is simply a unit of comparison, a ratio, between two sound pressures. In general, it is not a unit of measurement with an absolute value, such as an inch or a pound. The concept of the decibel is based on the pressure of one sound or reference level, with which the pressure of another sound is compared. Thus, a sound of 60 dB is a sound that is 60 dB more intense than a sound that has been standardized as the reference level. The reference level must be either implied or specifically stated in all sound measurement, for without the reference level, the expression of intensity in terms of decibels is meaningless. It would be the same as saying that something is "twice," without either implying or specifically referring to the other object with which it is being compared.

Two Reference Levels

For the purpose of this book, two important reference levels are used. In making physical noise measurements, as in a noisy industry or an orchestra hall, the base used is the sound pressure of 0.0002 μbar (one millionth of one barometric pressure or of one atmosphere), which is known as acoustical zero decibels. Sound-measuring instruments such as sound-level meters and noise analyzers are calibrated with this reference level. Several other terms have been used to describe acoustical zero. They include 0.0002 dyne/cm^2, 20 μN/m^2, and 20 μPA. Now, 0.0002 μbar has been accepted. When a reading is made in a room and the meter reads so many decibels, the reading means that the sound-pressure level in that room is so many decibels greater than acoustical zero. The designation SPL means that the measurement is sound-pressure level relative to 0.0002 μbar. When SPL is written, it tells us both the reference level and the phenomenon is being measured.

The other important reference level that is used in audiometry is known as zero decibels (0 dB) of hearing loss or average normal hearing. This level is not the same as that used as a base for noise measurement. Rather, it is known as hearing threshold level, or HTL. In the middle-frequency range (around 3000 Hz), it is 10 dB above the reference level known as acoustical zero. In testing hearing with an audiometer, 40-dB loss in hearing on the audiogram means that the individual requires 40 dB more of sound pressure than the average normal person to be able to hear the tone presented.

Since the baseline or reference level is different for the audiometer than it is for noise-measuring devices, it should be clear now that a noise of say 60 dB in a room is not the same intensity as the 60 dB tone on the audiometer. The noise will sound less loud because it is measured from a weaker reference level.

Formula for the Decibel

With these reference levels established, the formula for the decibel is worked out. To compare the two pressures, we have designated them as Pressure 1 and Pressure 2, with Pressure 2 being the reference level. The ratio can be expressed as P_1/P_2.

Another factor that must be taken into account is that in computing this ratio in terms of decibels, the computation must be logarithmic. A logarithm is the exponent or the power to which a fixed number or base (usually 10) must be raised in order to produce a given number. For instance, if the base is 10, the log of 100 is 2, because $10 \times 10 = 100$. In such a case, 10 is written with the exponent 2 as 10^2. Similarly, if 10 is raised to the fourth power and written as 10^4, the result is $10 \times 10 \times 10 \times 10$, or 10000; the logarithm of 10000 is, therefore 4. If only this logarithmic function is considered, the formula has evolved as far as $dB = P_1/P_2$. But it is not yet complete.

When the decibel was borrowed from the engineering field, it was a comparison of sound powers and not pressures and it was expressed in bels and not decibels. The decibel is 1/10 of a bel, and the sound pressure is proportional to the square root of the corresponding sound power. It is necessary, therefore, to multiply the logarithm of the ratio of pressures by 2 (for the square root relationship) and by 10 (for the bel-decibel relationship). When this is done, the decibel formula is complete and the decibel in terms of sound-pressure levels is defined thus:

$$dB = \frac{(20 \log P_1)}{P_2}$$

For instance, if the pressure designated as P_1 is 100 times greater than the reference level of P_2, substitution in the formula gives $dB = 20 \times \log 100/1$. Since it is known that the log of 100 is 2 (as $10^2 = 100$), it can be seen that the formula reduces to $dB = 20 \times 2$, or 40 dB. Therefore, whenever the pressure of one sound is 100 times greater than that of the reference level, the first sound can be referred to as 40 dB. Likewise, if P_1 is 1000 times greater, then the number of decibels would be 60, and if it is 10000 times greater, the number of decibels is 80. A few other relationships are convenient to remember. If sound intensity is multiplied by 2, sound pressure increases by 6 dB. If intensity is multiplied by 3.16 (the square root of 10), sound pressure increases by 10 dB. When intensity is multiplied by 10, sound pressure increases by 20 dB. These relationships can be seen clearly in Fig 1–8.

In actual sound measurement, if P_1 is 1μbar, being a pressure of 1 dyne/cm², then the ratio is 1/0.0002, or 5000. By the use of a logarithmic table or a special table prepared to convert pressure ratios to decibels, the pressure level in such a case is found to be 74 dB, based on a reference level of 0.0002 μbar (Fig 1–8). Table 1–1 shows where a number of common sounds fall on this decibel scale in relation to a 0.0002-μbar reference level. This base level is used for calibrating standard sound-measuring instruments.

In audiometric testing, which uses a higher reference level than that for noise measurement, the tester does not need to concern himself or herself with additional mathematical formulas, because the audiometer used in testing is calibrated to take into account the increase above acoustical zero to provide the necessary reference level for audiometry of average normal hearing (0 dB of hearing loss).

Important Points

The important thing to remember is that the decibel is a logarithmic ratio. It is a convenient unit, because 1 dB approaches the smallest change in intensity between two sounds that the human ear can distinguish.

An important aspect of the logarithmic ratio is that as the ratio of the pressures becomes larger because the sound becomes more intense, the rate of increase in decibels becomes smaller. Even if the ratio of the pressures is enormous, such as one pressure being 10 million times that of another, the number of decibels by which this ratio is expressed does not become inordinately large, being only 140 dB. This is the principal reason for using the decibel scale. From the psychoacoustic aspect, it takes comparatively little increase in sound pressure to go from 0 to 1 dB, and the normal ear can detect this. However, when an attempt is made to increase the

Table 1–1. The Physics of Sound at a Given Distance from Noise Source

	Environmental Decibels Re 0.0002 Microbar	
	-140-	
F-84 at take-off (80' from tail)		
Hydraulic press (3')	-130-	Boiler shop (Maximum level)
Large pneumatic riveter (4')		
Pneumatic chipper (5')		
	-120-	
Multiple sandblast unit (4')		Jet engine test control room
Trumpet auto horn (3')		
Automatic punch press (3')	-110-	
Chipping hammer (3')		Woodworking shop
Cut-off saw (2')		Inside DC 6 Airliner
		Weaving room
Annealing furnace (4')	-100-	
Automatic lathe (3')		Can manufacturing plant
		Power lawn mower (Operator's ear)
Subway train (20')		Inside subway car
Heavy trucks (20')		
Train whistles (500')		Inside commercial jet
	-90-	
10 HP outboard (50')		
		Inside sedan in city traffic
Small trucks accelerating (30')		
	-80-	
Light trucks in city (20')		Garbage disposal (3')
		Heavy traffic (25' to 50')
Autos (20')		
	-70-	Vacuum cleaner
		Average traffic (100')
		Accounting office
Conversational speech (3')		Chicago industrial areas
	-60-	Window air conditioner (25')
15000 KVA, 115 KV Transformer 3 (200')		
	-50-	Private business office
Light traffic (100')		
		Average residence
	-40-	Quiet room
		Minimum levels for residential areas at night
	-30-	Broadcasting studio (Speech)
		Broadcasting studio (Music)
	-20-	Studio for sound pictures
	-10-	
Threshold of hearing—Young men 1000 to 4000 cps		
	-0-	

sound pressure from 140 to 141 dB, also an increase of 1 dB, which the ear can barely detect, it takes an increase of about 10 million times as much in absolute pressure.

A point to be remembered is that the effect of adding decibels together is quite different from that of adding ordinary numbers. For example, if one machine whose noise has been measured as 70 dB of noise is turned on next to another machine producing 70 dB, the resulting level is 73 dB and not 140 dB. This is obtained as follows: When combining decibels, it is necessary to use an equation that takes into account that energy or power exerted by the sound sources, rather than the sound pressure exerted by this energy. The equation is:

$$dB_{power} = 10 \log_{10} \frac{E_1}{E_0}$$

where E_1 is known power (energy) and E_0 is the reference quantity
(there were two machines operating rather than one, resulting in a 2:1 ratio)

$$dB_{power} = 10 \log_{10} \frac{2}{1}$$

$$= (10)(0.3010) \text{ (the logarithm of 2 is 0.3010)}$$
$$= 3.01$$

Fig 1–9 is a chart showing the results obtained from adding noise levels. It may be used instead of the for-mulas. On this chart, it will be seen that if 70 db and 76 dB are being added, the difference of 6 dB is located on the graph, and this difference is found to produce an increase of 1 dB, which is added to the higher number. Therefore, the combined level of noise produced by the two machines is 77 dB above the reference level.

dBA Measurement

Most sound level meters that are used to measure noise levels do not simply record sound pressure level relative to 0.0002 μbar (dB SPL). Rather, they are generally equipped with three filtering networks: A, B, and C. Use of these filters allows one to approximate the frequency distribution of a given noise over the audible spectrum (Figs 1–10 and 1–11). In practice, the frequency distribution of a noise can be approximated by comparing the levels measured with each of the frequency ratings. For example, if the noise level is measured with the A and C networks and they are almost equal, then most of the noise energy is above 1000 Hz, because this is the only portion of the spectrum where the networks are similar. If there is a large difference between A and C measurements, most of the energy is likely to be below 1000 Hz. The use of these filters and other capabilities of sound level meters are discussed in other literature.[3]

The A network is now used when measuring sound to estimate the risk of noise-induced hearing loss, because it more accurately represents the ear's response to loud noise. It is not possible to describe a noise's damaging effect on hearing simply by stating its intensity.

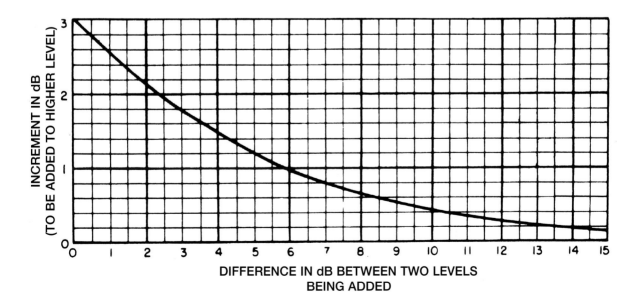

Fig 1–9. Results obtained from adding noise levels.

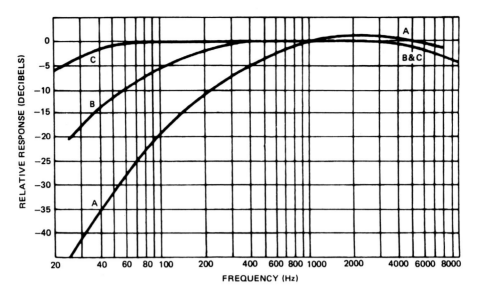

Fig 1–10. Frequency-response characteristics of a sound-level meter with A, B, and C weighting.

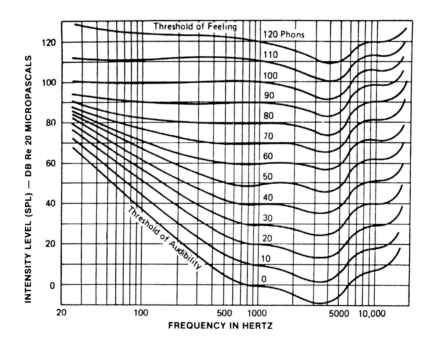

Fig 1–11. Fletcher-Munson curves showing the sensitivity of the ear to sounds of various frequencies.

For instance, if one noise has a spectrum similar to that shown in curve A in Fig 1–10, with most of its energy in the low frequencies, it may have little or no effect on hearing. Another noise of the same overall intensity, having most of its sound energy in the higher frequencies (curve C), could produce substantial hearing damage after years of exposure. Examples of low-frequency noises are motors, fans, and trains. High-frequency noises are produced by sheet metal work, boiler making, and air pressure hoses. Although the human ear is more sensitive in the frequency range 1000 Hz to 3000 Hz than it is in the range below 500 Hz and above 4000 Hz (Fig 1–11), this frequency-specific differential sensitivity does not fully explain the ear's vulnerability to high-frequency sounds. Various explanations have been proposed involving everything from teleology to redundancy of low-frequency loci on the cochlea to cochlear shearing mechanics, but the phenomenon is not completely understood. Mechanisms of noise-induced hearing loss are discussed in other literature.[3]

Summary

Sound is a form of motion. Consequently, the laws of physics that govern all moving bodies apply to sound. Sound is the propagation of pressure waves radiating from the vibrating body through an elastic medium.

Sound requires energy. It is important to understand various components of sound and the methodologies used to measure and describe them.

References

1. Van Bergeijk WA, Pierce JR, David EE. *Waves and the Ears*. New York, NY: Doubleday; 1960:44.
2. Lipscomb DM. Noise and occupational hearing impairment. *ENT-J*. 1980;59:13–23.
3. Sataloff RT, Sataloff J. *Hearing Loss*. 3rd ed. New York, NY: Marcel Dekker; 1993:371–402.

2

Music and the Brain

Thomas Swirsky-Sacchetti, Kelly Gilrain, Elisabeth Mandel, Joseph Tracy, and Steven Mandel

Neuropsychology is the science of brain-behavior relationships. Neuropsychologists are interested in understanding the neural or brain-related underpinnings of all forms of human behavior, including memory, problem solving, motor coordination, language, emotional functioning, and, more recently, musical behavior. With advances in functional neuroimaging techniques that allow us to view the brain at work, more is being understood about many aspects of music, including perfect pitch, musical imagery, the tune versus the lyric of music, memory for music, and our emotional responses to music. All of these topics will be covered, but first we will provide some general basic principles of how the brain works. We will then share what we have learned from individuals with acquired or inherited brain abnormalities that render their musical skills defunct or leave them intact. Last, we will present an overview of the rapidly changing landscape of music and the brain arising from advances in technology that are contributing to our knowledge base at an astounding rate.

The first attempt to localize human behavior to specific brain regions was known as the science of phrenology. Gall and Spurzheim,[1] the two anatomists credited with founding of phrenology, attributed large and complex aspects of human behavior (eg, music, religiosity, and humor) to various parts of the brain based on the superficial features of the skull. As you can see from Figure 2–1, music was thought to be localized to a small region of the brain above the left eye. Gall identified this particular site by palpation of the head of several talented musicians and first recognized it in Mozart's head.[2] Today, we understand that a series of physiological interactions occurs within interconnected brain regions as any specific behavior is accomplished. This pattern of activations was termed a "functional loop" by Luria[3] and more recently a "neural network" by others who have devoted themselves to teasing apart the sequential or simultaneous pattern of activations that occur as one engages in behavior.

The Lesion-Deficit Approach

One basis for the original identification and growing understanding of music-specific neural networks has been the study of individuals with lesions or brain anomalies that to varying degrees interrupt or, conversely, spare, musical behavior. It is far more difficult to understand neural circuitry in an intact brain. Lesions that result in specific musical deficits provide clues as to the role of that particular brain region in the neural circuit. This approach to teasing apart the neural network underlying musical skill is known as the lesion-deficit approach. In autism, brain abnormalities can be so pervasive and severe as to render the individual incapable of independent living or normal social discourse. It is typical, however, for autistic individuals to have an intact or even high level of musical ability despite severely disrupted language capabilities. These individuals, referred to as music-savants, provide strong support for the notion of specialized pathways in the brain that subserve music.[4] Peretz[5] describes an autistic young woman with an IQ of 70 (intellectually deficient range) who is dependent on her parents. Although language was delayed, she started to play piano informally at 2 years of age. Her level of achievement was described by Peretz as equivalent to that of an amateur pianist. However, she possesses absolute pitch and has an exceptional memory for music, being able to reproduce a conventional

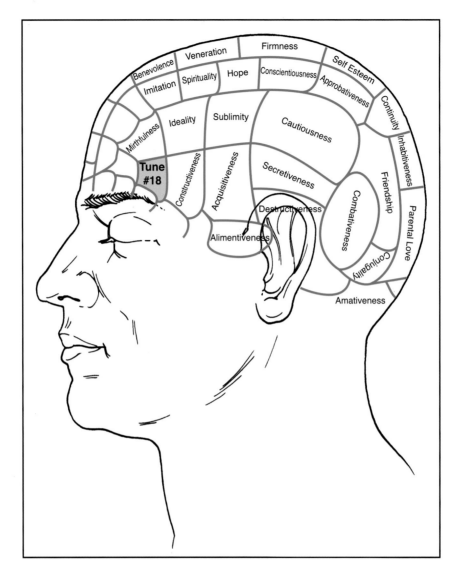

Fig 2–1. Gall's original system had 27 faculties that were later expanded by Spurzheim and called phrenology. This figure shows the location of faculties according to Spurzheim.

piece of music composed for experimental purposes after hearing it only once.

Epilepsy is another disorder that supports the notion of music-specific neural networks. In musicogenic epilepsy, music can trigger the firing of neurons that culminates in a seizure. When abnormalities in brain waves are recorded from electrodes attached to the scalp, the locus often involves the temporal lobes,[6] regions that are frequently involved in various aspects of music processing (see Fig 2–2). Depth electrodes allowed Penfield and Perot[7] to stimulate specific regions of the brain, triggering circuits involved in musical memory. These stimulated musical experiences are more frequent in response to stimulation of

the left temporal lobe; although, as we shall see, involvement of the right or left temporal lobe depends on the specific nature of the musical task, musical training, and even gender. A unique method to study hemispheric lateralization is the intracarotid amobarbital test, which is used for assessment of language dominance and memory functions in patients being considered for surgery to control epileptic seizures. During this procedure, one hemisphere is anesthetized and rendered incapable of activity for a brief period during which the "awake" hemisphere can be tested. Borchgrevink[8] reported that his subjects lost control of pitch and tonality (although rhythm was preserved) during right hemisphere anesthetization.

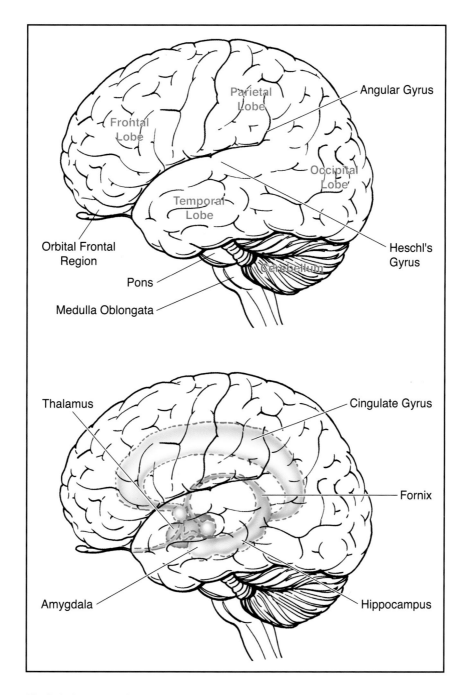

Fig 2–2 Anatomy of the brain depicting cortical and subcortical structures.

During left hemisphere anesthetization, subjects lost speech production and comprehension as well as singing ability.

The study of stroke patients has also provided insight regarding the neural networks subserving musical abilities. Luria et al[9] described Shebalin, a famous composer who, after a stroke involving the left temporal region, was unable to distinguish the sounds of speech or to comprehend language yet continued to compose significant musical works. According to Shostakovich, one of his peers, Shebalin's musical production after his stroke (14 chorales, 2 sonatas, 2 quatuors, 11 songs, and 1 symphony) was indistinguishable from what he had composed before the stroke. Vignolo[10] studied the dissociation between auditory agnosia (ie, inability to recognize environmental sounds) and musical agnosia (ie, impaired recognition of music) in stroke patients. Patients with right hemisphere stroke tended to have either auditory agnosia, or both auditory and musical agnosia with rhythm remaining intact. Patients with left hemisphere stroke tended to have preserved music and impaired rhythm, a pattern that occurred in isolation or with the additional deficit of semantic misidentification of environmental sounds (eg, a crying baby was confused with a laughing baby but not with a meowing cat). These results reflect the complexity of the neural networks that subserve music. Neither auditory agnosia nor music agnosia is subserved by completely independent neural networks. Rather, specific dimensions of these processes may involve overlapping and differing brain regions. The results of this study support the findings of others: Different aspects of music recognition (eg, melody and rhythm) have divergent results in the face of stroke, with melody (pitch) being more disrupted by right hemisphere stroke and rhythm by left hemisphere stroke. The identification of environmental sounds has a similar dissociation, with acoustic sound impairment (eg, the inability to distinguish the sound of an engine from an animal cry) being more vulnerable to right hemisphere lesions and semantic environmental sound impairment (eg, confusing the sound of two different animal noises) being more vulnerable to left hemisphere stroke.

Musically "learning-disabled" individuals have also provided fresh insights into the neural underpinnings of music. Individuals born with a musical deficiency, despite normal intelligence, adequate exposure to music, and normal interpersonal skills, suffer from what has historically been referred to as "tone deafness" and more recently termed "congenital amusia."[11] These musically learning-disabled individuals are, in a sense, a mirror image of the music-savant syndrome characteristic of autism. Peretz reports that these individuals have a specific deficit in pitch perception that does not involve lyrics or recognition of environmental sounds. The term "congenital amusia" is preferable to tone deafness because these individuals have musical deficits that extend beyond pitch discrimination. Bella and Peretz[12] demonstrated that the ability to tap in synchronization with music of varying types is significantly impaired in individuals with congenital amusia when compared to a control group. However, the same individuals were no different from controls when synchronized tapping to noise bursts was required.

Functional Neuroimaging Studies

Our understanding of music-specific neural networks has been greatly facilitated by advanced technology

that allows us, for the first time, to view the brain while it is engaged in a particular behavior. Two of these advanced technologies are the positron emission tomography (PET) and functional magnetic resonance imaging (fMRI). The fMRI takes advantage of the physiologic fact that when neurons activate their metabolic needs increase and blood perfuses the local region of brain activity to meet the increased need. With this influx of blood, the proportion of oxygenated hemoglobin increases; and this causes a change in the local magnetic field. When placing a person's head in a large magnet (ie, brain scanner) and sending out a series of precise electromagnetic pulses, this change in the magnetic field can be detected and its exact location identified relative to the less active surrounding tissue. In contrast, PET involves injection of radioactive drug in a very small dose that is readily eliminated. This radiopharmaceutical is absorbed by active neurons to a much greater degree than by silent, inactive neurons. As the drug decays, it sends out pulses of gamma rays that can be measured; and through computer algorithms, the exact origin of these gamma ray emissions in the brain can be detected. Both PET and fMRI yield brain maps of regional brain activity, although the spatial resolution of fMRI is superior to that of PET.

Pitch

Pitch is defined as the property of sound that varies with the frequency of a vibration. It can be thought of as the quality of a sound and is associated with a tone or a harmony via a musical instrument or human voice. The combination of sounds results in the formation of chords, harmonic structure, and the sequencing of these sounds. When these sounds are grouped together, they form melodies. The brain's ability to process pitch and subsequent pitch patterns is crucial to musical ability and has been studied more than any other aspect of music from a neuropsychological perspective. The neural networks involved in pitch have recently been captured in functional imaging studies.

The brain's ability to detect pitch occurs in various stages. According to Zatorre,[13] pitch is first encoded in the brainstem; but the individual's conscious perception of the tone takes place in the auditory cortex. As tones are sequenced to become melodies and occur over time, activation is seen more often in the temporal and frontal lobes.

Thus, the auditory cortex (ie, superior temporal lobe) is involved in the early stages of pitch processing, while additional brain regions become involved in complex abilities such as the perception of melodies. Zatorre indicates that underlying neural areas in the temporal lobe most likely account for one's ability to engage in the analysis of these melodies. Utilizing PET scans, Lauter et al[14] found activation in the superior temporal lobe in response to pure tones. Lockwood et al[15] reported activation of the medial and lateral Heschl's gyrus in the left hemisphere when a pure tone was presented to the right ear. Wessinger et al[16] studied the effect of harmonic tones presented to both ears of participants. Activation was again found in the left hemisphere with high-frequency tones activating the medial superior temporal plane more than low-frequency tones. Talavage et al[17] identified activation in Heschl's gyrus after presentation of a low-frequency stimulus and activation of areas lateral and medial to this after presentation of a high-frequency stimulus.

While listening to music, the brain appears to employ the same neuronal network that is used to process language, suggesting that these areas may not be as specifically dedicated to language as first thought.[18] When experiencing music, the activation in these standard language areas is often bilateral (involving both hemispheres), although music processing clearly activates more right (nondominant) hemisphere structures and language processing more left (dominant) hemisphere structures. Zatorre[19] demonstrated that the left hemisphere region involved in hearing responds directly to legitimate speech and the comparable right hemisphere area responds to the tonal patterns. Another good example of this laterality comes from a study examining linguistic versus musical breaches where the expected grammar, in the case of language, or chord progression, in the case of music, is violated.[20] A left hemisphere region (Broca's area) responded more strongly to the language breaches, and a comparable right hemisphere region responded more strongly to the musical breaches. An area of the brain called the supramarginal gyrus (left side) appears to be critically involved in remembering pitch information,[21] suggesting that the areas that process pitch are not where the final memory for pitch is stored.

Absolute Pitch

The study of absolute pitch has far-reaching implications for our understanding of brain-behavior relationships. Because there is growing evidence that absolute pitch has a genetic component, but also appears to be dependent on the age when musical training is begun, Zatorre[22] points out that absolute pitch provides a paradigm to understand the interactions between genetics, the role of brain development, and how environmental factors modify and influence

behavior. Zatorre et al[23] examined the regional cerebral blood flow of individuals with absolute pitch and those with relative pitch to determine "normal" brain activity. He had both groups engage in two activities. First, they were asked to listen to pairs of tones with no explicit instructions. Second, they were asked to listen to pairs of tones and to determine the musical interval formed by the tones. Zatorre found that individuals with absolute pitch had increased brain activity in the frontal cortex while listening to tones with no instruction; whereas individuals with relative pitch did not. However, on an explicit interval judgment task, both groups showed a similar pattern of frontal activation. Thus, it appears that the frontal activation may reflect the more general cognitive task of labeling or decision-making regarding musical interval rather than an area of "absolute pitch" discrimination per se. Interestingly, differences in brain anatomy between these groups have been found. Individuals with absolute pitch have relatively reduced volume in the right-hemisphere auditory cortical area. It is not clear whether this difference is due to a relatively greater growth of the left hemisphere auditory cortex in possessors of absolute pitch.

Many factors, such as musical skill and experience, however, will alter these basic patterns of brain activation. For example, during a pitch discrimination task musicians with absolute pitch showed greater activation in a region of the left temporal lobe compared to musicians with relative pitch, with the latter showing more right hemisphere activation in the superior parietal cortex.[24] Another interesting finding is that, when nonmusicians are trained on pitch discrimination, the brain regions involved come to resemble those of experienced musicians by showing increased left temporal lobe activation in primary and secondary auditory regions.[24]

According to Griffiths,[25] there is also support for the idea of a "pitch center" in the lateral area of Heschl's gyrus. Based on fMRI research completed by Penagos et al,[26] when harmonic stimuli were resolved and the salience of the pitch was greater, activation in the lateral Heschl's gyrus was noted. When the harmonics were unresolved and pitch salience was weaker, the same activation was not found.

Timbre

Similar to pitch is the study of musical timbre. *Timbre* is the property of sound that allows an individual to distinguish one instrument from another and can be thought of as a combination of various acoustic parameters. Previous research[27] found that nonmusicians are better able to distinguish between changes in timbre than musicians. In terms of lateralization, research supports the idea of a right-hemisphere priority for timbre perception (for a review, see Samson[28]). For instance, in previous research[29] larger electrical activity was recorded on the right rather than the left hemisphere in the perception of timbre. Recent fMRI research[30] supports previous findings that judgment of timbre is mediated by right temporal lobe structures. Interestingly, research of skilled musicians[31] found that activation of both the left and right hemispheres was noted when their instrument of expertise, rather than a simple tone, was presented. As noted by Samson,[28] this finding implicates the possibility of neural plasticity (ie, any particular behavior can be accomplished by more than one neural network) for timbre in accomplished musicians. It also reflects a basic principle in brain-behavior relationships: the neural networks responsible for any given behavior are subject to a variety of individual differences including innate ability, training, and gender.

Musical Imagery

Musical imagery can be defined as "hearing music in one's mind." Studies examining the idea of musical imagery are difficult to complete due to its internal nature. However, research by Halpern[32] suggests that judgments of imagined music are similar to judgments of heard music. This research further suggests that we have internal representations of sounds that are similar in temporal relationship to external presentations of music. In other words, we will "imagine" melodies or rhythms within the same time frame as if they were actually presented to us. To determine a shared underlying neural component of perception and imagery, Halpern utilized the lesion-deficit approach. Individuals who had lesions that disrupted perception (damage to the superior temporal gyrus, particularly in the right temporal lobe) also had difficulty with imagery. Furthermore, functional neuroimaging revealed activity within the superior temporal gyri in both hemispheres while listening to music and while imagining music. According to Zatorre,[33] these findings support the idea that neural activity within sensory areas is accountable for the subjective experience of imagery.

In terms of the lateralization of this phenomenon to the right hemisphere, Halpern[34] completed another neuroimaging experiment that required participants to imagine the continuation of a familiar tune when provided with the beginning notes. Again, the superior temporal gyrus was activated when imagery was involved compared to when it was not. Because the tunes selected for this research were chosen to avoid verbal components, Halpern[34] was able to show a pattern of lateralization to the right hemisphere. This study provides further confirmation of right hemisphere involvement in the processing of melody. When music contains lyrics, however, different findings are evident. Flanders et al[35] found that distinctly different areas of the brain were recruited when imagining lyrical and nonlyrical music. Imaging lyrical music required activation of the left inferior frontal area, which the nonlyrical music did not, consistent with the notion that this frontal area plays a role in word retrieval.

Future research in this area should focus on explanations of the pathways and sources of the imagery process. Zatorre[33] noted that the mechanism of action underlying the activation of neural substrates in the sensory cortex remains unknown, and that this is an important area for future study. Finally, the difference between an individual who has highly developed musical imagery skills and one who does not is another aspect of musical imagery available for further examination.

Tune Versus Lyric

Brain studies focusing on singing versus speaking have been of interest in recent years. Research on the integration of words and music allows us to study issues such as stuttering and aphasias, in which singing can assist the individual with more fluent verbalization. As hypothesized by Cadalbert et al,[36] this phenomenon may be attributed to right hemisphere involvement, as certain mechanisms may allow one to articulate language that is otherwise thought to be subserved by the left hemisphere.

Previous lesion-deficit research[37] indicated that individuals with right hemisphere lesions were likely to be impaired in musical perception and imagery; whereas individuals with left hemisphere lesions had preservation of these abilities. Neuroimaging research completed by Jeffries et al[38] provides evidence for varying neural activity when comparing speaking and singing. In their research, Jeffries et al[38] compared cerebral activity patterns with nonmusician participants speaking and singing words to a well-known song (eg, Happy Birthday). Left hemisphere (posterior superior temporal gyrus, supramarginal gyrus, and frontal region) activity increases were found when a participant was speaking. When the participant engaged in singing, relative right hemisphere increases were found. These findings allow us to conclude that when singing lyrics we may call upon the right hemisphere more than the left, and vice versa when speaking the same words.

Memory for Music

Memory for music has been another very interesting area of research. Zatorre[13] maintains that short-term memory for music requires mainly right hemispheric abilities. His research demonstrates that right temporal-lobe lesions affect short-term memory for pitch. He additionally indicates that individuals with right frontal-lobe damage will display impaired pitch retention. Based on these findings, it seems that the right hemisphere plays a large role in musical memory.

Distinct neural networks for different aspects of verbal and nonverbal memory have been previously demonstrated in functional neuroimaging studies. Platel et al[39] sought to determine the neural substrates underlying semantic and episodic components of music and found distinct activation patterns. Semantic memory can be thought of as our ability to identify a familiar song or melody. Tasks utilizing semantic memory were linked to bilateral activation of the medial and orbital frontal cortex, the left angular gyrus, and the left anterior part of the middle temporal gyri. Thus, although right hemispheric activation is found in tasks requiring one to perceive unfamiliar music, left middle temporal activations are seen during semantic musical memory. Furthermore, frontal regions are activated when one is categorizing presented melodies.

In contrast, episodic memory for music is defined by Platel et al[39] as the ability to recognize a musical piece in the context of where it was encountered previously. During episodic memory tasks for music, bilateral activations were noted in the middle and superior frontal gyri and precuneus (more predominant on the right side). Platel et al[39] interpreted this right-sided precuneus activation to be the result of mental imagery utilized by participants to recall the presented musical piece. However, the bilateral activation of the frontal region should not be neglected as an insignificant finding. Because this area was activated particularly during unfamiliar melody tasks, these findings may reflect an increase in retrieval demands as the task became more difficult.

Emotion and Music

The extremely interesting area of music and emotion is difficult to study for various reasons. Most simply stated, the experience and enjoyment of music is subjective and what sounds "good" and elicits a positive emotion from one person may not elicit the same response in another. Additionally, an emotional response to music is typically unique to an individual and his or her sociocultural, educational, and histori-

cal background. In a unique study, Blood et al[40] attempted to identify the specific regions of the brain responsible for an emotional reaction to music. Because positive responses to music may be more variable, they presented participants with highly dissonant sounds thought to be unpleasant. While listening to these dissonant sounds, participants reported their evaluation of the sound as pleasant or unpleasant. Activation was seen in the parahippocampal region with increasing dissonance and in the orbitofrontal region with decreasing dissonance. These paralimbic cortical areas are believed to mediate both perceptual and cognitive representations and emotions (see Fig 2–2). Activation of these areas is similar to that seen when emotion is elicited by other stimuli or events. Furthermore, Blood et al[40] report that there seems to be a reciprocal relationship between positive and negative emotions and corresponding increase and decrease in brain activity. Thus, it may be concluded that music can evoke one reaction while inhibiting an incompatible one.

In another study, Blood et al[41] examined the experience of musical "chills." The "chills" were defined as a positive reaction to music explained as a euphoric experience. Using PET, several brain areas were found to be active during this experience. Most interestingly, activation was found in brain areas known to respond to highly rewarding or motivational events. According to Blood et al[41] activation of the dorsal midbrain, ventral striatum, insula, and orbitofrontal cortex all correlated with subjective experience of the "chills." Additionally, as the "chills" experience intensified, decreased activity was noted in the amygdala, which has been implicated in fear and negative emotion. Thus, it seems that the emotional experience of music engages brain regions similar to those used in the evolutionary drive for pleasant stimuli.

Conclusion

It is clear that the complexities associated with the generation, interpretation, and emotional response to music call on various areas of the brain. During generation of a melody, fine motor control subserved by the frontal regions is utilized for intonation, pitch, and volume. Self-monitoring of one's pitch, volume, and rhythmic phrasing requires auditory feedback from the temporal regions; and melodic memory requires the use of temporal and medial frontal regions. Emotional responses to the music experience involve limbic regions of the brain. The characteristics of the music and the musical background of the individual will alter the exact pattern of the brain's response.

Clearly, acquiring musical experience dramatically changes brain involvement; and musical experience may even alter the brain, perhaps increasing brain volume in certain regions.[42]

Although the role of genetics and innate musical ability has been demonstrated, the environment also plays a role in how the brain and the underlying neural pathways develop. Music is a fruitful area for future study and contribution to the nature-versus-nurture debate. Much remains to be learned about brain function, and music may be a window through which to view some very important processes. For instance, music may help us understand the way the brain generates positive versus negative emotions or how we process aesthetic or aversive experiences. Studies of musical composition and generation will contribute to our understanding of the neurobiology underlying creativity. Our knowledge of how sensory feedback influences and optimizes learning will certainly be enhanced by studies investigating mistakes made while playing music (eg, the left hand errs while the right hand continues to play correctly). Brain studies of music may also help us understand what exactly the infant brain is wired to do. For years we thought only language was "hard wired" in the brain, but perhaps we are all also musical creatures from birth.

Finally, as our understanding of the specific neural networks utilized in the perception and creation of music grows, we can formulate strategies to assist musicians in strengthening specific musical abilities.

References

1. Zola-Morgan S. Localization of brain function: the legacy of Franz Joseph Gall (1758–1828). *Ann Rev Neurosci.* 1995;18:359–383.
2. Bentivoglio M. Musical skills and neural functions: the legacy of the brains of musicians. *Ann N Y Acad Sci.* 2003;999:234–243.
3. Luria AR. *The Working Brain.* New York, NY: Basic Books; 1973.
4. Heaton P, Hermelin B, Pring L. Autism and pitch processing: a precursor for savant musical ability? *Music Perception.* 1998;15:291–305.
5. Peretz, I., Brain specialization in music. *The Neuroscientist.* 2002;8(4):372–380.
6. Wieser H. Lessons from brain diseases and some reflections on the emotional brain. *Ann N Y Acad Sci.* 2003;999:76–94.
7. Penfield W, Perot P. The brain's record of auditory and visual experience: a final summary and discussion. *Brain.* 1963;86:595–696.
8. Borchgrevink H. Prosody and musical rhythm are controlled by the speech hemisphere. In: Clynes M, ed. *Music, Mind and Brain.* New York, NY: Plenum Press; 1982:151–157.
9. Luria AR, Tsvetkova LS, Futer DS. Aphasia in a composer (V. G. Shebalin). *J Neurol Sci.* 1965;2(3):288–292.
10. Vignolo LA Musical agnosia and auditory agnosia: dissociation in stroke patients. *Ann N Y Acad Sci.* 2003;999:86,50–57.
11. Peretz I, Ayotte J, Zatorre RJ, et al. Congenital amusia: a disorder of fine-grained pitch discrimination. *Neuron.* 2002;33(2):185–191.
12. Bella DS, Peretz I. Congenital amusia interferes with the ability to synchronize with music. *Ann N Y Acad Sci.* 2003;999:166–169.
13. Zatorre R. Hemispheric specialization of human auditory processing: perception of speech and musical sounds. In: Christman S, ed. *Cerebral Asymmetries in Sensory and Perceptual Processing.* New York, NY: Elsevier Science; 1997:299
14. Lauter J, Herscovitch P, Formby C, Raichle ME. Tonotopic organization in the human auditory cortex revealed by positron emission tomography. *Hear Res.* 1985;20:199–205.
15. Lockwood A, Salvi RJ, Coad ML, et al. The functional anatomy of the normal human auditory system: responses to 0.5 and 4.0 Hz tones at varied intensities. *Cereb Cortex.* 1999;9:65–76.
16 Wessinger C, Buonocore MH, Kussmaul CL, Mangun GR. Tonotopy in human auditory cortex examined with functional magnetic resonance imaging. *Hum Brain Mapp.* 1997;5:18–25.
17. Talavage T, Ledden PJ, Benson RR, et al. Frequency-dependent responses exhibited by multiple regions in human auditory cortex. *Hear Res.* 2000;150:225–244.
18. Koelsch S, Gunter TC, von Cramon DY, et al. Bach speaks: a cortical "language-network" serves the processing of music. *Neuroimaging.* 2002;17:956–966.
19. Zatorre RJ. Neural specializations for tonal processing. *Ann N Y Acad Sci.* 2001;930:193–210.
20 Maess BS, Koelsch S, Gunter TC, Friederici AD. Musical syntax is processed in Broca's area: an MEG study. *Nat Neurosci.* 2001;4:540–545.
21. Gaab N, Gaser C, Zaehle T, et al. Functional anatomy of pitch memory—an fMRI study with sparse temporal sampling. *Neuroimaging.* 2003;19:1417–1426.
22. Zatorre RJ. Absolute pitch: a model for understanding the influence of genes and development on neural and cognitive function. *Nat Neurosci.* 2003;6:692–695.
23. Zatorre R, Perry D, Beckett C. Functional anatomy of musical processing in listeners with absolute pitch and relative pitch. *Proc Nat Acad Sci.* 1998;95:3172–3177.
24. Gaab N, Schlaug G. Musicians differ from non-musicians in brain activation despite performance matching. *Ann N Y Acad Sci.* 2003;999:385–388.
25. Griffiths TD. Functional imaging of pitch analysis. *Ann N Y Acad Sci.* 2003;999:40–49.
26. Penagos H, Oxenham A, Melcher J. Effects of harmonic resolvability on the cortical activity produced by complex tones. *J Assoc Res Otolaryngol.* In press.
27. Pitt MA. Perception of pitch and timbre by musically trained and untrained listeners. *J Exp Psychol Hum Percept Perform.* 1994:20:876–986.

28. Samson S. Neuropsychological studies of musical timbre. *Ann N Y Acad Sci.* 2003;999:144–151.
29. Jones SJ, Longe O, Vaz Pato M. Auditory evoked potentials to abrupt pitch and timbre change of complex tones: electrophysiological evidence of 'streaming'? *Electroencephalogr Clin Neurophysiol.* 1998;108(2):131–142.
30. Samson S, Zatorre R, Ramsay J. Deficits of musical timbre perception after unilateral temporal-lobe lesion revealed with multidimensional scaling. *Brain.* 2002;125:1–13.
31. Plomp R. Timbre as a multidimensional attribute of complex tones. In: Plomp E, Smoorenburg GF, eds. *Frequency Analysis and Periodicity Detection in Hearing.* Driebergen, The Netherlands: Sijthoff, Lieden; 1970:397–414.
32. Halpern AR. Mental scanning in auditory imagery for tunes. *J Exp Psychol Learn Mem Cogn.* 1998;14:434–443.
33. Zatorre RJ. Music and the brain. *Ann N Y Acad Sci.* 2003;999:4–14.
34. Halpern AR, Zatorre RJ. When that tune runs through your head: a PET investigation of auditory imagery for familiar melodies. *Cereb Cortex.* 1999;9:697–704.
35. Flanders AE, Tracy A, Enochs W, et al. Imagining a tune: discrimination of lyrical and non-lyrical musical imagery with functional MR imaging. Presented at the annual meeting of the *American Society of Neuroradiology*; June 5–11, 2004; Seattle, Wash.
36. Cadalbert A, Landis T, Regard M, Graves RE. Singing with and without words: hemispheric asymmetries in motor control. *J Clin Exp Neuropsychol.* 1994;16:664–670.
37. Samson S, Zatorre RJ. Contribution of the right temporal lobe to musical timbre discrimination. *Neuropsychologia.* 1994;31:231–240.
38. Jeffries KJ, Fritz JB, Braun AR. Words in melody: an H(2)15O PET study of brain activation during singing and speaking. *Neuroreport.* 2003;14(5):749–754.
39. Platel H, Baron JC, Desgranges B, Bernard F, Eustache F. Semantic and episodic memory of music are subserved by distinct neural networks. *Neuroimage.* 2003;20(1):244–256.
40. Blood AJ, Zatorre RJ, Bermudez P, Evans AC. Emotional responses to pleasant and unpleasant music correlate with activity in paralimbic brain regions. *Nat Neurosci.* 1999;2:382–387.
41 Blood AJ, Zatorre RJ. Intensely pleasurable responses to music correlate with activity in brain regions implicated in reward and emotion. *Proc Natl Acad Sci.* 2001;98:11818–11823.
42. Schlaug G, Jancke L, Huang V, Steinmetz H. In vivo evidence of structural brain asymmetry in musicians. *Science.* 1995;267:699–670.

3

Genetics of the Voice

Robert Thayer Sataloff

The genetics of voice is a fascinating subject for speculation. Unfortunately, it has been a challenging area of research, and exciting progress has been made only in the last few years. When this chapter was written for the second edition of this book, a computer search of 8,009,307 references in four databases (MEDLINE, Health, AIDS line, and Cancer Lit) was carried out using the key words: hereditary, genetics, voice, voice disorders, and familial. The MEDLINE database indexed articles from 1966 to 1996. The computer search produced only five references,[1-5] only three of which really discussed hereditary voice disorders.[2,3,5] The rest of the conditions discussed in this chapter were identified through the author's clinical experience and a review of the content and references contained in numerous speech-language pathology textbooks and reference texts on human genetics. There still appears to be no other published review on the subject of genetics of voice, although a valuable text available on genetic aspects of speech and language is available.[6] Although there has been no striking progress in traditional medical genetics of voice disorders, remarkable achievements have begun in voice-related molecular genetics and genomics. These are reviewed in detail in chapter 4 and mentioned only briefly in this chapter.

Normal Voice

Genetic factors do influence vocal quality. This has been recognized anecdotally in families and even nationalities (Italians, Welsh, Russians, and others). If one assumes that function is related to structure, the association of voice quality and genetic factors is intuitively comfortable. It is generally accepted that physical characteristics are genetically determined. If these include the size of the laryngeal cartilages, vocal fold length and structure, size and shape of the supraglottic vocal tract, and phenotypic similarities elsewhere in the vocal mechanism, then one might expect similarities in voice quality. If we postulate additional similarities in brain development, musical perception, and neuromotor control, the notion becomes even more attractive. However, in order to be credible, these issues require further study, and careful separation of genetic factors from environmental influences on development.

Some of the most interesting studies to date have looked at voice function in twins. In general, monozygotic twins have very similar voices. Dizygotic twins appear to show the same differences that would be expected among any children of the same age.[7] Coon and Cary[8] studied genetic and environmental determinants of musical ability in twins. Because there is more to vocal quality and ability than vocal fold structure alone, such studies are relevant when studying the genetics of voice. Coon and Cary examined monozygotic and dizygotic twins and found evidence of hereditable variation, although environment appeared to be a more important factor than heredity. Kalmus and Fry[9] studied dysmelodia (inability to sing on tune) and found it to be hereditable as an autosomal dominant trait with imperfect penetrance. They speculated that their findings seemed to indicate the existence of some deep structure of tonality perception, comparable with Chomsky's deep language structure.

Although Bernstein and Schlaper[10] began looking at the genetic influences on the voice as early as 1922, and Schilling,[11,12] Seeman,[13] Gedda, Bianchi, and Bianchi-Neroni,[14] and others carried out subsequent work, the complexities of genetic research in humans have left most of the relevant questions unanswered.

Pathological Voice and Syndromes

In addition to the voice quality characteristics that appear to be genetically transmitted in healthy individuals, many pathological conditions are associated with specific genetic voice dysfunctions.[15] For example, raspy voice quality has been recognized in hyalinosis cutis et mucosae,[16-18] Opitz BBB/G compound syndrome,[19-22] pachyonychia congenita syndrome,[23-25] Werner syndrome,[26,27] William syndrome,[28-31] and other conditions. High-pitched voice occurs in Bloom syndrome,[32-35] chondrodystrophic myotonia,[36-39] deletion (5p) syndrome,[40] Dubowitz syndrome,[41-43] Seckel syndrome, Silver-Russell syndrome, and Werner syndrome.[26,27] Low-pitched voice has been observed in cutis laxa syndrome,[44-46] de Lange syndrome,[47-49] deletion (18q) syndrome,[50-53] mucopolysaccharidoses (types I-H, II, III, VI), and Weaver syndrome.[54,55] Other voice abnormalities have been observed in myotonic dystrophy syndrome,[15,56] and in hereditary dystonias that may be associated with spasmodic dysphonia. A dominant form of spinal muscular atrophy associated with distal muscle atrophy, vocal fold paralysis, and sensorineural hearing loss has been reported. Familial vocal fold dysfunction associated with digital anomalies also exists. Verma et al described familial male pseudohermaphroditism with female external genitalia, male habitus, and male voice.[2] Urbanova reported familial dysphonia,[3] and Friol-Vercelletto et al reported familial oculopharyngeal muscular dystrophia with associated abnormal voice.[5] A variety of other genetic conditions have been associated with voice abnormalities, including Cri du Chat syndrome.[57,58] Plott syndrome,[59] Ehlers-Danlos syndrome,[60] Huntington's chorea,[61,62] von Reckinghausen's neurofibromatosis[63] (hoarseness and dysphagia), Hunter's and Hurler's syndromes (hoarseness due to laryngeal deposition of mucopolysaccharide metabolites),[64] a variety of craniofacial anomalies (Down syndrome, Crouzon's disease and others), and various short stature syndromes.[65] Hence, evidence for the existence of a genetic component to vocal quality is compelling.

Molecular Genetic Considerations

Developments in genetic research in recent years are exciting and have largely moved from clinical to molecular studies. Unfortunately, although substantial progress is being made, close scrutiny still reveals discouraging complexities. Much of today's genetic research is involved with gene mapping. This methodology is elegant, but of limited clinical value for broad questions like vocal quality. Traditionally, genetic markers have been useful for conditions associated with one major gene. They used to require an extremely specific phenotypic description. Indeed, without specification of not only a phenotype but also a candidate gene, linkage studies used to be extraordinarily difficult and time consuming. Recent technological advances such as the development of microassay technology have facilitated this process greatly, as discussed in chapter 6.

Because the basement membrane matrix proteins are found on the long arm of chromosome 1, and other materials may be localized to specific chromosomes, locating genes responsible for voice phenomena was recognized as practical in selected cases even before the development of newer techniques. For example, Mace et al[66] described a family with hereditary, congenital, bilateral adductor vocal fold paralysis inherited as an autosomal dominant, with linkage with HLA, a syndrome localized to chromosome 6, position 21.[3-23] However, for many questions regarding voice traits and problems, gene mapping remains to be done. Important research in this and other areas of molecular genetics and genomics is ongoing, as reviewed in chapter 6; but acquiring all of the information needed will take many years. In the meantime, it appears worthwhile to continue the study of pathological conditions known to be hereditary and associated with voice abnormalities. This research should include genetic, structural, physiologic, and epidemiologic studies. Such investigations, together with advances in molecular genetic research, should eventually lead us to the kind of information we seek about normal and exceptional voices. Later research efforts are likely to be facilitated by building a database of pedigree information now. A national registry to coordinate this information may even be appropriate, as suggested by Dr Stephen Gray (personal communication, June 1993). Clinicians should be encouraged to acquire much more meticulous family histories focusing on voice quality, skills, peculiarities, and other nonvoice-distinguishing features and diseases. This type of clinical research is also likely to provide information that will help us clarify the genetic nature of voice traits, not just pathology. In addition, it may give us insight into disease susceptibility. This has been recommended in the past for cancer. However, questions about benign disease still remain to be answered. For example, in families with vocal nodules, we have always assumed that environmental factors were causal. Perhaps there are also genetic deficiencies in healing patterns in response to phonotrauma that can be identified. If so, preventive measures may be possible and may guide medical, genetic, and surgical therapy.

Conclusion

Despite many exciting breakthroughs, much remains to be learned about how the voice functions, what causes phonatory dysfunction, and how voice characteristics (normal and abnormal) are transmitted within families and larger groups. Genetic research has barely begun to address these problems.

Considerable additional study should be encouraged to elucidate the genetics of voice. This research should investigate not only vocal tract structure and function, but also genetic aspects of cortical function, perception, and neurological control, which are so inextricably involved in voice production.

Although questions involving heredity are associated with somewhat discouraging difficulties in research design and implementation, they must be addressed along with the more limited anatomic and physiologic questions studied to date. Clinical and molecular genetic research should provide important new insights into healthy and pathological phonation, the relationship between vocal tract structure (such as basement membrane ultrastructure) and function, and valuable contributions to the physician's armamentarium for treating voice disorders.

References

1. Rudiger RA, Schmidt W, Loose DA, Passarge E. Severe developmental failure with coarse facial features, distal limb hypoplasia, thickened palmar creases, bifid uvula, and ureteral stenosis: a previously unidentified familial disorder with lethal outcome. *J Pediatr.* 1971;79(6):977–981.
2. Verma IC, Sansi PK, Kumar V, Ahuja MM. Familial male pseudohermaphroditism with female external genitalia, presence of labial testes, male habitus and voice, and complete absence of Muellerian structures and lack of breast development. *Birth Defects.* 1975;11(4):145–152.
3. Urbanova O. Familial occurrence of dysphonia [Czech]. *Cesk Otolaryngol.* 1973;22(3):180–183.
4. Shriberg LD. Four new speech and prosody-voice measures for genetics research and other studies in developmental phonological disorders. *J Speech Hear Res.* 1993;36(11):105–140.
5. Friol-Vercelletto M, Mussini JM, Dumas-Guillemot A, Denis G, Lavenant-Oger F, Feve JR. Familial cases of oculopharyngeal muscular dystrophy. A case. [Czech]. *Rev Otoneuroophtalmol.* 1983;55(4):329–336.
6. Ludlow CL, Cooper JA. *Genetic Aspects of Speech and Language Disorders.* New York, NY: Academic Press; 1983:3–218.
7. Luchsinger R, Arnold GE, eds. Genetics of the voice. In: *Voice-Speech-Language.* Belmont, Calif: Wadsworth Publishing Co; 1965:122–130.
8. Coon H, Carey G. Genetic and environmental determinants of musical ability in twins. *Behav Genet.* 1989;19(2):183–193.
9. Kalmus H, Fry DB. On tone deafness (dysmelodia): frequency, development, genetics and musical background. *Ann Hum Genet.* 1980;43:369–382.
10. Bernstein F, Schlaper B. Über die Tonlage der menschlichen Singstimme. Sitzungsberichte der Preuss. Akad Wiss, Math-physikal. Klasse; Berlin, Germany; 1922.
11. Schilling R. Über die Stimme erbgleicher Zwillinge. *Klin Scher.* 1936;15:756 [cited in Luchsinger and Arnold, see reference 7].
12. Schilling R. Über die Stimme erbgleicher Zwillinge. *Folia Phoniatr.* 1950;2:98–119.
13. Seeman M. Die Bedeutung der Zwillingspathologie für die Erforschung von Sprachleiden. *Arch Sprach-Stimmheilk.* 1937;1:88.
14. Gedda L, Bianchi A, Bianchi-Neroni L. La voce dei gemelli I: prova di identificazione intrageminale della voce in 104 coppie (58 Mz e 46 Dz). *Acta Gerontol* (Milano). 1955;4:121–130.
15. Gorlin R, Cohen MM, Levin LS. *Syndromes of the Head and Neck.* 3rd ed. New York, NY: Oxford University Press; 1990:48, 53, 99, 106, 108, 113, 143, 298, 300, 304, 314, 316, 339, 423, 446, 485, 507, 632, 792.
16. Finkelstein MW, Hammond HL, Jones RB. Hyalinosis cutis et mucosae. *Oral Surg Oral Med Oral Pathol.* 1982;54:49–58.
17. Hofer P-Å, Öhman J. Laryngeal lesions in Urbach-Wiethe disease. *Acta Pathol Microbiol Scand.* 1974;82A:547–558.
18. Ward WQ, Bianchine J, Hambrick GW. Lipoid proteinosis. *Birth Defects.*1971; 7(8):288–291.
19. Cordero JF, Holmes LB. Phenotypic overlap of the BBB and G syndromes. *Am J Med Genet.* 1978;2:145–152.
20. Funderburk SJ, Stewart R. The G and BBB syndromes: case presentations, genetics, and nosology. *Am J Med Genet.* 1978;2:131–144.
21. Opitz JM. G syndrome (hypertelorism with esophageal abnormality and hypospadias or hypospadias-dysphagia, or "Opitz-Frias" or "Opitz-G" syndrome)—perspective in 1987 and bibliography. *Am J Med Genet.* 1987;28:275–285. Editorial Comment.
22. Opitz JM, Summit RL, Smith DW. The BBB syndrome. Familial telecanthus with associated congenital anomalies. *Birth Defects.* 1969;5(2):86-94.
23 Cohn AM, McFarland JR. Pachyonychia congenita with involvement of the larynx. *Arch Otolaryngol.* 1976;102:233–235.
24. Jackson ADM, Lawler SK. Pachyonychia congenita: a report of six cases in one family. *Ann Eugen.* 1951–1952;16:142–146.
25. Laing CR, Hayes JR, Scharf G. Pachyonychia congenita. *Am J Dis Child.* 1966;111:649–652.
26. Epstein CJ, Martin GM, Schultz AL, Motlusky AG. Werner's syndrome. *Medicine.* 1966;45:177–221.
27. Zucker-Franklin D, Rifkin H, Jacobson HG. Werner's syndrome. An analysis of ten cases. *Geriatrics.* 1968;23(8):123–135.

28. Beuren AJ, Apitz J, Harmjanz D. Supravalvular aortic stenosis in association with mental retardation and a certain facial appearance. *Circulation.* 1962;26:1235–1240.

29. Beuren AJ, Schultz C, Eheril P, Harmjanz DM, Apitz J. The syndrome of supravalvular aortic stenosis, peripheral pulmonary stenosis, mental retardation and similar facial appearance. *Am J Cardiol.* 1964;13:471–483.

30. Jones KL, Smith PW. The Williams' elfin facies syndrome: a new perspective. *J Pediatr.* 1975;86:718–723.

31. Kivalo E, Autio L, Palo A, Amnell G. Mental retardation, typical facies and aortic stenosis syndrome. *Ann Med Intern Fenn.* 1965;54:81–87.

32. Bloom F. The syndrome of congenital telangiectatic erythema and stunted growth. *J Pediatr.* 1966;68:103–113.

33. German J. Bloom's syndrome. VIII. Review of clinical and genetic aspects. In: Goodman RM, Motulsky AG, eds. *Genetic Diseases Among Ashkenazi Jews.* New York, NY: Raven Press; 1978:121–139.

34. Katzenellenbogen I, Laron Z. A contribution to Bloom's syndrome. *Arch Dermatol.* 1960;82:609–616.

35. Keutel J, Marghesco S, Teller W. Bloom-Syndrom. *Z Kinderheilkd.* 1967;101:165–180.

36. Aberfeld DC, Hinterbuchner LP, Schneider M. Myotonia, dwarfism, diffuse bone disease and unusual ocular and facial abnormalities (a new syndrome). *Brain.* 1965;88:313–322.

37. Aberfeld DC, Namba T, Vye MV, Grob D. Chondrodystrophic myotonia: report of two cases. Myotonia, dwarfism, diffuse bone disease and unusual ocular and facial abnormalities. *Arch Neurol.* 1972;22:455–462.

38. Mereu TR, Porter IH, Hug G. Myotonia, shortness of stature, and hip dysplasia. Schwartz-Jampel syndrome. *Am J Dis Child.* 1969;117:470–478.

39. Pavone L, LaRosa M, LiVolti S, Mallica F. Immunologic abnormalities in Schwartz-Jampel syndrome. *J Pediatr.* 1981;98:512.

40. Manning KP. The larynx in the cri-du-chat syndrome. *J Laryngol Otol.*1977;91:887–892.

41. Müller W, Frisch H, Gassner I, Kofler J. Seckel-Syndrom. *Monatsschr Kinderheilkd.* 1978;126:454–456.

42. Wilheim OL, Méhes K. Dubowitz syndrome. *Acta Paediatr Hung.* 1986;27:67–75.

43. Wilroy RS Jr. Tipton RE, Summitt RL. The Dubowitz syndrome. *Am J Med Genet.* 1978;2:275–284.

44. Beighton P. The dominant and recessive forms of cutis laxa. *J Med Genet.* 1972;9:216–221.

45. Goltz RW, Hult A, Goldfarb M, Gorlin RJ. Cutis laxa, a manifestation of generalized elastolysis. *Arch Dermatol.* 1965;92:373–387.

46. Wilsch L, Schnmid G, Haneke E. Spätmanifeste Dermatochalasis. *Dtsch Med Wochenschr.* 1977;102:1451–1454.

47. Berg JM, McCreary BD, Ridler MAC, Smith GF. *The de Lange Syndrome.* New York, NY: Pergamon; 1970.

48. Breslau EJ, Disteche C, Hall JG, Thuline H, Cooper P. Prometaphase chromosomes in five patients with the Brachmann-de Lange syndrome. *Am J Med Genet.* 1981; 10:179–186.

49. Fraser WI, Campbell BM. A study of six cases of de Lange Amsterdam dwarf syndrome, with special attention to voice, speech and language characteristics. *Dev Med Child Neurol.* 1978;20:189–198.

50. Gorlin RJ. 18q-syndrome. In: Yunis JJ, ed. *New Chromosomal Syndromes.* New York, NY: Academic Press; 1977: 72–74.

51. Rethoré MO. Deletions and ring chromosomes. In: Vinken JP, Bruyn GW, eds. *Handbook of Clinical Neurology.* Amsterdam: North-Holland Publishing Co; 1977: 26–27.

52. Schinzel A, Hayashi K, Schmid W. Structural aberrations of chromosome 18 II. The 18q-syndrome. Report of three cases. *Humangenetik.* 1975;26:123–132.

53. Wilson MG, Towner JW, Forsman I, Siris E. Syndromes associated with deletion of the long arm of chromosome 18[del(18q)]. *Am J Med Genet.* 1979;3:155–174.

54. Bosch-Banyeras JM, Saleedo S, Lucaya J, Laverde R, Boronat M, Marti-Henneberg C. Acceleration du developpement postnatal, hypertome, elargissement des phalanges médianes et des metaphyses distales du femur, facies particuliar: s'agit-il d'un syndrome de Weaver? *Arch Fr Pédiatr.* 1978;35:177–183.

55. Weisswichert PH, Knapp G, Willich P. Accelerated bone maturation syndrome of the Weaver type. *Eur J Pediatr.* 1981;137:329–333.

56. Salomonson J, Kawamoto H, Wilson L. Velopharyngeal incompetence as the presenting symptoms of myotonic dystrophy. *Cleft Palate J.* 1988;25:296–300.

57. Joan K I. *Smith's Recognizable Patterns of Human Malformation.* 5th ed. Philadelphia: WB Saunders; 1997:44–46.

58. Aronson A. *Clinical Voice Disorders: An Interdisciplinary Approach.* New York, NY: Thieme-Stratton;1980:57–61.

59. Plott D. Congenital laryngeal abductor paralysis due to nucleus ambiguus dysgenesis in three brothers. *N Engl J Med.* 1964;271:593–596.

60. Scott-Brown WG. *Scott-Brown's Otolaryngology.* Vol 5. 5th ed. London: Butterworth's; 1987:119–144.

61. Darley F, Aronson A, Brown J. Differential diagnostic patterns of dysarthria. *J Speech Hear Res.* 1969;12:246–269.

62. Darley F, Aronson A, Brown J. Clusters of deviant speech dimensions in the dysarthrias. *J Speech Hear Res.* 1969;12:462–496.

63. Ramig LA, Scherer RC, Titze IR, Ringel SP. Acoustic analysis of voices of patients with neurological disease: rational and preliminary data. *Ann Otol Rhinol Laryngol.* 1988;97:164–172.

64. Ramig, LA. Acoustic analyses of phonation in patients with Huntington's disease: preliminary report. *Ann Otol Rhinol Laryngol.* 1986;95:288–293.

65. Heuer RJ, Sataloff RT, Spiegel JR, et al. Voice abnormalities in short stature syndromes. *Ear Nose Throat J.* 1995;74:622–628.

66. Mace M, Williamson E, Worgan D. Autosomal dominantly inherited adductor laryngeal paralysis—a new syndrome with a suggestion of linkage to HLA. *Clin Genet.* 1978;14:265–270.

4

Genomics and Proteomics in Voice

*Steven D. Gray,[†] Susan L. Thibeault,
and Riitta Ylitalo*

In the analysis of voice disorders, an understanding of genes, their expression, and the regulation of proteins is important. As clinicians, most often our understanding of genetics and voice disorders is limited to those fields in which selective genetic deficiencies responsible for a syndrome lead to a voice problem. These syndromes are discussed in chapter 3. Although knowledge of syndromes, mutations, and genetic deficiencies is important, genes have a much broader role in normal and abnormal voice production. Additionally, environmental effects on health are important in nearly every organ system; and this is true in voice. This chapter introduces the various roles that genes and environment play in the production of normal voice and voice disorders. There is much complimentary information and some overlap with chapter 8, Vocal Fold Injury and Repair. However, after reading these chapters, it is likely that readers will be impressed primarily with how much knowledge we lack and with the fact that our understanding of these areas is really quite meager.

The tissues that compose the vocal folds are made up of cells and the extracellular matrix (ECM).[1] The ECM is an organized meshwork of macromolecules that varies depending on the function of the organ. The cells in the surrounding area of the ECM generally control, maintain, or govern its composition. In vocal folds, the lamina propria is filled with proteins, glycoproteins, proteoglycans, carbohydrates, lipids, and other molecules that allow the tissue to perform the functions required such as phonation, resistance to injury, and providing a barrier to damaging inhalation agents. To maintain or create an ECM, the cells need to assess the ECM around them, determine if it is correct for the tissue's current needs, and then maintain or change it. The cells do this by using their genes.

Genes, located in chromosomes, are made up of deoxyribonucleic acid (DNA), which consists of amino acids lined up in particular sequences. The DNA in each nucleus of a cell in an organism is called the genome, and the study of this field is *genomics*. DNA cannot be used directly to make the components of the ECM. The DNA sequences are transcribed first into mRNA (messenger ribonucleic acid), and this mRNA contains the template for the production of a protein. The process of converting the message contained in the DNA to the mRNA is called *transcription*. The cell uses mRNA to make the proteins, and this is called *translation*.[2]

The field of the study of proteins is called *proteomics*. Proteins, being the products of the expression of genes, are the tools that a cell uses to accomplish the functions of a tissue. Thus, measuring or manipulating proteins can be a powerful way to diagnosis or treat diseases. Physicians are very aware of the numerous medications that have emerged recently through the field of proteomics. The antiarthritic medications (etanercept, infiximab), insulin, growth hormone, and botulism toxin are common examples of medications developed through proteomics. Studying the production and the function of proteins important in voice disorders will hopefully lead us to better treatments.

Gene expression refers to the amount a gene is actually being used. It describes a state of activity and is determined by identifying mRNA made from that gene.[3] For example, if mRNA for fibronectin is identified in a cell or tissue sample, then we know that the gene that codes for fibronectin is being used. When a

†Deceased.

gene is expressed more than its baseline activity, it is said to be *upregulated*; and discounting any other translational regulatory mechanisms, the protein for which it codes is produced at a higher quantity. When a gene is *downregulated*, less mRNA is produced from that gene. Many different cell types, such as neurons, fibroblasts, and myocytes, live in the vocal folds and nervous system and are ultimately involved in voice production. These cells, although performing different functions, have the same genes. However, the genes being used (gene expression) and the proteins in each cell type and ECM may differ depending on the function that is being performed by the cell.

Scientists are constantly studying whether or not certain factors will upregulate or downregulate the expression of a particular gene. Through these studies, factors that regulate gene expression have become classified into three general areas: (1) *microenvironment*, (2) *soluble factors*, and (3) *mechanical forces*. The first area is the microenvironment in which the cell lives. For instance, taking a liver cell and placing it in the muscle results in that cell no longer performing normal liver functions. Likewise, taking a living human cell from the vocal folds and placing it in a Petri dish will also change the function of that cell. Cells can be quite sensitive to changes in their microenvironment. There are many clinical examples of this, such as sun exposure leading to tanned skin or extraesophageal reflux leading to laryngeal tissue changes. The second major area is that of soluble factors. Soluble factors refer to factors that are soluble in serum and thus are circulating around the cell (eg, hormones and pharmaceutical agents). An example of soluble factors leading to gene expression differences with phenotypic changes is the use of corticosteroids and the development of Cushing's syndrome.[4] The third important area that effects gene expression is that of mechanical forces. It is well known that when cells are exposed to certain mechanical forces, they will change their gene expression.[4-5] Figure 4–1 shows an example. Experiencing mechanical forces arranges the cells in certain directions as well as changing the cell morphology. The exposure of cells to mechanical forces most likely changes the composition of the ECM, although this is not yet proven in clinical voice work.

In the study of gene expression in various organ systems, the above three categories may not maintain the same relative importance. For example, in the study of eye disease, the effect of mechanical forces may be negligible and not interesting. However, in the study of voice disorders, each of the above three areas has importance. Because of the location of the vocal folds and their exposure to inhalants, reflux, and changes in temperature and humidity, the microenvironment is important. Similarly, it is well documented that

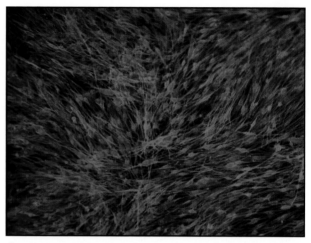

A

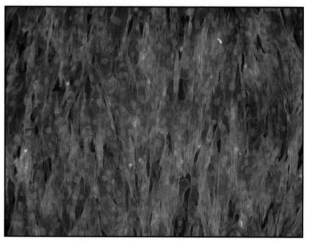

B

Fig 4–1. Human fibroblasts subjected to no strain (increase in length, stretch) in **A** and 50% strain in **B**. Strain was delivered by linearly stretching the substrate upon which the cells grow over a 1-week period until 50% strain was accomplished. Pictures were taken at 10× magnification. Note the disorganized and near-random arrangement in the nonstrained sample. The strained sample shows robust cells that are organized.

numerous changes in hormones and the exposure to medications can affect voice.[8-10] Lastly, the exposure to mechanical forces is very important in voice disorders.

Gene-Environment Interaction

It is now becoming quite obvious that voice production is the product of the genes and the environment to which those genes are exposed. Individuals probably carry genes that provide a certain genetic endowment for voice ability. However, exposing individuals (vocal folds) to an environment such as singing training or exercises also can lead to voice ability improvement. This improvement may be due to a combination of factors such as improved tissue, better neuromotor control, optimization of the vocal physiology, and so on. Studies in other fields may shed some light on voice ability. Drayna et al have now shown genetic disposition towards perfect pitch. This suggests that some individuals have the inherent genetic capability of recognizing certain pitches.[11] On the other hand, individuals can be trained to improve their recognition of pitch. Many of us have personally participated or know of individuals who, through exposure to music, have improved their abilities to recognize pitches and harmonics. Athletes often are described as being endowed with certain capabilities such as reaction time. For example, among other abilities, great sprinters can cycle their legs (termed stride rate) faster than others.[12] Although training may improve leg cycle rotation, this particular characteristic has been described as "something you are born with." Nevertheless, training does improve performance in even the best athletes.[13,14] Similar processes probably are active in voice abilities. This again reiterates the role of both genes and environment on the production of normal voice.

Genomics and Normal Voice Production

Very little information is available about gene expression in normal vocal folds. We have more information about the products of gene expression (proteins). Hirano has described the normal vocal fold architecture using histologic methods. His work divided the vocal fold into three lamina propria layers, and deeper to these layers was the thyroarytenoid muscle.[15] The division of these layers was based on the relative presence of the fibrillar proteins, collagen and elastin. Figure 4–2

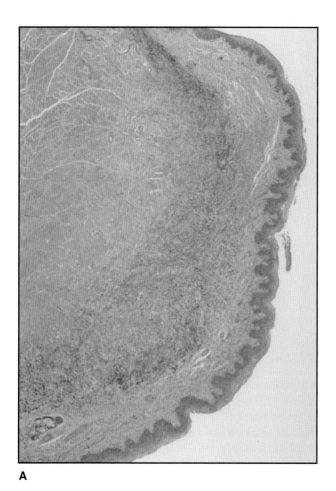

A

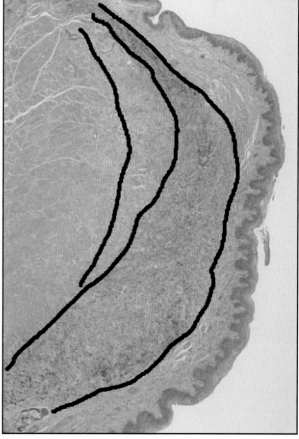

B

Fig 4–2. An adult male vocal fold stained with a Van Gieson stain. This stains the elastin fibers black. **A** shows the histologic stain as a cross-section through the mid-portion of the vocal fold. **B** shows the same section with the superficial, intermediate and deep layers of the vocal fold marked (using Photoshop; Adobe Systems Inc, San Jose, Calif). Note the many dark black dots in the intermediate layer that represent elastin fibers.

shows an example of this division. Studies of other proteins that compose the lamina propria demonstrate that their concentrations do not necessarily have a three-layer division, as collagen and elastin do.[16]

By the early 1990s, a fairly decent understanding of fibrillar proteins that made up the lamina propria had been secured. Attention then turned to the regulation of these proteins. *Regulation* refers to the events by which a protein is produced or destroyed and the balance between the two. It should be mentioned that proteins age. As proteins become old, they lose function.[17] As an elastin fiber becomes old, it becomes less elastic; whereas a collagen fiber becomes more stiff and brittle.[18] Tests of elastin or collagen fibers show that with age they are more likely to rupture or break with less force.[19] As humans, we commonly experience this phenomenon when we get back or knee injuries while doing the same activities that we could do at a younger age. The same process of aging occurs in the vocal folds. For this reason, it is important for the cells that are maintaining the tissue to constantly enzymatically destroy old proteins and replace them with new, better performing, proteins.

Studies that measure gene expression reflect in part the regulation of ECM proteins in human vocal folds. Figure 4–3 shows an example of studies measuring the mRNA for various proteins found in the ECM of the false vocal fold. It is apparent in this figure that both the mRNA that codes for the production of the protein and the mRNA that codes for the enzyme that destroys the protein are included. Also note that the small chain proteoglycans, such as decorin and fibromodulin, are produced quite abundantly; whereas the interstitial fibers, such as collagen and elastin, are produced in small amounts comparatively. This type of

study, when combined with protein studies, yields important information about regulation of the proteins.[20] Why there is so much more production of the small chain proteoglycans is not known. Are decorin and fibromodulin short-lived proteins that require constant production as opposed to collagen or elastin, which may have longer half-lives? What is the function of these proteins? Compared to our knowledge about the function of elastin and collagen fibers, our knowledge about the role of fibronectin, fibromodulin, and decorin is meager. Part of this is because these proteins are complex and multifunctional in their biologic roles. It is known that decorin and fibromodulin both are involved in collagen organization.

In the study of genomics and proteomics, the term "interesting" is used frequently. An interesting gene or an interesting protein is a gene or protein that shows variability in the disease or normal biologic function being studied. For example, collagen does not show much variation by age. Collagen density and elastin density across age groups are shown in Figure 4–4.[21,22] Therefore, in the study of effect of age on protein concentration, collagen is not very interesting. However, elastin does show quite a bit of variation across age groups. Both groups show variation by depth. Therefore, scientists looking at aging would call elastin an interesting protein; whereas collagen is not *in that study*. The term interesting is applied because, if a protein shows variation in the disease process, then it is likely to be involved in that disease process. Therefore, manipulating or intervening in the processes that cause the variation in the protein or gene may lead to treatment of the disease or a change in the symptoms of the disease.

Abnormal Gene Expression in Voice Disorders

Thibeault et al showed that fibronectin and perhaps fibromodulin are two very interesting gene expression profiles in both Reinke's edema and vocal polyps.[23] Furthermore, their work illustrated that the presence of fibronectin may have an effect on the biomechanical properties of the vocal fold as determined by mucosal wave motion. This was a significant study, because it starts to link up protein deposition with actual conditions encountered by clinicians and opens up avenues for treatment. In another study, Thibeault et al showed that fibronectin is an important determinant in scarring.[24] Although performed on a rabbit model, her results are consistent with human scarring studies. They showed that a likely determinant in stiffness from scar is not from increased collagen but rather from increased fibronectin.

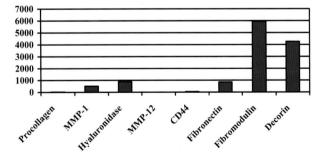

Fig 4–3. An example of gene expression studies examining the mRNA for various genes that influence the ECM proteins. This example is of the normal human false vocal fold. Similar profiles can be taken of laryngeal lesions. MMP1 = metalloproteinase 1, also known as collagenase; MMP12 = metalloproteinase 12, also more commonly known as elastase; CD44 = cellular receptor for hyaluronic acid.

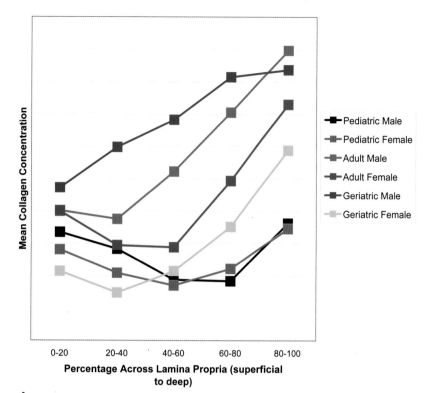

A

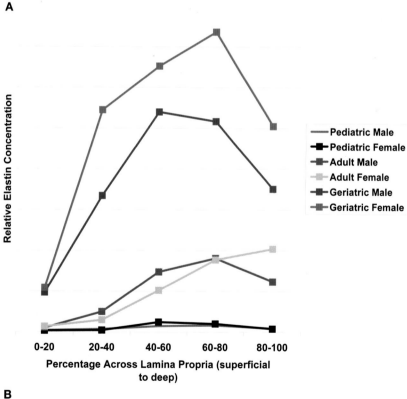

B

Fig 4–4. The concentration of the fibrillar proteins by age and gender. The x-axis is the percent depth starting at the basement membrane zone (0%) and finishing at the thyroarytenoid muscle (100% depth). **A** shows the concentration of collagen, **B** the concentration of elastin.

Studies in the early and mid-1990s provide some support of the effect of mechanical forces on gene expression. People with vocal fold nodules were found to have increased fibronectin and increased collagen type IV in their lamina propria and as a predominant component of the nodules.[25,26] Although these findings are in response to phonotrauma, the spectrum of injury from vocal abuse may range from actual mucosal tear or lamina propria tear to just increased mechanical forces causing overproduction of selected proteins that interfere with normal lamina propria viscosity and oscillatory motion. Frank mucosal tear, basement membrane zone, or lamina propria injury may result in a wound healing response, but changes in lamina propria proteins may also result from simple exposure to excessive mechanical forces. Please see chapter 8 on vocal fold response to injury for a more complete discussion.

There is a concern that the proteins in the vocal folds that are being currently studied are not indicative of the entire process of normal voice production and voice disorders. A new research methodology called microarray processing allows us to cast a much wider net and assay thousands of genes in the cells or tissues being studied. Using microarray processing, we can compare the gene expression across voice disorders. Figure 4–5 shows an example. In this example, 4612 genes were assayed to see if their gene expression was elevated or

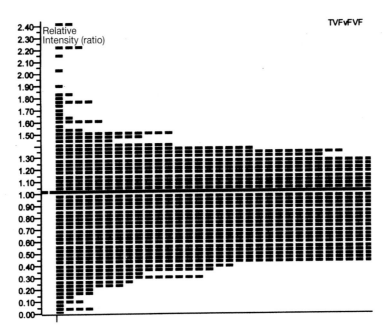

Fig 4–5. Results from microarray analysis show a comparison of mRNA levels for 4612 genes performed using true and false vocal fold tissue. Each box represents a gene. The x-axis shows the number of genes at that expression level. The x-axis is arbitrarily terminated, because the number of genes at the 1.0 expression level may number in the hundreds. The y-axis shows the expression level. A value of 1.0 is considered equal gene expression level in both tissues. In other words, if a collagen gene showed an expression level of 1.0, it would indicate that the gene is being equally expressed (at the same level or amount of expression) in both the true vocal fold and false vocal fold tissue. Gene expression levels above 2.0 ($2\times$ upregulated) or below 0.5 (50% downregulated) are generally considered significant. The y-axis is terminated at about 2.5 for purposes of this display, although many genes are expressed at higher levels and not shown here. Note the number of genes that are suppressed or downregulated (below 0.5) in true vocal folds compared to false folds, and those upregulated (>2.0). This illustrates some of the genes expressed that make true folds different than false folds. This type of analysis is a very powerful research tool and holds promise of helping us better diagnose and treat diseases. (Analysis performed using GeneSpring software; Silicon Genetics, Redwood City, Calif.)

decreased in a false vocal fold compared to true vocal folds. One can see that many genes are upregulated in the various conditions and then downregulated in the other conditions. This confirms the idea that vocal tissues are likely the product of particular genes being up- or downregulated in given the condition.

We have applied this analysis to the pathologic conditions of vocal process granuloma and vocal polyp.[27] Knowing which genes are up- or downregulated allows us to consider possible therapies targeted to modulate this gene expression. By determining which genes are up- or downregulated, we can also investigate the proteins produced, again providing us another avenue for therapeutic intervention. For example, in the list of genes that are upregulated or downregulated, collagen genes are not found. This indicates that trying to interfere with collagen production by using protein products to stimulate or decrease collagen may not be useful in these two disease processes. Collagenlike products perhaps are helpful in other diseases not described. Further work along these avenues is needed.

Genomics and Future Therapy

As the information that the human genome provides becomes more precise and detailed, increased knowledge of the genes that are implicated in vocal fold biology is inevitable. Combined with rapidly emerging technologies–DNA microarray and protein array (arrays that can be used to screen for interaction of proteins with other proteins, DNA, antibodies, cells, or small molecules), this offers a future research environment that will be expanding rapidly. Consequently, with an enhanced understanding of normal and disease vocal fold states, amplification of future diagnostic and therapeutic targets is foreseeable. Improved diagnostic capabilities could include the use of gene and protein quantification. Therapeutic directions may include new molecular-targeted drug discoveries, alteration of lamina propria through gene and protein transfection, and voice therapy approaches validated to alter the molecular composition of the lamina propria. The application of genomics and proteomics to the study of voice biology offers great potential for future clinical diagnosis and treatment.

Acknowledgment This work was supported by NIH Grant RO1 DC04336-01 from the National Institute on Deafness and Other Communicative Disorders (NIDCD).

References

1. Gray SD, Hirano M, Sato K. Molecular and cellular structure of vocal fold tissue. In: Titze IR, ed. *Vocal Fold Physiology: Frontiers in Basic Science.* San Diego, Calif: Singular Publishing Group; 1993.
2. Alberts B, Bray D, Lewis J, Raff M, Roberts K, Watson JD. Macromolecules: structure, shape and information. In: Alberts B, Bray D, Lewis J, Raff M, Roberts K, Watson JD, eds. *Molecular Biology of the Cell.* 3rd ed. New York, NY: Garland Publishing; 1994.
3. Alberts B, Bray D, Lewis J, Raff M, Roberts K, Watson JD. Basic genetic mechanisms and control of gene expression. In: Alberts B, Bray D, Lewis J, Raff M, Roberts K, Watson JD, eds. *Molecular Biology of the Cell.* 3rd ed. New York, NY: Garland Publishing; 1994.
4. Product information: Prelone. Muro Pharmaceutical. *In: Physicians' Desk Reference.* 55th ed. Albany, NY: Thomson Healthcare; 2001:2110.
5. Grodzinsky AJ, Levenston ME, Jin M, Frank EH. Cartilage tissue remodeling in response to mechanical forces. *Annu Rev Biomed Eng.* 2000;2:691–713.
6. Margolis LB, Popov SV. Induction of cell processes by local force. *J Cell Sci.* 1991:98:369–373.
7. Harris RC, Haralson MA, Badr KF. Continuous stretch-relaxation in culture alters rat mesangial cell morphology, growth characteristics, and metabolic activity. *Lab Invest.* 1992:66(5):548–554.
8. Baker J. A report on alterations to the speaking and singing voices of four women following hormonal therapy with virilizing agents. *J Voice.* 1999;13(4):496–507.
9. Abitbol J, Abitbol P, Abitbol B. Sex hormones and the female voice. *J Voice.* 1999;13(3):424–446.
10. Thompson AR. Pharmacological agents with effects on voice. *Am J Otolaryngol.* 1995;16(1):12–18.
11. Drayna D, Manichaikul A, de Lange M, Snieder H, Spector T. Genetic correlates of musical pitch recognition in humans. *Science.* 2001;291(5510):1969–1972.
12. Mero A, Komi PV. Force-, EMG-, and elasticity-velocity relationships at submaximal, maximal and supramaximal running speeds in sprinters. *Eur J Appl Physiol Occup Physiol.* 1986;55(5):553–561.
13. van Ingen Schenau GJ, de Koning JJ, de Groot G. Optimisation of sprinting performance I running, cycling and speed skating. *Sports Med.* 1994;17(4):259–275.
14. Mero A, Komi PV, Gregor RJ. Biomechanics of sprint running. A review. *Sports Med.* 1992;13(6):376–392.
15. Hirano M. Structure of the vocal fold in normal and disease states. Anatomical and physical study. *ASHA Reports.* 1981;11:11–30.
16. Pawlak AS, Hammond T, Hammond E, Gray SD: Immunocytochemical study of proteoglycans in vocal folds. *Ann Otol Rhinol Laryngol.* 1996;105(1):6–11.
17. Mohan S, Radha E. Age-related changes in rat muscle collagen. *Gerontology.* 1980;26:61–67.
18. Braverman IM, FonferkoE. Studies in cutaneous aging: I. The elastic fiber network. *J Invest Dermatol.* 1982;78:434–443.
19. Nielsen HM, Skalicky M, Viidik A. Influence of physical exercise on aging rats. III. Life-long exercise modifies the aging changes of the mechanical properties of limb muscle tendons. *Mech Ageing Dev.* 1998;100(3):243–260.
20. Ding H, Gray SD. Senescent expression of genes coding collagens, collagen-degrading metalloproteinases, and tissue inhibitors of metalloproteinases in rat vocal folds: comparison with skin and lungs. *J Gerontol A Biol Sci Med Sci.* 2001;56(4):B145–152.

21. Hammond TH, Gray SD, Butler JE. Age- and gender-related collagen distribution in human vocal folds. *Ann Otol Rhinol Laryngol.* 2000;109(10 Pt 1):913–920.

22. Hammond TH, Gray SD, Butler J, Zhou R, Hammond E: Age- and gender-related elastin distribution changes in human vocal folds. *Otolaryngol Head Neck Surg.* 1998; 119(4):314–322.

23. Thibeault SL, Gray SD, Li W, Ford CN, Smith ME, Davis RK. Genotypic and phenotypic expression of vocal fold polyps and Reinke's edema. *Ann Otol Rhinol Laryngol.* 2001;111(4):302–309.

24. Thibeault SL, Bless DM, Gray SD. Interstitial protein levels in rabbit vocal fold scarring. *J Voice.* 2003;17(3):377–383.

25. Courey M, Shohet J, Scott M, Ossof RH. Immunohisto-chemical characterization of benign laryngeal lesions. *Ann Otol Rhinol Laryngol.* 1996;105:525–531.

26. Gray SD, Hammond E, Hanson DF. Benign pathologic responses of the larynx. *Ann Otol Rhinol Laryngol.* 1995; 104(1):13–18.

27. Thibeault SL, Hirschi W, Gray SD. DNA microarray gene expression analysis of a vocal fold polyp and granuloma. *J Speech Lang Hear Res.* 2003;46(2):491–502.

5

Laryngeal Embryology and Vocal Development

David H. Henick and Robert Thayer Sataloff

The larynx is an anatomically complex structure. Familiarity with laryngeal embryology is helpful in understanding adult anatomy and vocal function throughout life. The available literature is confusing, and several different concepts of human laryngeal development have been proposed. The confusion can be attributed to several factors: (1) Previous authors have labeled various anatomic sites inconsistently. (2) Wax models, which are created from postmortem human fetal histologic sections, are the mainstay of our current understanding of laryngeal development. Observations that are made based on these models are subject to individual interpretation. (3) Prior to the existence of the Carnegie collection, there was no centralization of the specimens and wax-model reconstructions for each subsequent scientist to analyze and compare. Hence, one can only speculate as to the reason for the contrasting conclusions made in the literature.

This chapter is divided into two sections. The first section discusses the existing theories of the prenatal development of the laryngeal vestibule, cartilage framework, and musculature. In addition, the contributions of the branchial arch apparatus to the supporting structures of the larynx are discussed. The second section describes the postnatal anatomic differentiation of the larynx with respect to its role as a voice-producing organ.

Prenatal Development

The Carnegie system of classification represents the standard nomenclature for defining critical stages in embryologic development. It has been arranged in 23 stages. The term *stage* is used to designate subsequent levels of development by the appearance of specific morphologic features that did not exist at the previous level of development. This classification is useful because neither embryonic age nor the length of an embryo accurately coincides with the level of morphologic development.[1] A summary of the developmental stages of the human embryo according to O'Rahilly,[2,3] O'Rahilly and Boyden,[4] Muller, O'Rahilly, and Tucker,[5] and O'Rahilly and Muller[6] is outlined in Table 5–1. Although the following discussion of laryngeal development deviates from the features shown in Table 5–1, it is useful for comparison purposes.

Laryngeal Vestibule Function

Fleischmann (1820) provided the first documented treatise that described laryngeal development (cited by Walander[7]). Since that time there have been several important studies on the origin and development of the larynx.[8–14] Probably the most influential work performed in the late nineteenth century was contributed by His (1885), in his description of the developing gastrointestinal tract and the pharyngeal arches.[8] He proposed that the respiratory primordium (RP) appeared as an outpouching from the cephalic portion of the pharynx by the third week of gestational age. In his anatomic drawings (Fig 5–1), he demonstrated that the groove behind the lung primordium ascended toward the pharyngeal floor (or the level of the fourth pharyngeal pouch) by an "ascending notch," thus separating the foregut into a ventral trachea and a dorsal esophagus. Smith[12] called the ana-

TABLE 5–1. Developmental Stages of the Human Embryo.

Stage	Pairs of Somites	Length (mm)	Age (days)	Features
9	1–3	1.5–2.5	20	Foregut appears
10	4–12	2.0–3.5	22	Oropharyngeal membrane appears; laryngotracheal sulcus and pulmonary primordium
11	13–20	2.5–4.5	24	Oropharyngeal membrane ruptures
12	21–29	3.0–5.0	26	Oropharyngeal membrane disappears; lung bud develops
13	30–?	4.0–6.0	28	Cervical sinus becomes apparent; lung bud separates from digestive tube; trachea and esophagus may become recognizable; stomach begins to develop
14		5.0–7.0	32	Arytenoid swellings and epithelial lamina form in larynx: lung sacs curve dorsally and embrace esophagus
15		7.0–9.0	33	Pharyngotracheal duct connects digestive and respiratory tubes; lobar buds develop
16		8.0–11.0	37	Cervical sinus is disappearing; epithelial lamina is complete and separates digestive from respiratory tube; embryonic vestibule of larynx appears; primary palate begins to form
17		11.0–14.0	41	Vestibule of larynx deepens; skeleton of pharyngeal arches and larynx is dense mesenchyme; segmental bronchial buds develop
18		13.0–17.0	44	Hyoid chondrification begins; some subsegmental bronchial buds appear
19		16.0–18.0	47½	Mescenchymal epiglottis and several cartilages appear; infraglottic cavity is expanding
20		18.0–22.0	50½	Cricoid lamina develops; ventricle of larynx begins to appear
21		22.0–24.0	52	Epithelial lamina begins to disintegrate
22		23.0–28.0	54	Oral cavity and pharynx increase in width and height
23		27.0	56½	Oral cavity is still increasing in width and height; most individual laryngeal muscles are identifiable; secondary (hard) palate is forming; soft palate has not fused; connection occurs between vestibule and infraglottic cavity; large parts of epithelial lamina are still present; ventricle of larynx opens; vocal ligament may appear

Source: (From O'Rahilly et al,[6] with permission.)

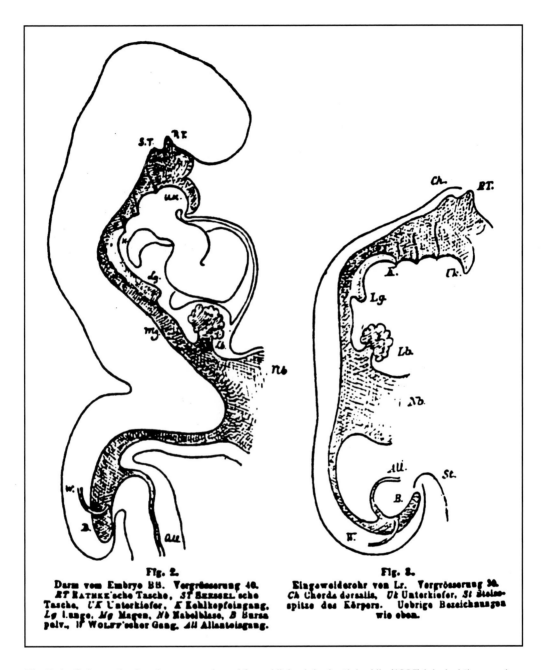

Fig 5–1. Schematic drawings reproduced from His' original article. His (1885) labeled the respiratory primordium as the "lung" primordium *(Lg)*. Note the faint stippled line that travels caudocranially from just behind the *Lg* to the level of the pharyngeal floor, or fourth pharyngeal pouch, theoretically dividing the foregut into ventral and dorsal halves. This represents his concept of the tracheo-esophageal septum or "ascending notch." His incorrectly assumed that the trachea develops cephalic to the origin of the respiratory primordium and therefore concluded that the respiratory primordium gave rise only to the lungs. However, subsequent authors have shown that the respiratory primordium gives rise to the larynx, trachea, bronchi, and lungs.[11,13,14] (From His W. *Anatomie menschlicher Embryonen*. III. *Zur Geschichte der Organe*. Leipzig: Vogel; 1885.)

tomic structure responsible for separating the trachea and esophagus the "endodermal septum" based on contrasting histologic findings to His. His' and Smith's theories, however, were similar because both assumed that the trachea developed cephalad to the origin of the respiratory primordium *(RP)*, and that an ascending process was required to separate the trachea from the esophagus.[8,12]

His' theory implied that the distance between the pharyngeal floor and the tracheo-esophageal separation would gradually decrease as time progressed. However, Zaw-Tun's findings disagreed.[13] Zaw-Tun (1982) used the histologic serial sections at both the Carnegie collection of human embryos in Davis, California, and the Shatner collection at the University of Alberta to create a complete chronologic sequence of laryngeal development using wax-model reconstructions. He classified the foregut segment that separated the pharyngeal floor (at the level of the fourth pharyngeal pouch) from the origin of the respiratory primordium *(RP)* as the primitive laryngopharynx *(PLPh)*. Contrary to His' thesis, Zaw-Tun found that the PLPh lengthened as the embryo matured. Furthermore, Zaw-Tun showed that the trachea developed as a result of the continued lengthening of the respiratory primordium *(RP)* from its site of origin from the foregut, which he called the primitive pharyngeal floor (Fig 5–2).[14] Eventually, the PLPh devel-

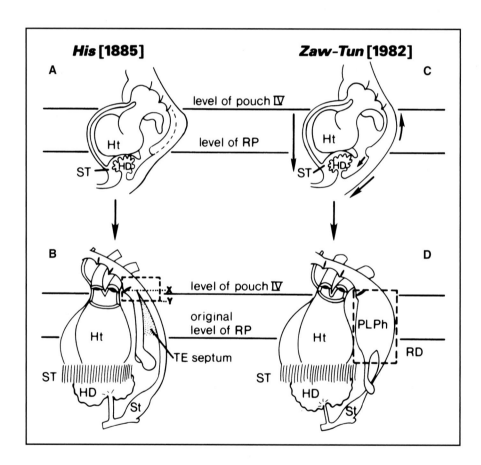

Fig 5–2. Depiction of the concepts of His[8] and Zaw-Tun[13] of the origin of the trachea and esophagus. The two constant landmarks are the level of the fourth pharyngeal pouch *(IV)* and the level of the respiratory primordium *(RP)*. According to His, the distance between *IV* and *RP* should decrease over time as seen in **B**. Kallius,[9] Soulie and Bardier,[23] and Walander[7] believed that the larynx developed from the stippled box seen in **B**. However Zaw-Tun[13] showed that the distance between *IV* and *RD* remains constant, and labeled this region of the foregut the primitive laryngopharynx *(PLPh)*, as seen in **C** and **D**. The *PLPh* would eventually become the supraglottis, stippled box in **D**. *ST* = septum transversum; *Ht* = heart; *St* = stomach; *HD* = hepatic diverticulum; TE septum = tracheo-esophageal septum. (From Zaw-Tun HA, Burdi AR. Re-examination of the origin and early development of the human larynx. *Acta Anat.* 1985;122:165. Used by permission.)

oped into the laryngeal vestibule, or supraglottis; the primitive pharyngeal floor developed into the glottic region; and the cephalic portion of the descending respiratory primordium developed into the infraglottis. Whereas His[8] concluded that the respiratory primordium gave rise to the lungs and bronchi, Zaw-Tun[13,14] demonstrated that it gave rise to the larynx, trachea, bronchi, and lungs.

Negus[11] described conclusions similar to Zaw-Tun's in his study of comparative anatomy among fish and mammals. Negus discussed the evolutionary changes seen in the development of the respiratory apparatus as a simple muscle sphincter surrounding the glottis (*Lepidosiren*) to the gradual development of cartilages that surround the sphincter (in mammals). His diagrams (Fig 5–3) depict the respiratory apparatus as developing from a ventral outpouching of the foregut to give rise to the tracheobronchial tree (simi-

lar to the respiratory primordium described by previous authors). Zaw-Tun expanded on this theory by showing that the cephalic end of the "ventral outpouching" gave rise to the glottis and infraglottis with cartilages developing around it.[14] The intrinsic muscles of the larynx, first apparent as a circular layer of cells,[10,15] represent the sphincter that in fish surrounds the glottis.

The laryngeal developmental sequence of stages 11 through 14 that was proposed by Zaw-Tun[16] is shown in Fig 5–4. Figure 5–4A depicts a stage 11 specimen seen from a lateral perspective. The hepatic primordium *(HP)* is initially contiguous with the respiratory primordium *(RP)*, and both are embedded within the septum transversum *(ST—the stippled region)*. Due to the rapid proliferation of the hepatic primordium *(HP)* on the undersurface of the septum transversum *(ST)*, the foregut lengthens and the res-

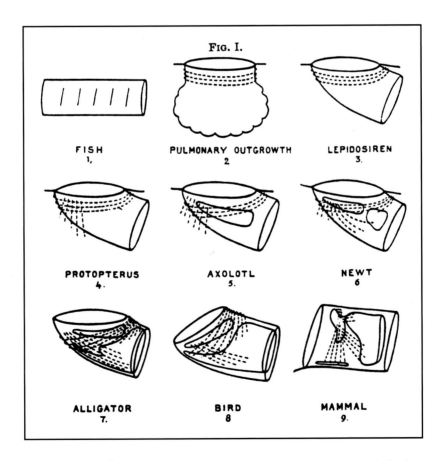

Fig 5–3. Negus[11] demonstrated the phylogenetic changes occurring in the larynx. Acquisition of a muscular sphincter (seen in *Polypterus*, as it functions to guard against entrance of water), lateral cartilages (seen in amphibians, and structurally similar to the human arytenoids), and a cartilaginous ring (seen in reptiles, and structurally similar to the human cricoid cartilage) are depicted as one ascends the evolutionary scale.

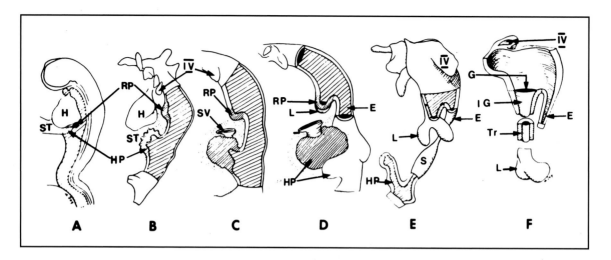

Fig 5–4. Developmental stages of the respiratory primordium, shown in reconstruction. **A.** Stage 11. **B.** Stage 12, early. **C.** Stage 12, late. **D.** Stage 13, early. **E** and **F.** Stage 13, late. *H* = heart; *ST* = septum transversum; *RP* = respiratory primordium; *HP* = hepatic primordium; *IV* = fourth pharyngeal pouch; *SV* = sinus venosus; *L* = lung; *E* = esophagus; *S* = stomach; *G* = glottis; *IG* = infraglottis; *Tr* = trachea. (From Zaw-Tun HA. Development of congenital laryngeal atresias and clefts. *Ann Otol Rhinol Laryngol.* 1988;97:354. Used by permission.)

piratory primordium *(RP)* separates from the hepatic primordium *(HP)*. This separation permits the respiratory primordium to dilate and bifurcate ventrocaudally into lug buds (Fig 5–4, B–F). As the respiratory primordium descends, it gives rise to a funnel-shaped structure. The cephalic end of the funnel becomes the infraglottis *(IG)*, and the caudal end (or tubular shape) becomes the developing trachea *(Tr)*. Concurrently, the foregut segment between the levels of the original sites of the hepatic primoridium *(HP)* and respiratory primordium *(RP)* stretches to give rise to the esophagus *(E)*, stomach *(S)*, and cephalic half of the duodenum (Fig 5–4E).

According to Zaw-Tun, the primitive laryngopharynx *(PLPh)*, that segment of foregut above the level of the original site of the respiratory diverticulum, is subject to the compressive forces of the proliferating pharyngeal mesoderm.[14] This causes its lateral walls to merge together ventrodorsally to form the epithelial lamina, a temporary obliteration of the laryngeal lumen (stage 15). Eventually, recanalization of the epithelial lamina will give rise to the laryngeal vestibule, or supraglottis (stages 19 to 23). Congenital laryngeal stenosis can be attributed to the incomplete recanalization of the epithelial lamina.[16]

Arey[17] demonstrated the laryngeal developmental sequence viewed by unroofing the dorsal aspect of the pharyngolaryngeal region (Fig 5–5). From this perspective, the laryngeal inlet is presented as a median slit in the pharyngeal floor, as shown in Figure 5–5A. Starting in stage 13, the continued proliferation of the surrounding pharyngeal mesoderm and

the fourth branchial arch arteries gives rise to the arytenoid swellings, which flank the entrance to the median slit (Fig 5–5B). Continued growth of the third branchial arch artery gives rise to a median epiglottic swelling that is derived from the dorsal aspect of the hypobranchial eminence. This changes the shape of the median vertical slit to a T-shaped laryngeal outlet (Fig 5–5, C and D). The transverse pouch of the T descends along the ventral aspect of the epithelial lamina to the glottis region by stage 14 to form the laryngeal cecum and eventually the laryngeal ventricles.[14] Recanalization of the epithelial lamina in stages 19 to 23 to form the supraglottis is represented by the separation of the arytenoid swellings in Figure 5–5E.

Controversy exists in the literature concerning the anatomic interpretation of the median slit seen in the pharyngeal floor. Based on His'[8] premise of an ascending tracheo-esophageal separation, Kallius[9] and Frazer[10] believed that the median pharyngeal slit represented the level at which the trachea and esophagus separated. Furthermore, Kallius demonstrated it would develop into the cephalic portion of the trachea, whereas Frazer demonstrated it would develop into the future glottic region. Zaw-Tun, however, demonstrated that the median slit in the pharyngeal floor was the entrance to the primitive laryngopharynx *(PLPh)*, and hence represented the eventual opening into the adult supraglottis.[14]

Computer technology has enabled scientists to analyze complex anatomical relationships as they change over space and time. A recent study[18] utilized

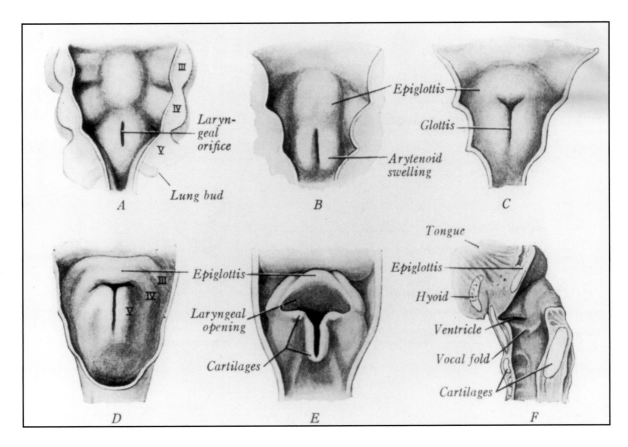

Fig 5–5. Development of the human larynx, as seen by unroofing the embryo to show the floor of the pharyngeal cavity. **A.** At 5 mm. **B.** At 9 mm. **C.** At 12 mm. **D.** At 16 mm. **E.** at 40 mm (×7). **F.** Sagittal hemisection, at birth (×15). In **A**, His[8] assumed the "ascending notch" reached the level of the pharyngeal floor, and the tracheo-esophageal separation would be at the level shown. Hence, according to His, level **A** would represent the cephalic end of the trachea. According to Zaw-Tun[13] level **A** represents the entrance to the primitive laryngopharynx, which eventually becomes the supraglottis. (From Arey LB. *Developmental Anatomy.* 7th ed. Philadelphia: WB Saunders; 1965. Used by permission.)

computer-generated, three-dimensional solid-model reconstructions to portray critical stages in the development of the murine larynx. The mouse was chosen as an animal model because (1) laryngeal development is essentially uniform in all mammals, (2) the genetic analysis for murine development is well defined, and (3) embryos of a predetermined age can be easily and accurately staged. The results of this developmental study were in close correlation with the findings of Zaw-Tun and will be described in further detail.

Serial histological sections of the laryngopharyngeal region of mice embryos were obtained from day 9 of gestation to day 18. STERECON, a computer graphics system designed to allow three-dimensional tracings of structural contours from three-dimensional images, was used to generate the three-dimensional models.[19,20] Photographic transparencies of each histological section were then projected onto a screen that was the same size as a high-resolution computer monitor. By means of a digitizing tablet, color-coded lines were drawn on the monitor, outlining the structures of interest, for example, the epithelial lining of the foregut, foregut lumen, muscles, cartilages, and arteries. The resulting contours were stored in a database and used to form wire-framed models. Wireframe models were then transferred to a Silicon Graphics workstation and rendered as solid, shaded reconstructions with Wavefront Technologies software. This allowed anatomic structures to be viewed in continuity, in any desired orientation, and in relation to any other given structure. In addition, internal structures could be visualized by sectioning models in various planes.

Figure 5–6 is a lateral view of a three-dimensional reconstruction of the epithelial lining of the developing laryngopharyngeal region. The first sign of the respiratory system is seen as an epithelial thickening along the ventral aspect of the foregut known as the respiratory primordium. The respiratory primordium is separated from the hepatic primordium (HP) by the

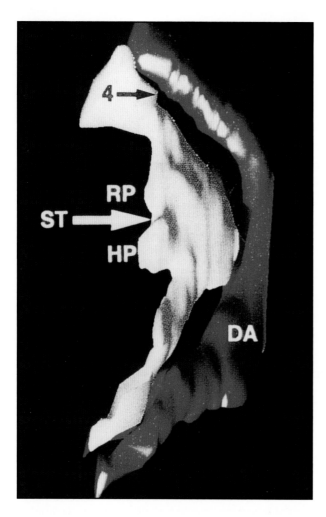

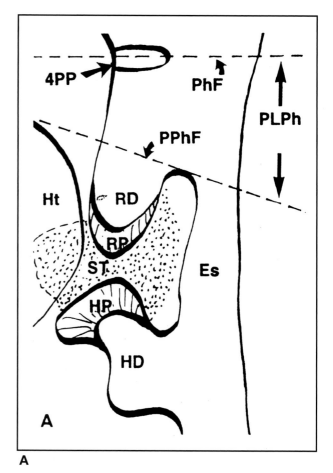

A

Fig 5–6. Stage 11 (17-somite mouse embryo). Lateral view of 3-D reconstruction of epithelial lining for foregut. First evidence of respiratory system is indicated by epithelial thickening along ventral aspect of foregut called respiratory primordium *(RP)*. Respiratory primordium is separated from hepatic primordium *(HP)* by septum transversum *(ST)*, which is indicated by solid white arrow. Septum transversum will eventually develop into central tendon of the developing diaphragm. *4* = site of developing pharyngeal pouch; *DA* = dorsal aorta. (Courtesy of John S Rubin, MD, Robert T Sataloff, MD, DMA, Gwen S Korovin, MD, and Wilbur James Gould, MD, from the book *Diagnosis and Treatment of Voice Disorders*. New York: Igaku-Shoin Medical Publishers; 1995.)

Fig 5–7. Stage 12 (22-somite mouse embryo). **A.** Schematic representation of midsagittal section through laryngopharyngeal region. Respiratory diverticulum *(RD)* is ventral outpocketing of foregut lumen that extends into respiratory primordium *(RP)*. Similarly, hepatic diverticulum *(HD)* results from extension of foregut lumen into hepatic primordium *(HP)*. Cephalic portion of *RD* will eventually develop into infraglottic region of adult larynx. Site of origin of *RD* is called primitive pharyngeal floor *(PPhF)*; it will eventually develop into glottic region of adult larynx. Esophagus *(Es)* separates from *RD* at level of *PPhF*. Primitive pharyngeal floor is separated from fourth pharyngeal pouch *(4PP)* by segment of foregut called primitive laryngopharynx *(PLPh)*. Pharyngeal floor *(PhF)* is at same level as *4PP*. Primitive laryngopharynx will eventually develop into supraglottic region of adult larynx. *Ht* = heart; *ST* = septum transversum. *(continues)*

septum transversum, a structure that will eventually develop into the central tendon of the diaphragm.

Figure 5–7A is a schematic representation of the laryngopharyngeal regions of a stage 12 embryo in comparison with the mature fetal larynx in a midsagittal plane. The respiratory diverticulum is a ventral outpocketing of foregut lumen that extends into the respiratory primordium. The site of origin of the respiratory diverticulum is called the primitive pharyngeal floor and eventually develops into the glottic region of the adult larynx. The cephalic portion of the

respiratory diverticulum eventually develops into the infraglottic region of the adult larynx. The primate pharyngeal floor is separated from the pharyngeal floor, or the level of the fourth pharyngeal pouch, by a segment of foregut originally classified by Zaw-Tun as the primitive laryngopharynx, as discussed above. This will eventually become the adult supraglottic larynx.

Figure 5–7B is a ventral view of a three-dimensional reconstruction of the epithelial lining of the laryngopharyngeal region of a stage 12 embryo. The respi-

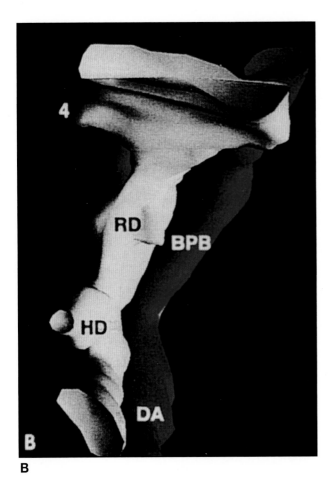

B

Fig 5–7. *(continued)* **B.** Ventral view of 3-D reconstruction of epithelial lining of laryngopharyngeal region. Respiratory diverticulum has given rise to bilateral projections called bronchopulmonary buds *(BPB)*; they will eventually develop into lung parenchyma. *DA* = dorsal aorta; *4* = fourth pharyngeal pouch. (Courtesy of John S Rubin, MD, Robert T Sataloff, MD, DMA, Gwen S Korovin, MD, and Wilbur James Gould, MD, from the book *Diagnosis and Treatment of Voice Disorders*. New York: Igaku-Shoin Medical Publishers; 1995.)

In stages 13 and 14 (Fig 5–8), the bronchopulmonary buds are drawn caudally and dorsally because they are tethered to the septum transversum and the cephalic aspect of the foregut and the respiratory diverticulum migrates superiorly. As a result, (1) two primary main-stem bronchi develop and (2) the carina is seen as a distinct region that develops from the caudal aspect of the respiratory diverticulum, and it is the site of origin of the two primary bronchi.

Figure 5–9 shows the distance between the carina and the respiratory diverticulum by two white solid arrows in a stage 14 embryo. The lengthening of this foregut segment will eventually give rise to the devel-

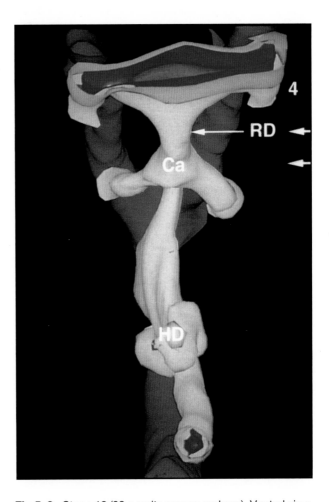

Fig 5–8. Stage 13 (28-somite mouse embryo). Ventral view of epithelial lining of foregut. Bronchopulmonary buds have continued to be drawn dorsocaudally from carina *(Ca)* due to cephalic rotation of embryo and because bronchopulmonary buds are tethered to septum transversum. Carina *(Ca)* develops from caudal aspect of respiratory diverticulum *(RD)*. Two white solid arrows indicate distance between *RD* and *Ca. HD* = hepatic diverticulum. (Courtesy of John S Rubin, MD, Robert T Sataloff, MD, DMA, Gwen S Korovin, MD, and Wilbur James Gould, MD, from the book *Diagnosis and Treatment of Voice Disorders*. New York: Igaku-Shoin Medical Publishers; 1995.)

ratory diverticulum has given rise to bilateral projections called bronchopulmonary buds, which will eventually develop into the lower respiratory tract. The buds are tethered to the superior aspect of the septum transversum.

Dynamic changes to the developing foregut region are occurring at this and subsequent stages. For example, the heart and the hepatic primordium are proliferating at a rapid rate on opposing surfaces of the septum transversum. These differential forces are exerted on the adjacent foregut region, which leads to a dramatic lengthening of the foregut in a cephalocaudal plane. The result can be seen as the distance between the respiratory primordium and the hepatic primordium increases over time.

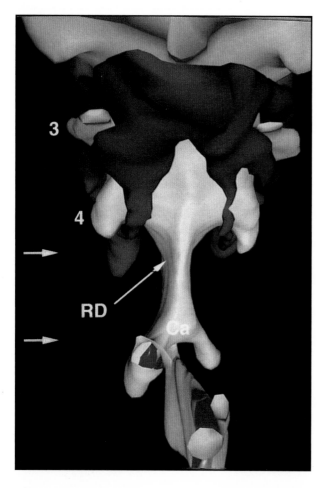

Fig 5–9. Stage 14 (35-somite mouse embryo). Ventral view of 3-D reconstruction of epithelial lining of laryngopharyngeal region. Compared with Fig 7-8, lengthening of *Ca* from *RD* is demonstrated with two white solid arrows. Lenthening of this foregut segment will eventually give rise, in part, to developing trachea. Carina *(Ca)* continues to descend from site of respiratory diverticulum *(RD)*. Numerals 3 and 4 are the third and fourth pharyngeal pouches. (Courtesy of John S Rubin, MD, Robert T Sataloff, MD, DMA, Gwen S Korovin, MD, and Wilbur James Gould, MD, from the book *Diagnosis and Treatment of Voice Disorders*. New York: Igaku-Shoin Medical Publishers; 1995.)

oping trachea. At this point in development, dramatic lengthening of the trachea and esophagus occurs. Anatomically, the esophagus is in close proximity to the region of the carina. Vascular compromise to the developing esophagus may give rise to esophageal atresia or the spectrum of tracheo-esophageal anomalies seen in Figure 5–10.

Esophageal atresia in a newborn infant usually presents clinically with increased salivation requiring frequent suctioning, with the pulmonary triad of coughing, choking, and cyanosis. These symptoms are the result of saliva pooling in the blind proximal esophageal pouch with subsequent overflow into the infant's airway. Aspiration is greater in infants who have a direct airway connection because of an associated tracheo-esophageal fistula.

Tracheoesophageal fistula with a distal esophageal pouch occurs in 80% to 85% of affected patients and results in gastric distention due to the air ingested with each breath. The stomach distention, associated with increased gastric acid production, results in respiratory symptoms due to (1) direct tracheal aspiration of the mixture of refluxed air or gastric acid and (2) decreased diaphragmatic excursion. If the diagnosis is delayed or missed and feeding is begun, choking episodes occur, with the potential for further airway soilage.

Vascular compromise to the developing trachea at this stage of development may give rise to complete tracheal agenesis, atresia, or tracheal stenosis with complete tracheal rings (Fig 5–11). Both of these anomalies are associated with normal laryngeal and pulmonary development because the insult is limited to the region of the developing trachea.

Figure 5–12 demonstrates a coronal section through a reconstruction of a late stage 14 embryo. The infraglottis, which is the most cephalic portion of the respiratory diverticulum, has the characteristic shape of an upright triangle when sectioned in the coronal plane; this is characteristic of the adult conus elasticus. The primitive laryngopharynx, which extends from the infraglottis to the level of the fourth pharyngeal pouch, has become compressed bilaterally along its ventral aspect, called the epithelial lamina. This compression is due to forces exerted by the proliferating triangular-shaped, laryngeal mesodermal anlage and branchial arch arteries. The laryngeal mesodermal anlage eventually develops into the laryngeal cartilages and muscles. An elevation of median pharyngeal floor gives rise to the arytenoid swellings. This occurs at the same level as the fourth pharyngeal pouch. The trachea is seen as the uniformly circular lumen separating the infraglottis from the carina.

In stage 15, the epithelial lamina continues to obliterate the primitive laryngopharynx from a ventral to dorsal direction until obliteration is essentially complete by stage 16. Figure 5–13 is a lateral view of a three-dimensional reconstruction of the laryngopharyngeal region of a stage 16 embryo. A glass simulation is used to represent the epithelial lining of the foregut so that the internal changes to the lumen *(blue)* can be seen. The primitive laryngopharynx is seen as the segment of the foregut between the infraglottis, which has a characteristic shape of an inverted triangle when sectioned in the sagittal plane, and

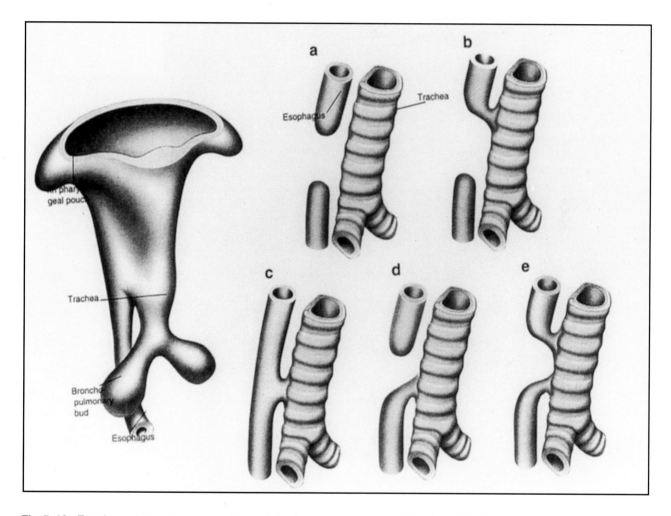

Fig 5–10. Esophageal atresia and spectrum of tracheo-esophageal fistulae. **A.** Esophageal atresia (8%). **B.** Esophageal atresia, proximal tracheo-esophageal fistula (<1%). **C.** Tracheo-esophageal H-Fistula, no atresia (4%). **D.** Esophageal atresia, distal tracheo-esophageal fistula (87%). **E.** Esophageal atresia, proximal and distal tracheoe-sophageal fistula (<1%). (Courtesy of John S Rubin, MD, Robert T Sataloff, MD, DMA, Gwen S Korovin, MD, and Wilbur James Gould, MD, from the book *Diagnosis and Treatment of Voice Disorders*. New York: Igaku-Shoin Medical Publishers; 1995.)

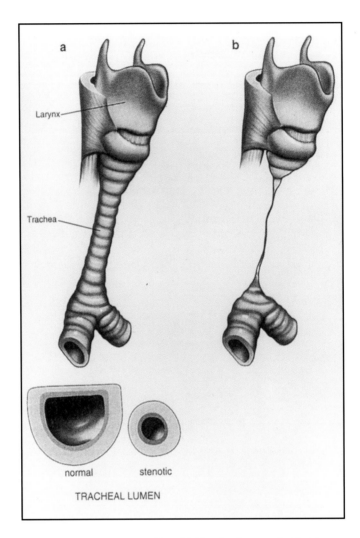

Fig 5–11. Tracheal anomalies. (**a**) Tracheal stenosis. Axial sections demonstrate the concentric circular tracheal cartilage with the loss of the membranous trachea posteriorly. (**b**) Tracheal atresia. Relatively normal laryngeal and pulmonary development is seen in both of these anomalies. (Courtesy of John S Rubin, MD, Robert T Sataloff, MD, DMA, Gwen S Korovin, MD, and Wilbur James Gould, MD, from the book *Diagnosis and Treatment of Voice Disorders.* New York: Igaku-Shoin Medical Publishers; 1995.)

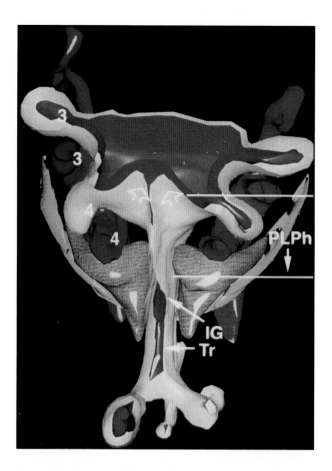

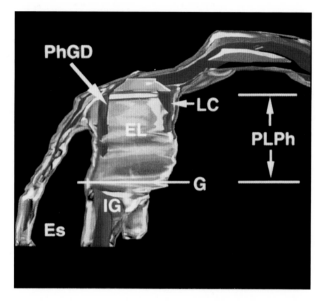

Fig 5–12. Stage 14 (36-somite mouse embryo). Coronal section of a 3-D reconstructed embryo. Region of primitive laryngopharynx (PLPh) has become compressed bilaterally, probably because of forces exerted by the (purple) laryngeal mesodermal anlage and fourth branchial artery (4, red). Infraglottis (IG) has characteristic shape of upright triangle when sectioned in this coronal plane. Infraglottis is separated from carina by ovoid-circular lumen of trachea (Tr). Also, at level of fourth pharyngeal pouch (4), elevation of median pharyngeal floor, as indicated by open white arrows, will give rise to developing arytenoid swelling. (Courtesy of John S. Rubin, MD, Robert T. Sataloff, MD, DMA, Gwen S. Korovin, MD, and Wilbur James Gould, MD, from the book *Diagnosis and Treatment of Voice Disorders*, Igaku-Shoin Medical Publishers, New York, NY; 1995.)

Fig 5–13. Stage 16 (50-somite mouse embryo). Lateral view of 3-D reconstruction of foregut epithelial lining. Glass simulation was used so that internal *(blue)* luminal anatomy could be visualized. Primitive laryngoharynx *(PLPh)* extends from floor of pharynx (level of AS; *yellow*) to infraglottic region below *(IG*; previously cephalic end of respiratory diverticulum). Glottis *(G)* is just cephalic to *IG*. Primitive laryngopharynx is completely obliterated except for narrow pharyngoglottic duct *(PhGD)* dorsally and developing laryngeal cecum *(LC)* ventrally. (Courtesy of John S Rubin, MD, Robert T Sataloff, MD, DMA, Gwen S Korovin, MD, and Wilbur James Gould, MD, from the book *Diagnosis and Treatment of Voice Disorders*. New York: Igaku-Shoin Medical Publishers; 1995.)

the arytenoid swellings *(yellow).* Complete obliteration of the primitive laryngopharynx is seen except for a ventral laryngeal cecum and a dorsal pharyngoglottic duct *(PhGD).* The dorsal pharyngoglottis is the last remnant of the patent communication between the hypopharynx and the infraglottis.

The laryngeal cecum originates as a triangular-shaped lumen along the ventral aspect of the arytenoid swellings and progresses caudally along the ventral aspect of the primitive laryngopharynx until

it reaches the level of the glottis in stage 18 (Fig 5–14). In stage 19, the epithelial lamina begins to recanalize from a dorsocephalad to a ventrocaudal direction. In the process, communication is reestablished between the ventral laryngeal cecum and the dorsal pharyngoglottis. The last portion of the primitive laryngopharynx to recanalize is at the glottic level, as indicated by the white broken line in Fig 5–15. It is the incomplete recanalization of the epithelial lamina that can give rise to the full spectrum of supraglottic

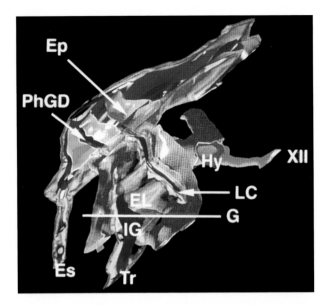

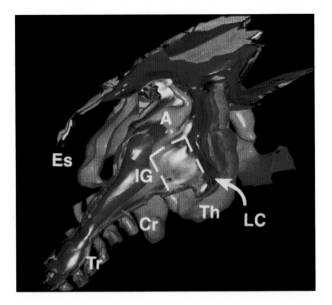

Fig 5–14. Stages 17 and 18 (62-somite mouse embryo). Lateral view of 3-D reconstruction of foregut epithelial lining of laryngopharyngeal region with its surrounding laryngeal mesodermal anlagen (purple). Glass simulation was used to enhance visualization of internal luminal anatomy (blue). Compared to Fig 5–13, (stage 16), primitive laryngopharynx is still obligterated except for pharyngoglottic duct *(PhGD)* dorsally and laryngeal cecum *(LC)* ventrally, which has, at this stage, descended to glottic *(G)* region *(white line)*. Eventually, recanalization of epithelial lamina *(EL)* will bring dorsal PhGD into communication with ventral LC to give rise to laryngeal vestibule, or supraglottic larynx. *Ep* = epiglottis anlage, Hy = hyoid anlage, XII = 12th cranial nerve, Tr = trachea, Es = esophagus. (Courtesy of John S Rubin, MD, Robert T Sataloff, MD, DMA, Gwen S Korovin, MD, and Wilbur James Gould, MD, from the book *Diagnosis and Treatment of Voice Disorders*, Igaku-Shoin Medical Publishers, New York, NY; 1995.)

Fig 5–15. Stages 19 through 23. 3-D reconstruction of laryngopharyngeal region, sectioned in midsagittal plane exposing right medial aspect of embryo. Glass simulation is used to view luminal (dark blue) anatomy. White broken lines indicate area in which epithelial lamina has not completely recanalized. It has been suggested that incomplete recanalization of epithelial lamina can give rise to full spectrum of supraglottic stenosis and glottic webs seen clinically. *Es* = esophagus; *A* = arytenoid cartilage; *Th* = thyroid cartilage; *Cr* = cricoid cartilage; *Tr* = trachea; *IG* = infraglottis; *LC* = laryngeal cecum. (Courtesy of John S Rubin, MD, Robert T Sataloff, MD, DMA, Gwen S Korovin, MD, and Wilbur James Gould, MD, from the book *Diagnosis and Treatment of Voice Disorders*. New York: Igaku-Shoin Medical Publishers; 1995.)

and glottic atresias seen clinically. In stage 21, the laryngeal cecum gives rise bilaterally to the two laryngeal ventricles.

Figure 5–16 is a schematic representation of a stage 18 embryo prior to the recanalization of the epithelial lamina. Complete failure of the epithelial lamina to recanalize would give rise to a type I atresia (Fig 5–16A). Complete recanalization of the epithelial lamina except at the glottic level would give rise to a type III atresia, or a glottic web (Fig 5–16C). Partial recanalization of the epithelial lamina would give rise to a type II atresia (Fig 5–16B). In types I and II atresia, there is associated subglottic stenosis because the insult in development occurred at an earlier point in development, preventing the complete development of the infraglottic region. In addition, there are no

signs of laryngeal ventricles, since they are among the last structures to develop normally.

Laryngeal Cartilage and Muscle Formation

The branchial arch apparatus is an important contributor to the composition and construction of the developing larynx. Branchial arches III, IV, V, and VI are of particular interest, although the fifth arch merges with the sixth branchial arch tissues. Each of the arches is composed of the three primary germ cell layers: an inner cell mass of endoderm, a core of middle cells of mesoderm, and outer cells of ectoderm.[21]

The endodermal derivatives of arches III, IV, and VI contribute to the formation of the pharynx, larynx, trachea, bronchi, and alveoli.

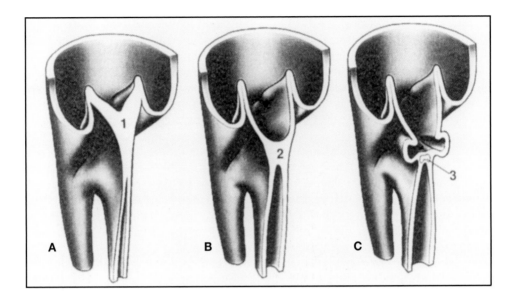

Fig 5–16. Stage 18 embryo prior to the recanalization of the epithelial lamina. **A.** Type I atresia results in a complete supraglottic stenosis. **B.** Type II atresia results in partial supraglottic stenosis. Communication between supraglottis and infraglottis is usually maintained through a patent pharyngoglottic duct. **C.** Type III atresia corresponds to formation of a glottic web. (Courtesy of John S Rubin, MD, Robert T Sataloff, MD, DMA, Gwen S Korovin, MD, and Wilbur James Gould, MD, from the book *Diagnosis and Treatment of Voice Disorders*. New York: Igaku-Shoin Medical Publishers; 1995.)

The mesodermal layer gives rise to the voluntary and involuntary musculature, the vascular and lymphatic systems, and the skeletal elements of the head and neck. The third arch supplies the stylopharyngeus muscle, the common and internal carotid arteries, and the body and greater cornu of the hyoid bone. The fourth arch gives rise to the inferior pharyngeal constrictor muscle, the cricothyroid, and cricopharyngeus muscles. Its arterial supply on the right is the proximal subclavian artery and on the left the aorta. The skeletal components are the thyroid cartilage and cuneiform cartilages. The sixth arch gives rise to all intrinsic muscles of the larynx, except the cricothyroid muscle. Its arterial supply is the pulmonary artery on the right and the ductus arteriosus on the left; and its skeletal components are the cricoid, the arytenoid, and corniculate cartilages, as well as the trachea.

The ectodermal derivatives give rise to the cranial and spinal nerves of all the arches. Innervation to the laryngeal skeletal musculature can be traced to its branchial arch of origin. The third arch gives rise to the glossopharyngeal nerve and its superior and inferior ganglia. The fourth arch gives rise to the jugular and nodose ganglia and superior laryngeal nerve, and the sixth arch gives rise to the recurrent laryngeal nerve. The left recurrent laryngeal nerve remains with the artery of the sixth arch (ductus arteriosus), and the right nerve moves cranially and laterally in association with the artery of the fourth arch (subclavian) because the right homologue of the sixth arch disappears. This explains the caudolateral to rostromedial course of the right recurrent laryngeal nerve.

The formation of laryngeal cartilages from the surrounding mesodermal anlage has been well established, although there are differing theories regarding the actual sequence of chondrification. At approximately 32 days of gestation of human laryngeal development (stage 14), laryngeal mesodermal anlage surrounds the primitive laryngopharynx (Fig 5–12). These sites of condensed mesoderm observed in transverse histologic sections appear as an isosceles triangle and represent the anlage of both the cartilage and the intrinsic muscles of the developing larynx.[14] Based on the shape and site of this wedge-shaped area, Zaw-Tun demonstrated that the ventrolateral margins were the anlage destined to become the thyroid cartilage, and that the caudal arch was anlage destined to become the cricoid cartilage. The first single chondrification site was identified at stage 16 along the ventral aspect of the cricoid anlage. Chondrification advanced dorsally and bilaterally along each side of the infraglottis during stages 19 to 21, until fusion occurred in the mid-dorsal cricoid lamina. Incomplete fusion can explain the full spectrum of laryngotracheal clefts seen clinically in the neonate.[16] Benjamin and Inglis classified laryngeal clefts into four types:[22] Type 1, interarytenoid area; Type 2, partial cricoid; Type 3, total cricoid: remains above the thoracic inlet; Type 4, laryngotracheoesophageal cleft.

Zaw-Tun's observations of cricoid chondrification are unlike those of Fleischmann (1820) and Arnold (1851), who reported that the cricoid developed from chondrifying halves that met dorsally first and ventrally later (cited by Zaw-Tun[14]). Kallius,[9] on the other hand, described chondrification of the cricoid as occurring from bilateral centers that met ventrally first and dorsally later. Furthermore, Soulie and Bardier[23] stated that cricoid chondrification occurred in both directions simultaneously from bilateral centers. An embryologic basis for the relative success of the anterior cricoid split operation for laryngeal stenosis can, in part, be attributed to these earlier theories that describe fusion occurring along the ventral aspect of the cricoid.

The anlagen of the arytenoid cartilages lie within the mesoderm lateral to the epithelial lamina, just above the glottic level.[14] The change from condensed mesoderm to a precartilaginous template with vocal, muscular, and apical processes is complete by stage 21. The vocal process is the last portion of the arytenoid to completely chondrify. Laryngeal hyaline cartilages develop from branchial mesoderm, whereas elastic cartilages are derived from mesoderm of the floor of the pharynx.[24] Most of the arytenoid is composed of hyaline cartilage. However, the vocal processes are developed separately in association with the vocal folds and consist of elastic cartilage. The arytenoid cartilages (from the Greek word *arytaineoeides* meaning ladle-shaped) are pyramidal in shape, consisting of an apex, base, and two processes. The base articulates with the cricoid cartilage. The apex attaches to the corniculate cartilage of Santorini and to the aryepiglottic fold. The vocal process projects anteriorly to connect with the vocal ligament, and the muscular process is the point of insertion of most of the muscles that move the arytenoid.[25] The cricoarytenoid facets are well defined, smooth, and symmetrical. Each arytenoid articulates with an elliptical facet on the posterior superior margin of the cricoid ring. The cricoid facet is about 6 mm long and is cylindrical.[26] Most of the cricoarytenoid motion has traditionally been described as rocking; and along the long axis of the cricoid facet, gliding has also been described.[27] Limited rotary pivoting has been

thought to occur, as well. More recent refinements in our understanding of arytenoid motion are described in chapter 7.

The arytenoid cartilages and the cricoarytenoid facets are extremely symmetrical and consistent.[26] The cricoarytenoid joint is an arthroidal joint, supported by a capsule lined with synovium. The capsule is strengthened posteriorly by the cricoarytenoid ligament.[28] This ligament is strong and ordinarily prevents subluxation. The axis of the joint is at an angle of 45° from the horizontal plane. The cricoarytenoid joint controls abduction and adduction of the true vocal folds, thereby facilitating respiration, protection of the airway, phonation, and other laryngeal functions.

The extrinsic laryngeal muscles develop from the epicardial ridge as part of the infrahyoid muscle mass. It separates into superficial and deep layers, and each layer eventually divides into two masses. The superficial layer splits longitudinally to form lateral and medial parts, resulting in the sternohyoid and omohyoid muscles. The deep layer attaches to the oblique line of the thyroid cartilage, separates into lower and upper parts, and forms the sternothyroid and thyrohyoid muscles. Arytenoid motion is controlled directly by intrinsic laryngeal muscles including the posterior cricoarytenoid, lateral cricoarytenoid, arytenoideus, oblique arytenoid, and thyroarytenoid. It is also affected by the cricothyroid muscle, which increases longitudinal tension on the vocal fold (which attaches to the vocal process of the arytenoid), and to a lesser degree by the thyroepiglottic muscle, which tenses the aryepiglottic fold.

Postnatal Development

Embryologically, the larynx develops most of its anatomical characteristics by the third month of fetal life. At birth, the thyroid cartilage and hyoid bone are attached to each other. The laryngeal skeleton then separates and the slow process of ossification begins. The hyoid bone starts to ossify by 2 years of age. The thyroid and cricoid cartilages ossify during the early 20s, and the arytenoid cartilages ossify in the late 30s. Except for the cuneiform and corniculate cartilages, the entire laryngeal skeleton is ossified by age 65. In the infant, the epiglottis is bulky and omega-shaped. It does not open to its normal adult configuration until puberty. At birth, the larynx is high in the neck, resting at about the level of the third and fourth cervical vertebrae (C3 and C4). It descends to about the level of C6 by the age of 5, and continues its gradual descent, lying at about the level of C7 between ages 15 and 20. Descent continues throughout life in both sexes. As the larynx descends, vocal tract length relationships change and average voice pitch tends to become lower. In infancy, the membranous (vibrating) and cartilaginous portions of the vocal folds are equal in length. By adulthood, the membranous portion accounts for approximately two-thirds of vocal fold length. Total vocal fold length is 6 to 8 mm in the infant, but increases to 12 to 17 mm in the adult female and to 17 to 23 mm in the adult male. The dimensions of all other aspects of laryngeal anatomy increase as well.

First vocalizations sometimes occur prior to birth, although the birth cry is normally the first sound uttered. Its frequency averages about 500 Hz (one octave above middle C). At this time, laryngeal mobility is limited primarily to vertical movements, and the appearance of the larynx is very similar to that of primates (monkeys). As the child grows, mean fundamental frequency of speech (the predominant pitch of the speaking voice) drops gradually. By 8 years of age, it is approximately 275 Hz. Until puberty, male and female larynges are about the same size. During childhood, the physiologic frequency range (the highest and lowest sounds the child can produce) remains fairly constant. However, the musical frequency range increases. That is, the child becomes able to produce musically acceptable sounds throughout an increasing percentage of the frequency range. Thus, between the ages of 6 and 16, the important developmental change is not the absolute range (constant at about 2½ octaves) but rather improved control, efficiency, and quality. Throughout life, mean fundamental frequency drops steadily in females from about 225 Hz in the 20- to 29-year-old group to about 195 Hz in the 80- to 90-year-old group.[29] In males, fundamental frequency of the speaking voice drops until roughly the fifth decade, after which it rises gradually.[30] Recent observations suggest that these aging changes may be less prominent, or may not occur at all, in professional voice users.

References

1. Tucker JA. Development of the human air and food passages. In: *Pediatric Otolaryngology*. 2nd ed. Philadelphia, Pa: WB Saunders; 1990:1041–1054.
2. O'Rahilly R. Developmental stages in human embryos, including a survey of the Carnegie collection. A. Embryos of the first three weeks (stages 1 to 9). Washington, DC: Carnegie Institution; 1973.
3. O'Rahilly R. The timing and sequencing of events in the development of the human digestive system and associated structures during the embryonic period proper. *Anat Embryol.* 1978;153:123–136.
4. O'Rahilly R, Boyden EA. The timing and sequencing of events in the development of the human respiratory system during the embryonic period proper. *Z Anat Engwgesch.* 1973;141:237–250.
5. Muller F, O'Rahilly R, Tucker JA. The human larynx at the end of the embryonic period proper. 1. The laryngeal and infrahyoid muscles and their innervation. *Acta Otolaryngol (Stockh).* 1981;91:323–336.
6. O'Rahilly R, Muller F. Chevalier Jackson Lecture. Respiratory and alimentary relations in staged embryos. *Ann Otol Rhinol Laryngol.* 1984;93:421.
7. Walander A. Prenatal development of the epithelial primordium of the larynx in rat. *Acta Anat.* 1950;10 (suppl 13).
8. His W. Anatomie menschlicher Embryoenen. III. *Zur Geschichte der Organe.* Leipzig: Vogel; 1885:12–19.
9. Kallius E. Beitrage zur Engwickelungsgeschichte des Kehlkopfes. *Anat Hft (Wiesbaden).* 1897;9:303–363.
10. Frazer JE. The development of the larynx. *J Anat Physiol.* 1910;44:156–191.
11. Negus VE. The mechanism of the larynx. *Lancet.* 1924;206:987–993.
12. Smith E. The early development of the trachea and esophagus in relation to atresia of the esohagus and tracheoesophageal fistula. *Contr Embryol.* 1957;36:41–57.
13. Zaw-Tun HA. The tracheo-esophageal steptum—fact or fantasy? Origin and development of the respiratory primordium and esophagus. *Acta Anat.* 1982;114:1–21.
14. Zaw-Tun HA, Burdi AR. Re-examination of the origin and early development of the human larnyx. *Acta Anat.* 1985;122:163–184.
15. Hast MH. Early development of the human laryngeal muscles. *Ann Otol Rhinol Laryngol.* 1972;81:524–531.
16. Zaw-Tun HA. Development of congenital laryngeal atresias and clefts. *Ann Otol Rhinol Laryngol.* 1988;97:353–358.
17. Arey LB. *Developmental Anatomy.* 7th ed. Philadelphia: WB Saunders; 1965:260–268.
18. Henick DH. Three-dimensional analysis of murine laryngeal development. *Ann Otol Rhinol Laryngol.* 1993;102(suppl 159):1–24.
19. Marko M, Leith A, Parsons D. 3-Dimensional reconstructions of cells from serial sections and whole cell mounts using multi-level countouring of stereo micrographs. *J Electron Microsc Tech.* 1988;9:395–411.
20. Leith A, Marko M, Parsons D. Computer graphics for cellular reconstructions. *IEEE Comput Graphic Applicat.* 1989;9:16–23.
21. Hast MH. The development of the larynx. *Otolaryngol Clin North Am.* 1970;3:413–438.
22. Benjamin B, Inglis A. Minor congenital laryngeal clefts: diagnosis and classification. *Ann Otol Rhinol Laryngol.* 1989;87:417–420.
23. Soulie A, Bardier E. Recherches sur le development du larynx chez l'homme. *J Anat Physiol* (Paris). 1907;43:137–240.

24. Langman J. *Medical Embryology*. 3rd ed. Baltimore: Williams and Wilkins; 1975:269–272.

25. Hollinshead WH. *Anatomy for Surgeons*. vol 1, 3rd ed. New York: Harper & Row.

26. Maue WM, Dickson DR. Cartilages and ligaments of the adult human larnyx. *Arch Otolaryngol*. 1971;94:432–439.

27. von Leden H, Moore P. The mechanics of the cricoarytenoid joint. *Arch Otolaryngol*. 1961;73:63–72.

28. Pennington CL. External trauma of the larynx and trachea. *Ann Otol Rhinol Laryngol*. 1972;81:546–554.

29. McGlone R, Hollien H. Vocal pitch characteristics of aged women. *J Speech Hear Res*. 1963;6:164–170.

30. Hollien H, Shipp T. Speaking fundamental frequency and chronologic age in males. *J Speech Hear Res*. 1972;15:155–159.

6

Clinical Anatomy and Physiology of the Voice

Robert Thayer Sataloff

Anatomy

The anatomy of the voice is not limited to the region between the suprasternal notch and the hyoid bone. Practically all body systems affect the voice. The larynx receives the greatest attention because it is the most sensitive and expressive component of the vocal mechanism, but anatomic interactions throughout the patient's body must be considered in treating voice disorders. It is helpful to think of the larynx as composed of four anatomic units: skeleton, mucosa, intrinsic muscles, and extrinsic muscles, as well as vascular, neurological, and other related structures. The glottis is the space between the vocal folds.

Laryngeal Skeleton: Cartilages, Ligaments, and Membranes

The most important parts of the laryngeal skeleton are the thyroid cartilage, the cricoid cartilage, and the two arytenoid cartilages (Fig 6–1). The laryngeal cartilages are connected by soft attachments that allow changes in their relative angles and distances, thereby permitting alterations in the shape and tension of the tissues extended between them. The intrinsic muscles of the larynx are connected to these cartilages. For example, one of the intrinsic muscles, the thyroarytenoid (TA), extends on each side from the arytenoid cartilage to the inside of the thyroid cartilage just below and behind the thyroid prominence. The medial belly of the TA is also known as the vocalis muscle, and it forms the body of the vocal fold.

The pyramidal, paired arytenoid cartilages sit atop the superior edge of the cricoid cartilage. They each include a muscular process, a vocal process and an apex, a body, and a complex, concave articular surface. They are hyaline cartilages, except for the vocal process, and the apices in some cases, which are composed of fibroelastic cartilage. The hyaline portions generally begin to ossify at around 30 years of age.[1]

Ossification of the thyroid cartilage begins earlier, usually at around 20 years of age, and usually begins posteriorly and inferiorly.[1] The two thyroid laminae join in the midline, forming an angle of approximately 120° in women and approximately 90° in men. The thyroid prominence is also more noticeable in men and is commonly known as the "Adam's apple." Just above the thyroid prominence, the thyroid laminae form a "V," the thyroid notch. Posteriorly, the laminae extend to form superior and inferior cornua (horns). The superior cornu connects to the hyoid bone via the thyrohyoid ligament. The inferior cornu is connected to the cricoid cartilage by a synovial cricothyroid joint. The joint is encased in a capsular ligament, which is strengthened posteriorly by a fibrous band. Movement of the paired cricothyroid joints is diarthrodial. The primary movement is rotary, with the cricoid rotating around a transverse axis passing through both joints. Gliding in various directions also occurs to a limited extent. This joint tends to move anteromedially during vocal fold adduction and posterolaterally during vocal fold abduction and permits the anterior aspects of the cricoid and thyroid cartilages to be brought more closely together to increase vocal fold length (and frequency of phonation, or pitch) in response to cricothyroid (CT) muscle contraction.

The perichondrium of the thyroid cartilage is thinner internally than externally. Externally, in the midline, there is a tiny landmark that can be helpful in identifying the position of the anterior commissure.[2] This small, diamond-shaped surface depression is

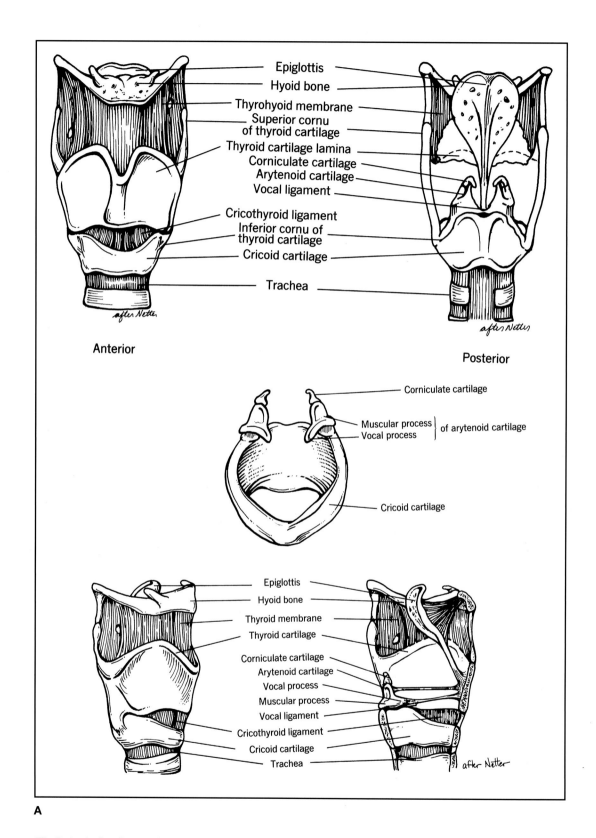

Fig 6–1. A. Cartilages of the larynx.

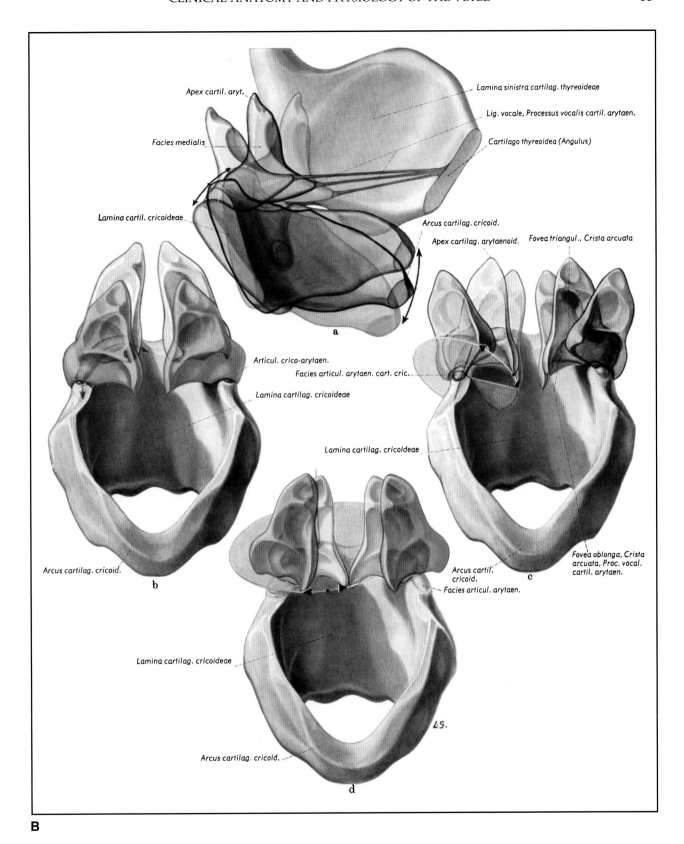

B

Fig 6–1. *(continued)* **B.** Schematic representation of position changes of laryngeal cartilages illustrating the most extreme positions achieved by each. (From Pernkopf E. *Atlas of Topographical and Applied Human Anatomy.* Munich: Urban & Schwarzenberg; 1963, with permission.)

associated with a slightly lighter color compared to the adjacent thyroid cartilage. It is found in the anterior midline, approximately halfway between the thyroid notch and the inferior border of the thyroid cartilage; and a small, unnamed artery travels through this tiny depression, as described by Adams et al.[2] At a corresponding location on the inner surface, there is a small protrusion that is devoid of perichondrium. This is the point of attachment of Broyle's ligament and the anterior commissure tendon. The rest of the thyroid cartilage is covered with fairly thick perichondrium; and the smooth, concave inner surface is covered by a mucosal membrane. Broyle's ligament is formed by the vocal ligament (which is also the upper border of the conus elasticus), the internal perichondrium of the thyroid cartilage, and the thyroepiglottic ligament.

The oblique line is another important external landmark of the thyroid cartilage. It runs anteroinferiorly from a superior thyroid tubercle located just inferior to the superior cornu, and it extends to the inferior thyroid tubercle located at the lower border of the thyroid lamina. The oblique line is actually a ridge to which the thyrohyoid, sternothyroid, and inferior pharyngeal constrictor muscles attach. Fibers from the palatopharyngeus and stylopharyngeus muscles attach to the posterior border of the thyroid cartilage.

The signet ring-shaped cricoid cartilage is the only circumferential cartilaginous structure in the airway. Its posterior lamina may rise to a height of approximately 30 millimeters (mm), and its anterior arch may be only a few millimeters in height. Not only is the anterior aspect of the arch thin, but it also ossifies later than the posterior aspect of the cricoid cartilage, which begins to ossify in the early to mid-twenties. Because the anterior portion of the arch is both thin and tends to ossify later, it is particularly prone to fracture during surgical manipulation. This should be remembered in procedures such as cricothyroid approximation; traction should always be centered laterally on the cricoid arch, rather than near the midline. The cricoid is connected to the thyroid cartilage not only through the cricothyroid joints, but also through the cricothyroid membrane and its midline thickening known as the cricothyroid ligament.

Internal dimensions of the cricoid cartilage and trachea vary substantially. Such information is important with regard to tracheal intubation, dilatation, stenting, endoscopy, anastomosis, and transplantation. The luminal cross sections vary between and among men and women. The smallest dimension occurs in the frontal plane.[3] In women, this measures approximately 11.6 mm, with a range of 8.9 to 17.0 mm. In men, it is about 15 mm, with a range of 11 to 21.5 mm. The distance between the cricoarytenoid joint facets varies from person to person, as well, as does the angle between longitudinal axes of the cricoarytenoid joint facets (42° to 74° in women, 37° to 75° in men).[3]

The cross section of the trachea is also highly variable, with a frontal diameter reported as narrow as 9.9 mm in women and 12 mm in men.[3] The marked variation in size and shape highlights the difficulty in creating a standardized rigid stent. It should also be noted that the diameter of the cricoid ring in some women is too narrow to permit the atraumatic passage of an endotracheal tube with a 7 mm internal diameter. Anatomic variation also must be taken into consideration during laryngotracheal replacement or transplantation.

In addition to the cricoid, thyroid and paired arytenoid cartilages, there are numerous other components of the laryngeal skeleton and the related structures. The superior aspect of the laryngeal skeleton is the hyoid bone, which is usually ossified by age 2. The hyoid bone attaches to the mylohyoid, geniohyoid, and hyoglossus muscles superiorly and inferiorly connects to the thyroid cartilage via the thyrohyoid membrane. This U-shaped bone has an inferiorly located lesser cornu and a superiorly located greater cornu on each side.

The epiglottis is a fibroelastic cartilage that is shaped like a leaf and narrows inferiorly where it becomes the petiole. The petiole attaches to the inner surface of the thyroid cartilage immediately below the thyroid notch by the thyroepiglottic ligament. The superior aspect of the epiglottis faces the base of the tongue anteriorly and the laryngeal inlet posteriorly. The hyoepiglottic ligament connects the posterior surface of the hyoid bone to the lingual surface of the epiglottis. On its laryngeal surface, the epiglottis contains a protuberance that sometimes obscures view of the anterior commissure. This is the epiglottic tubercle. Perichondrium is less densely adherent to the epiglottic cartilage on the lingual surface than on the laryngeal surface, explaining why epiglottic edema tends to be more prominent in the vallecula than in the laryngeal inlet. However, edema on the lingual surface can push the epiglottis posteriorly, resulting in airway obstruction. The pre-epiglottic space is formed by the mucosa of the vallecula superiorly, the thyroid cartilage and thyrohyoid membrane anteriorly, and the epiglottis posteriorly and inferiorly. Blood vessels and lymphatic channels course through this space.

There are several cartilages of less functional importance located above the thyroid cartilage. The cartilages of Santorini, or corniculate cartilages, are fibroelastic and are found above the arytenoid cartilages. They help improve the rigidity of the aryepiglottic folds. Like the epiglottis and many other elastic cartilages, they do not ossify. The cuneiform cartilages (cartilages of Wrisberg) also do not ossify, even though they consist of hyaline cartilage. They are located in the aryepiglottic folds and also improve rigidity, helping to direct swallowing toward the piriform sinuses. The triticeal cartilages are located laterally within the thyrohyoid ligaments. These structures are hyaline cartilages and often do ossify (as may the lateral thyrohyoid ligaments themselves). They may easily be mistaken on x-rays for foreign bodies. The lateral thyrohyoid ligaments are actually thickenings of the thyrohyoid membrane. There is also more central thickening called the medial thyrohyoid ligament. The laryngeal vessels and the internal branches of the superior laryngeal nerves enter the thyrohyoid membrane posterior to the lateral thyrohyoid ligaments. The thyrohyoid ligaments and membranes are among the structures that suspend the larynx directly or indirectly from the skull base. The other structures that do so include the stylohyoid ligaments, the thyrohyoid ligaments and membrane, the thyroepiglottic ligaments, the cricothy-

roid ligaments and membrane, the cricoarytenoid ligaments, and the cricotracheal ligament and membrane.

The arytenoid cartilages are capable of complex motion, as discussed in detail in the following chapter. Previously, it was believed that the arytenoids rock, glide, and rotate. More accurately, the cartilages are brought together in the midline and revolve over the cricoid. It appears as if individuals use different strategies for approximating the arytenoids, and these strategies may influence a person's susceptibility to laryngeal trauma that can cause vocal process ulcers and laryngeal granulomas.

The larynx contains two important, large, paired "membranes," the triangular membranes and the quadrangular membranes (Fig 6–2). The paired trian-

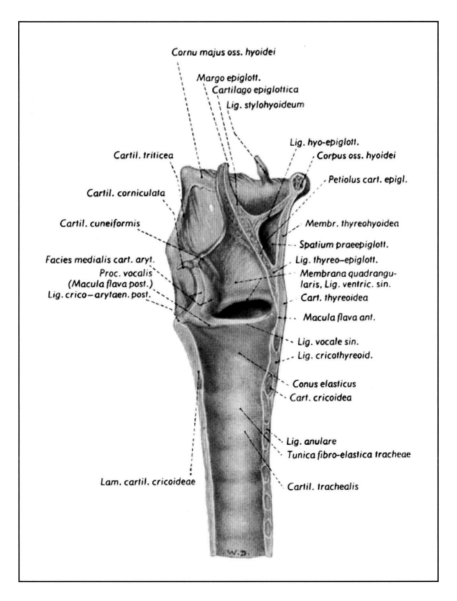

Fig 6–2. Internal view of the larynx illustrating the position of the quadrangular and triangular membranes. (From Pernkopf E. *Atlas of Topographical and Applied Human Anatomy.* Munich: Urban & Schwarzenberg; 1963, with permission.)

gular membranes form the conus elasticus. Each triangular membrane is attached to the cricoid and thyroid cartilages anteriorly (the base of the triangular membrane), to the cricoid cartilage inferiorly, and to the vocal process of the arytenoid cartilage posteriorly (the apex of the triangular membrane). The superior edge of each fibroelastic triangular membrane is the vocal ligament, forming the intermediate and deep layers of lamina propria of the vocal folds, as discussed below. These structures extend anteriorly to form a portion of Broyle's ligament. More anteriorly, a portion of the conus elasticus constitutes the cricothyroid ligament.

Like the upper border of the triangular membrane, the upper and lower borders of the quadrangular membrane are free edges. The upper border of each quadrangular membrane is the aryepiglottic fold, bilaterally. The lower border extends from the inferior aspect of the epiglottis to the vocal process of the arytenoid cartilages and forms part of the vestibular (or ventricular) fold, or false vocal fold. Superior and inferior thickenings in the quadrangular membrane form the aryepiglottic ligament and the vestibular ligament, respectively. The quadrangular membrane is shorter in vertical height posteriorly than anteriorly. Lateral to these structures is a region called the paraglottic space. It is bounded laterally by the thyroid lamina and medially by the supraglottic mucosa covering the vestibular fold from the ventricle to the aryepiglottic fold. There is a thin, elastic membrane that is contiguous above with the quadrangular membrane and below with the conus elasticus, forming an intermediate segment of elastic tissue that encloses the laryngeal ventricle. The paraglottic space is contiguous with the space between the cricoid and thyroid cartilages. The laryngeal inlet lies between the aryepiglottic folds.

The region formed by the paired ventricular and aryepiglottic folds is designated as "supraglottis." A pouch of mucosa between the under surface of the false vocal folds and the upper surface of the true vocal folds is called the ventricle of Morgagni, or the laryngeal ventricle. The superior aspect of the laryngeal ventricle is known as the saccule of Hilton. The supraglottis extends from the tip of the epiglottis to the junction between the floor and lateral wall of the laryngeal ventricle. Hence, most clinicians define the floor of the ventricle as part of the glottic larynx. The glottic larynx also includes the true vocal folds, anterior commissure, and interarytenoid region at the level of the vocal folds posteriorly (commonly, and incorrectly, referred to as the posterior commissure). The subglottis begins at the junction of squamous and respiratory epithelium under the vibratory margin of the vocal folds,

about 5 mm below the beginning of the vibratory margin. The subglottis ends at the inferior border of the cricoid cartilage.

Larynx: Mucosa

With the exception of the vocal folds, the epithelial lining of most of the vocal tract is pseudostratified, ciliated columnar epithelium, typical respiratory epithelium involved in handling mucous secretions. The vibratory margin of the vocal fold is covered with nonkeratinizing, stratified squamous epithelium, better suited than respiratory epithelium to withstand the trauma of vocal fold contact. Vocal fold lubrication is created by cells in several areas. The saccule, the posterior surface of the epiglottis, and the aryepiglottic folds contain seromucinous, tubuloalveolar glands that secrete serous and/or mucinous lubricant. There are also goblet cells within the respiratory epithelium that secrete mucus. These are especially common in the area of the false vocal folds. The goblet cells and glands also secrete glycoproteins, lysozymes, and other materials essential to healthy vocal fold function. The laryngeal mucosa also contains immunologically active Langerhans' cells.[4] In most people, secretory glands are not located near the vibratory margin.

The vibratory margin of the vocal folds is much more complicated than simply mucosa overlying muscle. It consists of five layers[5] (Fig 6–3). The thin, lubricated epithelium covering the vocal folds forms the area of contact between the vibrating vocal folds and acts somewhat like a capsule, helping to maintain vocal fold shape. The superficial layer of the lamina propria, also known as Reinke's space, is composed of loose fibrous components and matrix and lies immediately below the epithelial layer. It contains very few fibroblasts and consists of a network of mucopolysaccharides, hyaluronic acid, and decorin that provides for the flexibility required of the vocal fold cover layer.[6-9] In normal vocal folds the superficial lamina propria also contains fibronectin. Fibronectin is also thought to be deposited as a response to tissue injury.[10] The superficial lamina propria also contains elastin precursors (elaunin and oxytalin), but relatively few mature elastin or collagen fibers. Ordinarily, it has few or no lymphatics, secretory glands or capillaries. Myofibroblasts and macrophages were found in the superficial lamina propria in about one third of laryngeal specimens studied by Catten et al[9] and were more common in women than in men. The third layer of the vocal folds is the intermediate layer of the lamina propria. Mature elastin fibers make up most of the intermediate layer. They are arranged longitudinally. This layer also contains large quantities of hyaluronic

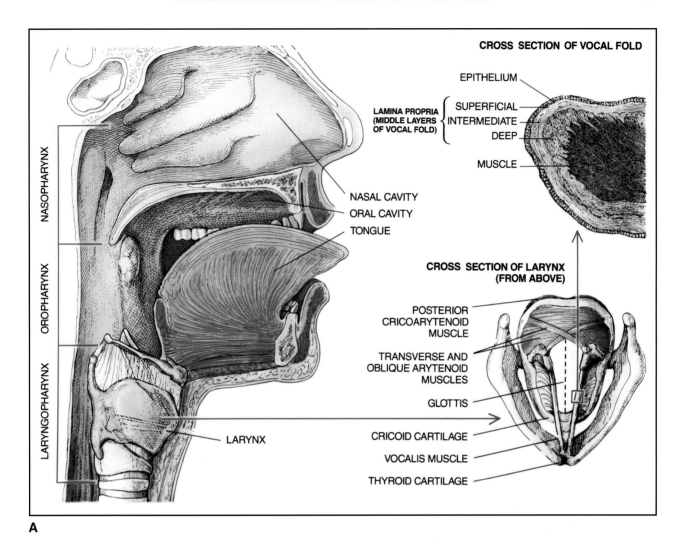

A

Fig 6–3. A. An overview of the larynx and vocal tract, showing the vocal folds, and the region from which the vocal fold was sampled to obtain the cross-section showing the layered structure. (Reprinted with permission from Sataloff, RT. The human voice. *Sci Am*. 1992;267:108-115.)

acid, a relatively inflexible space-filler that is hydrophilic and is believed to act as a shock absorber.[7] Fibromodulin also is present in the intermediate layer.[8] The deep layer of the lamina propria, the fourth layer, is composed primarily of longitudinally arranged collagenous fibers and is rich in fibroblasts. The TA or vocalis muscle constitutes the body of the vocal fold and is the fifth layer, as well as one of the intrinsic laryngeal muscles. The region that consists of the intermediate and deep layers of the lamina propria is called the vocal ligament and lies immediately below Reinke's space. It is important to note that this layered structure of the vocal folds is not present at birth, but rather begins developing at around the age of 7 or 8 years and is not completed until the end of adolescence.[11,12] There are other differences between the pediatric and adult larynx that are not reviewed in this chapter; but many are discussed elsewhere in this book in connection with relevant clinical entities. A great deal more information is available about the ultrastructure of human vocal folds and may be found in other literature.[13]

Although variations along the length of the membranous vocal fold are important in only a few situations, the surgeon, in particular, should be aware that they exist. The mucosa (epithelium and lamina propria, together) of the normal adult male has been described as being approximately 1.1 mm thick. The superficial layer is about 0.3 mm; the vocal ligament is about 0.8 mm;[14] and the epithelium is about 5 to 25 cells (about 50 microns) in thickness.[15] However, particularly interesting research by Friedrich et al shows

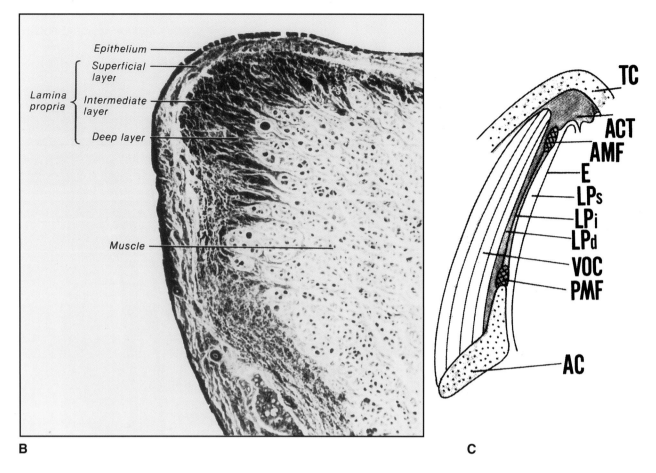

B

C

Fig 6–3. *(continued)* **B.** The structure of the vocal fold. (Reprinted with permission from Hirano M. *Clinical Examination of Voice*. New York: Springer-Verlag; 1981:5.) **C.** Schematic representation of a horizontal section of the vocal fold. TC, thyroid cartilage; ACT, anterior commissure tendon; AMF, anterior macula flava; PMF, posterior macula flava; AC, arytenoid cartilage; E, epithelium; LP, lamina propria; s, superficial layer; i, intermediate layer; d, deep layer; VOC, vocalis muscle. (From Gray S, Hirano M, Sato K. Molecular and cellular structure of vocal fold tissue. In: Titze IR: *Vocal Fold Physiology*. San Diego: Singular Publishing Group, Inc; 1993:4, with permission.)

additional interesting complexity and variation in the anatomy of the vocal fold.[16] Friedrich et al divided the vocal fold into five histological and functional portions. Three of the portions included the musculomembranous vocal fold, and the other two regions were divisions of the posterior glottic region and included the region of the vocal process of the arytenoids, which constitutes the cartilaginous portion of the vocal folds and the lateral wall of the posterior glottis. They also found significant differences between men and women in terms of not only absolute measurements, but also relative dimensions of various portions of the vocal fold. In particular, the middle portion of the musculomembranous vocal fold was twice as long in men (8.5 mm) as in women (4.6 mm), accounting for 37% of total glottic length in men and only 29% in women. The authors speculate that this difference in the length of the vibrating portions of the vocal folds may explain why the fundamental fre-

quency ratio between men and women is approximately 1:2, while the overall laryngeal dimensions are only 1:1.5. In addition to variations in length, Friedrich et al also found that the thickness of the lamina propria varied depending upon location along the length of the vocal fold and on gender. (Fig 6–4) Friedrich's elegant research should be interpreted in the historical context of earlier observations, some of which appear to provide data that are contradictory to his. Actually, the methods of observation and intent of the studies differed; and most of the findings in the various studies are reconcilable.

In 1986, Hirano et al[17] studied the posterior glottis in 20 specimens obtained from autopsy, photographing the larynges from above and below in neutral, adducted, and abducted conditions. They also studied the histology of the posterior glottis in the same three conditions. Hirano et al defined the posterior glottis as consisting of three portions: the posterior wall of the

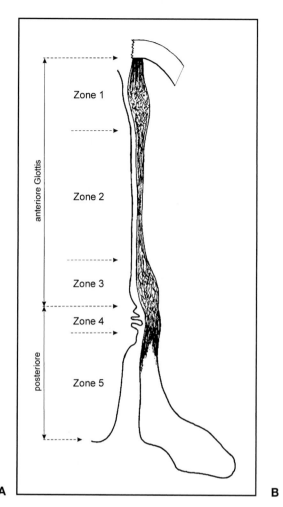

A

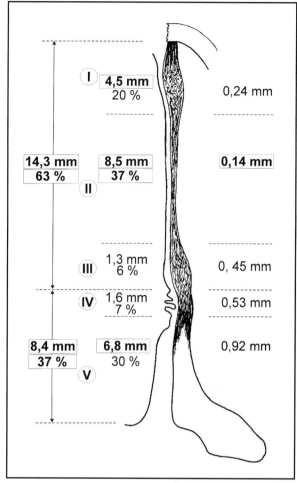

B

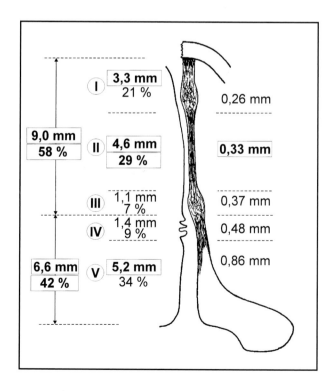

C

Fig 6–4. **A.** Vocal fold divided into zones. **B.** Proportions of the vocal fold constituted by each zone in men. **C.** thickness of the lamina propria in millimeters in women. Note that the European numbering system is used in which 0.45 mm is written as 0,45 mm. (Courtesy of Gerhardt Friederich, M.D.)

glottis, the lateral wall of the posterior glottis, and the cartilaginous portion of the vocal fold. They noted that the posterior larynx closes at the supraglottis during vocal fold adduction, rather than at the glottis, thus producing a conical space that can be seen only from below. Using this methodology, they calculated that the posterior glottis accounted for 35 to 45% of the entire glottic length, and 50 to 65% of the entire glottic area. The mucosa covering the posterior glottis consisted of ciliated epithelium, and the lamina propria consisted of only two layers. The superficial layer was looser in structure, and the deep layer was composed of dense elastic and collagenous fibers with numerous mucosecretory glands. Many of the fibers in the deep layer ran vertically in the region of the posterior wall of the glottis, but the fibers on the lateral wall were found to run obliquely. This study provided useful, interesting anatomic information. However, in interpreting its physiological significance, it should be remembered that abduction and adduction were accomplished by threads attached to the muscular processes of the arytenoid cartilages; and the results may or may not be identical to the complex motions that occur during phonation in a living human.[17]

It has long been recognized that particularly striking variations occur at the anterior and posterior portions of the musculomembranous vocal fold, the region between the vocal process and attachment of the vocal fold to the thyroid cartilage.[18] Anteriorly, the intermediate layer of the lamina propria becomes thick, forming an oval mass called the anterior macula flava. This structure is composed of stroma, fibroblasts, and elastic fibers. Anteriorly, the anterior macula flava inserts into the anterior commissure tendon (Broyle's ligament). The anterior commissure tendon is a mass of collagenous fibers, which is connected to the midpoint of the thyroid cartilage anteriorly, the anterior macula flava posteriorly, and the deep layer of the lamina propria laterally. As Hirano has pointed out, this arrangement allows the stiffness to change gradually from the pliable musculomembranous vocal fold to the stiffer thyroid cartilage.[18] Sato et al have described stellate cells in the macula flava that are related to fibroblasts, but which appear to constantly synthesize extracellular matrices that are required for normal human vocal fold mucosal function.[19-21] Changes in extracellular matrices alter vocal fold function, particularly viscoelasticity; and these changes are associated with some aspects of vocal aging. Aging changes in the vocal fold stellate cells in the macula flava may be responsible for some of the age-related extracellular matrices alterations.[22-25]

A similar gradual change in stiffness occurs posteriorly where the intermediate layer of the lamina propria also thickens to form the posterior macula flava, another oval mass that is structurally similar to the anterior macula flava. The posterior macula flava attaches to the vocal process of the arytenoid cartilage through a transitional structure that consists of chondrocytes, fibroblasts, and intermediate cells.[26] Thus, the stiffness progresses from the flexible musculomembranous vocal fold to the slightly stiffer macula flava, to the stiffer transitional structure, to the elastic cartilage of the vocal process, and to the hyalin cartilage of the arytenoid body. It is believed that this gradual change in stiffness serves as a cushion that may protect the vocal folds from mechanical damage caused by contact or vibrations.[26] It may also act as a controlled damper that smooths mechanical changes during vocal fold movements. This arrangement seems particularly well suited to vibration, as are other aspects of the vocal fold architecture. For example, blood vessels in the vocal folds begin posteriorly and anteriorly and run parallel to the vibratory margin, with very few vessels entering the mucosa perpendicular to the free edge of the vibratory margin or from the underlying muscle. Even the elastic and collagenous fibers of the lamina propria run approximately parallel to the vibratory margin, allowing them to compress against each other or pull apart from each other flexibly and parallel with the forces of the mucosal wave. The more one studies the vocal fold, the more one appreciates the beauty of its engineering.

Functionally, the five layers have different mechanical properties and are analogous to ball bearings of different sizes that allow the smooth shearing action necessary for proper vocal fold vibration. The posterior two fifths (approximately) of the vocal folds are cartilaginous, and the anterior three fifths are musculomembranous (from the vocal process forward) in adults. Under normal circumstances, most of the vibratory function critical to voice quality occurs in the musculomembranous portion.

Mechanically, the vocal fold structures act more like three layers consisting of the cover (epithelium and superficial layer of the lamina propria), transition (intermediate and deep layers of the lamina propria), and the body (the vocalis muscles). Understanding this anatomy is important because different pathologic entities occur in different layers and require different approaches to treatment. For example, fibroblasts are responsible for scar formation. Therefore, lesions that occur superficially in the vocal folds (eg, nodules, cysts, and most polyps) should permit treatment without disturbance of the intermediate and deep layers, where fibroblast proliferation, or scar formation occurs.

In addition to the five layers of the vocal fold, there is a complex basement membrane connecting the epithelium to the superficial layer of the lamina propria.[27] The basement membrane is a multi-layered, chemically complex structure. It gives rise to Type VII collagen loops which encircle Type III collagen fibers in the superficial layer of the lamina propria (Fig 6–5).

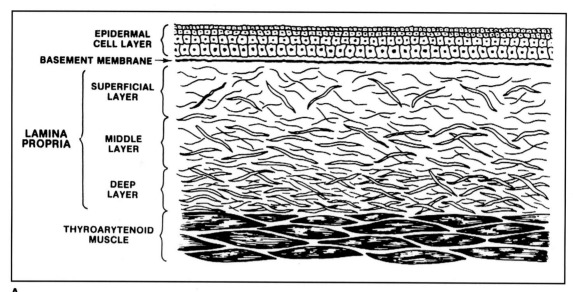

A

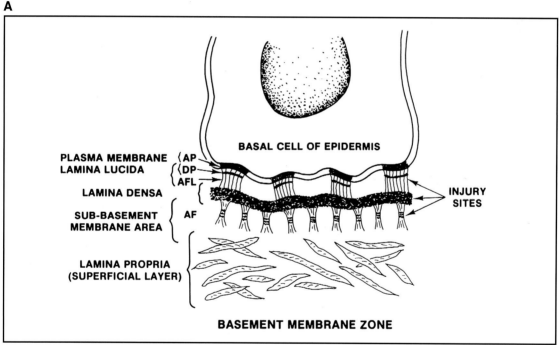

B

Fig 6–5. A. Structure of the vocal fold (not drawn to scale). The basement membrane lies between the epithelium and the superficial layer of the lamina propria. (From Gray S, Basement membrane zone injury in vocal modules. In: Gauffin, J, Hammarberg B. *Vocal Fold Physiology,* Singular Publishing Group; 1991, with permission.) **B.** Basement membrane zone. Basal cells are connected to the lamina densa by attachment plax (AP) in the plasma membrane of the epidermis. Anchoring filaments (AFL) extend from the attachment plax through the sub-basal densa plate (DP) and attach to the lamina densa (dark single-layer, electron-dense band just beneath the basal cell layer.) The sub-basement membrane zone consists of anchoring fibers (AF) that attach to the lamina densa and extend into the superficial layer of the lamina propria. Type VII collagen fibers attach to the network of the lamina propria by looping around Type III collagen fibers. (From Gray S. Basement membrane zone injury in vocal nodules. In: Gauffin, J, Hammarberg B, eds. *Vocal Fold Physiology.* Singular Publishing Group; 1991, with permission.)

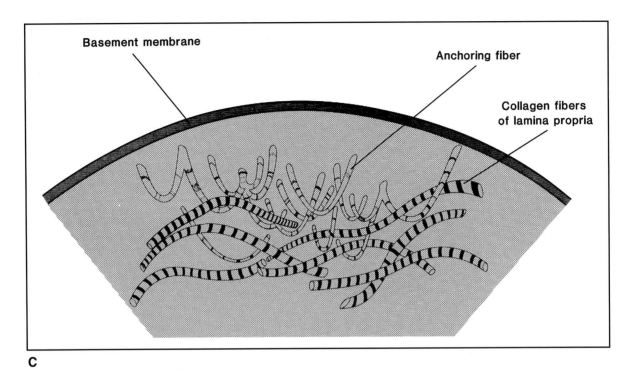

C

Fig 6–5. *(continued)* **C.** Type VII collagen anchoring fibers pass from the basement membrane, reinserting into it. Through the anchoring fiber loops pass Type III collagen fibers of the superficial layer of lamina propria (Courtesy of Steven Gray, MD)

Current research has changed substantially our understanding of vocal fold composition and function. For example, in his description of the basement membrane zone, Gray described a chain-link fence arrangement of anchoring fibers, which he believes permits tissue compression and bending.[6] The density of the anchoring fibers is greatest in the area of greatest vibration and shearing stresses, in the middle of the musculomembranous portion of the vocal folds. Knowledge of the basement membrane has already been important in changing surgical techniques, as discussed later in this book. It also appears important in other matters, such as the ability to heal following trauma, the development of certain kinds of vocal fold pathology, and in histopathologic differential diagnosis.

The vocal folds may be thought of as the oscillators of the vocal mechanism.[28] Above the true vocal folds are tissues known as the "false vocal folds." Unlike the true vocal folds, they do not make contact during normal speaking or singing. However, they may produce voice during certain abnormal circumstances. This phenomenon is called dysphonia plica ventricularis. Until recently, the importance of the false vocal folds during normal phonation was not appreciated. In general, they are considered to be used primarily for forceful laryngeal closure; and they come into play during pathological conditions. However, contrary to popular practice, surgeons should recognize that they cannot be removed without affecting phonation. The physics of airflow through the larynx is very complex, involving vortex formation and sophisticated turbulence patterns that are essential to normal phonation. The false vocal folds provide a downstream resistance, which is important in this process; and they probably play a role in vocal tract resonance, as well.

Laryngeal: Blood Supply and Lymphatic Drainage

The larynx receives its blood supply primarily from the inferior and superior laryngeal arteries and the cricothyroid artery. The superior laryngeal arteries arise from the superior thyroid arteries, which are branches of the external carotid arteries. The superior laryngeal arteries course with the superior laryngeal nerves, piercing the thyrohyoid membrane with the internal branch of the superior laryngeal nerve. The superior laryngeal arteries supply the structures related to the quadrangular membranes and piriform sinuses, primarily above the cricoid cartilage. These include the epiglottis, aryepiglottic fold, thyroarytenoid (TA) muscle, lateral cricoarytenoid (LCA) muscle, interarytenoid (IA) muscle, and vocal fold mucosa. There are anastomoses with the superior laryngeal artery on the contralateral side and with the inferior laryngeal artery. The cricothyroid (CT) artery also arises from the superior thyroid artery and supplies the CT muscle and membrane, some of the extrinsic laryngeal musculature, and portions of the subglottic pharynx (after penetrating the cricothyroid membrane). The inferior laryngeal arteries arise from the inferior thyroid arteries, branches of the thyrocervical trunk. On the left, the inferior thyroid artery may arise directly from the subclavian artery. The inferior laryngeal arteries travel with the recurrent laryngeal nerves to supply the posterior cricoarytenoid (PCA) muscle, and probably portions of the true vocal fold ventricles and false vocal folds, in some cases. The superior laryngeal veins join the internal jugular veins, and the inferior laryngeal veins empty into the thyrocervical trunks and from there communicate with the subclavian venous system.

The blood supply to the vocal fold mucosa deserves special attention. It is unusual in several ways. The vocal folds contain only small vessels including arterioles, venules, and capillaries. They run parallel to the vibratory margin of the vocal fold, entering from anterior or posterior; and they have frequent arteriovenous anastomoses.[29] This arrangement appears to optimize vessel patency and blood flow even in the presence of the substantial shearing forces encountered during high-pressure phonation. Although Franz and Aharinejad have suggested that there are venous connections between the mucosa and muscle,[29] other authors disagree.[30,31] There appear to be no direct communications between the microvasculature of the superficial lamina propria and the medial belly of the thyroarytenoid (vocalis) muscle. However, Franz and Aharinejad appear to have been correct in suggesting that the serpentine course of subepithelial vessels is engineered to accommodate safely the extreme changes in length and tension that may occur during phonation.[30]

The vessels along the vibratory margin have a different structure than those on the superior surface of the vocal fold or in the TA muscle.[12] For example, capillaries along the vibratory margin are lined by endothelial cells and encircled by pericytes with tight intercellular junctions. The endothelial cells have intermediate-thickness filaments near the cell nucleus and bundles of thick filaments adjacent to the luminal cell membrane.[31] These filaments, together with the lamellate structure of the basement membrane and its interspersed myocytes and pericytes, form a lattice that stabilizes the structure of the microvessels, helping them to tolerate the high shearing forces that can be generated during phonation.[31] This structure

enhances mechanical support and helps explain the relative infrequency with which vocal fold hemorrhage occurs, even during forceful phonation. The other vessels of the vocal fold and laryngeal muscles are composed mainly of simple, endothelial-lined capillaries of the continuous (nonfenestrated) variety (the most common type of capillary).[32]

Lymphatic drainage from the larynx occurs through superficial and deep systems, although the deep system is most important. The superficial lymphatic system communicates bilaterally and provides only intramucosal drainage. Each deep system is submucosal and drains its lateral structures. Lymphatic drainage from the larynx courses superiorly and inferiorly. Supraglottic lymphatic vessels travel with the superior laryngeal and superior thyroid vessels to deep cervical lymph nodes (levels II and III) associated with the internal jugular veins. This drainage may be bilateral. There are also lymphatic vessels from the laryngeal ventricles that course through the cricothyroid membrane and thyroid gland en route to the prelaryngeal, prethyroid, supraclavicular, pretracheal, and paratracheal lymph nodes. Inferiorly, lymphatic vessels from the glottic and subglottic larynx form two posterolateral pedicles and a middle pedicle. The posterolateral pedicles travel unilaterally with the inferior thyroid artery to the deep lateral cervical (levels III and IV), subclavian, paratracheal, and tracheoesophageal lymph nodes. The middle pedicle courses through the cricothyroid membrane, communicating with pretracheal and Delphian nodes, which drain into the deep cervical lymph nodes. There is scant lymphatic drainage from the true vocal folds.

Larynx: Intrinsic Muscles

The intrinsic muscles are responsible for abduction, adduction, and tension of the vocal folds (Figs 6–6 and 6–7). All but one of the muscles on each side of the larynx are innervated by the two recurrent (or inferior) laryngeal nerves, which are discussed in detail below. Because these nerves usually run long courses from the neck down into the chest and back up to the larynx (hence, the name "recurrent"), they are easily injured by trauma, neck surgery, and thoracic surgery. The left recurrent laryngeal nerve is more susceptible to injury during chest surgery because of its course around the aortic arch. The right recurrent laryngeal nerve, however, is more likely to have an oblique course laterally in the neck and thus may be at greater risk for injury in neck surgery. Such injuries may result in abductor and adductor paralysis of the vocal fold. The remaining muscle, the CT muscle, is innervated by the superior laryngeal nerve on each side, which is especially susceptible to viral and traumatic injury.

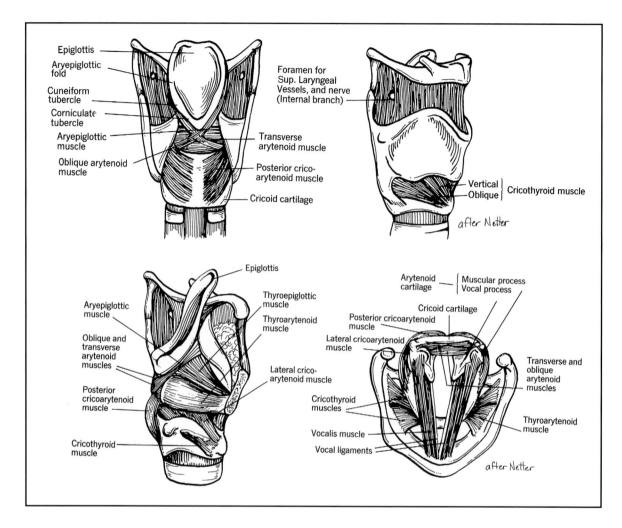

Fig 6–6. The intrinsic muscles of the larynx.

For some purposes, including electromyography and surgery, it is important to understand the function of individual laryngeal muscles in detail. The muscles of primary functional importance are those innervated by the recurrent laryngeal nerves including the thyroarytenoid (TA), posterior cricoarytenoid (PCA), lateral cricoarytenoid (LCA), and interarytenoid or arytenoideus (IA), and the superior laryngeal nerves including the cricothyroid (CT) (Figs 6–6, 6–7, and 6–8)

The TA muscle adducts, lowers, shortens, and thickens the vocal folds, thus rounding the vocal fold's edge. Thus, the cover (epithelium and superficial layer of lamina propria) and transition (intermediate and deep layers of lamina propria) are effectively made slacker, while the body is stiffened. Adduction from vocalis muscle (the medial belly of the TA) contraction is active, particularly in the musculomembranous segment of the vocal folds. Contraction of the vocalis muscle tends to lower vocal pitch. The thyroarytenoid

originates anteriorly from the posterior (interior) surface of the thyroid cartilage and inserts into the lateral base of the arytenoid cartilage, from the vocal process to the muscular process. More specifically, the superior bundles of the muscle insert into the lateral and inferior aspects of the vocal process and run primarily in a horizontal direction. The antero-inferior bundles insert into the anterolateral aspect of the arytenoid cartilage from its tip to an area lateral to the vocal process. (These fibers are associated primarily with the lateral belly.) The most medial fibers run parallel to the vocal ligament and insert onto the medial aspect of the vocal process. There are also cranial fibers that extend into the aryepiglottic fold. Anteriorly, the vertical organization of the muscle results in a twisted configuration of muscle fibers when the vocal fold is adducted. The neuromuscular organization of the medial belly of the TA muscle is more complex than previously believed. Research by Sanders is clarifying these complexities;

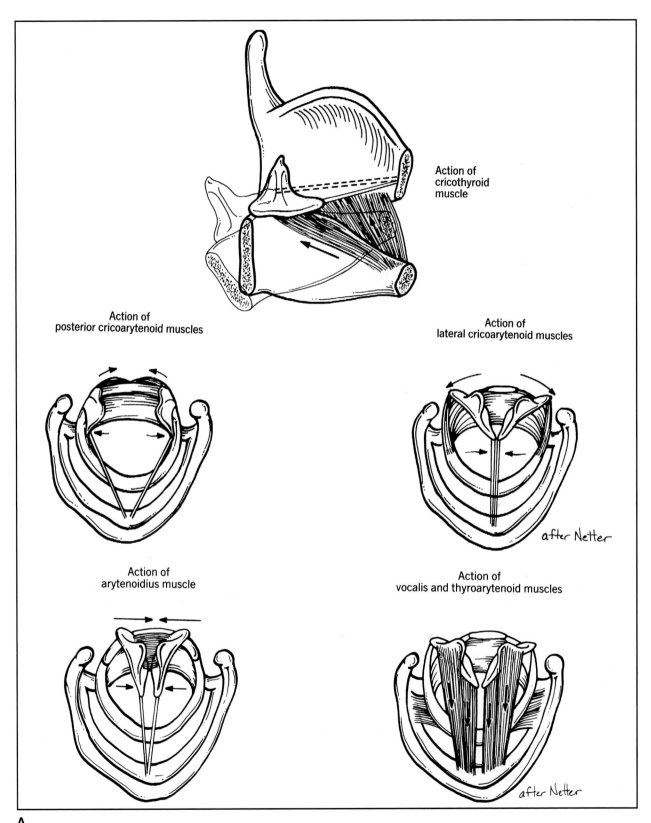

Action of
cricothyroid
muscle

Action of
posterior cricoarytenoid muscles

Action of
lateral cricoarytenoid muscles

after Netter

Action of
arytenoidius muscle

Action of
vocalis and thyroarytenoid muscles

after Netter

A

Fig 6–7. A. Action of the intrinsic muscles. In the bottom four figures, the directional arrows suggest muscle actions, but may give a misleading impression of arytenoid motion. These drawings should not be misinterpreted as indicating that the arytenoid cartilage rotates around a vertical axis. The angle of the long axis of the cricoid facets does not permit some of the motion implied in this figure, as discussed in chapter 7. However, the drawing still provides a useful conceptualization of the effect of individual intrinsic muscles, so long as the limitations are recognized.

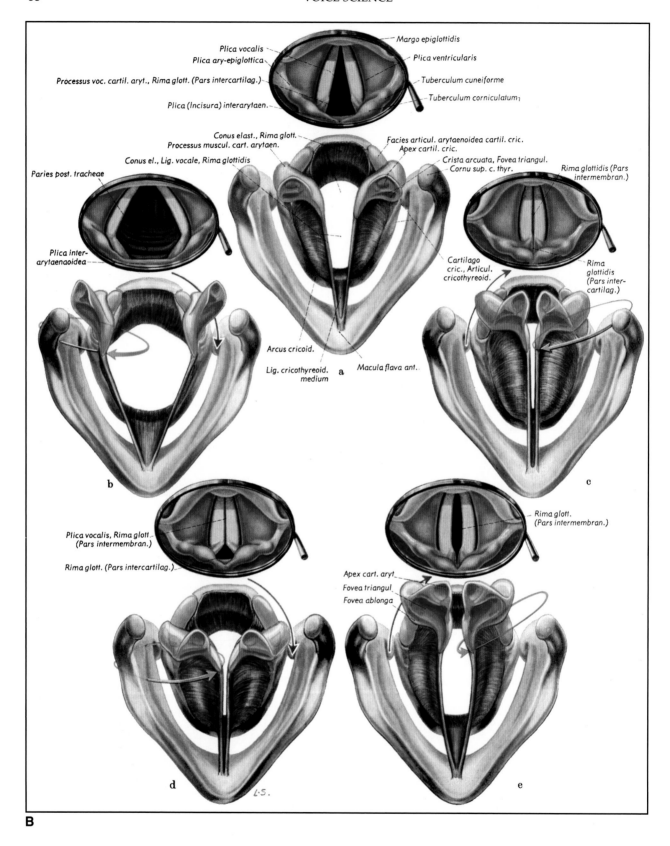

Fig 6–7. *(continued)* **B.** The shapes of the glottis as seen on mirror examination and on anatomic preparations during rest (a), inspiration (b), phonation (c), whispering (d), and falsetto singing (e). (From Pernkopf E. *Atlas of Topographical and Applied Human Anatomy.* Munich: Urban & Schwarzenberg; 1963, with permission.)

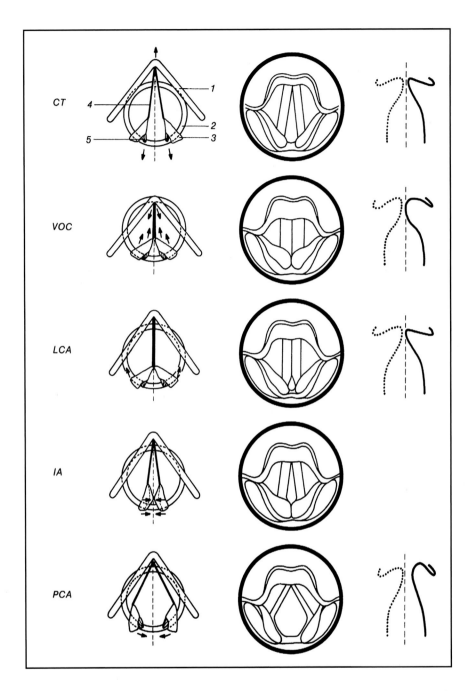

Fig 6–8. A. A schematic presentation of the function of the laryngeal muscles. The left column shows the location of the cartilages and the edge of the vocal folds when the laryngeal muscles are activated individually. The arrows indicate the direction of the force exerted. 1, thyroid cartilage; 2, cricoid cartilage; 3, arytenoid cartilage; 4, vocal ligament; 5, posterior cricoarytenoid ligament. The middle column shows the views from above. The right column illustrates contours of frontal sections at the middle of the musculomembranous portion of the vocal fold. The dotted line illustrates the vocal fold position when no muscle is activated. CT, cricothyroid; VOC, vocalis; LCA, lateral cricoarytenoid; IA, interarytenoid; PCA, posterior cricoarytenoid. (From Hirano M. *Clinical Examination of Voice.* New York: Springer-Verlag; 1981:8, with permission.)

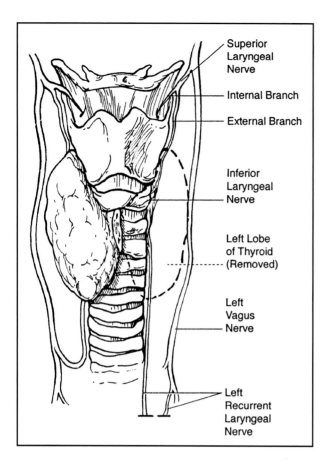

Fig 6–8. *(continued)* **B.** The superior and recurrent laryngeal nerve branch from the vagus nerve and enter the larynx.

and he has shown, for example, that muscle groups along the superior and inferior margin of the medial (contact) surface of the vocal folds function differently from one another.[33] The thyroarytenoid is the third largest intrinsic muscle of the larynx. The TA muscle is divided into two compartments. The medial compartment is also known as the vocalis muscle. It contains a high percentage of slow-twitch muscle fibers. The lateral compartment has predominantly fast-twitch muscle fibers. One may suspect that the medial compartment (vocalis) is specialized for phonation, whereas the lateral compartment (muscularis) is specialized for vocal fold adduction; but these suppositions are unproven.

The LCA muscle is a small muscle that adducts, lowers, elongates, and thins the vocal fold. All layers are stiffened, and the vocal fold edge takes on a more angular or sharp contour in response to LCA muscle contraction. It originates on the superior lateral border of the cricoid cartilage and inserts into the anterior lateral surface of the muscular process of the arytenoid.

It is an extremely important adductor and is especially important in the initial movement from abduction to adduction. The bilaterally innervated IA muscle (arytenoideus, or interarytenoid muscle, a medium-sized intrinsic muscle) primarily adducts the cartilaginous portion of the vocal folds. It is particularly important in providing medial compression to close the posterior glottis. It has relatively little effect on the stiffness of the musculomembranous portion. The interarytenoid muscle is the only unpaired laryngeal muscle. It is innervated by the recurrent laryngeal nerve and receives fibers from the internal branch of the superior laryngeal nerve (although there is no evidence that the internal branch of the superior laryngeal nerve provides motor innervation to this muscle. The IA muscle consists of transverse and oblique fibers. The transverse fibers originate from the lateral margin of one arytenoid and insert into the lateral margin of the opposite arytenoid. The oblique fibers originate posteriorly and inferiorly from the base of the cricoid cartilage, but they extend around the apex of the arytenoid cartilage to continue as the aryepiglottic musculature.

The PCA muscle abducts, elevates, elongates, and thins the vocal fold by rocking the arytenoid cartilage posterolaterally. All layers are stiffened, and the edge of the vocal fold is rounded during PCA muscle contraction. It is the second largest intrinsic muscle. It originates over a broad area of the posterolateral portion of the cricoid lamina and inserts on the posterior surface of the muscular process of the arytenoid cartilage, forming a short tendon that covers the cranial aspect of the muscular process.

When the superior laryngeal nerves are stimulated, the CT muscles move the vocal folds into the paramedian position. They also lower, stretch, elongate, and thin the vocal folds, stiffening all layers and sharpening the vocal folds' contours. It is the largest intrinsic laryngeal muscle and is largely responsible for longitudinal tension, a very important factor in control of pitch. Contraction of the CT muscles tends to increase vocal pitch through their lengthening effect on the vocal folds. The CT muscle originates from the anterior and lateral portions of the arch of the cricoid cartilage and has two bellies. The oblique belly inserts into the posterior half of the thyroid lamina and the anterior portion of the inferior cornu of the thyroid cartilage. The vertical (erect) belly inserts into the inferior border of the anterior aspect of the thyroid lamina.

Intrinsic laryngeal muscles are skeletal muscles. Skeletal muscles are composed primarily of three types of fibers. Type I fibers are highly resistant to fatigue, contract slowly, and utilize aerobic (oxidative) metabolism. They have low glycogen levels, high levels of oxidative enzymes, and are relatively smaller in diameter. Fast-contracting Type IIB fibers are subdivided into Types IIA, IIB, and IIX. The myosin heavy chain isoform in each fiber type is primarily responsible for determining contraction speed. Only Type I, IIA, and IIX fibers are present in humans. Type IIA fibers use principally oxidative metabolism but contain both a high level of oxidative enzymes and glycogen. They contract rapidly but are also fatigue resistant. Type IIB fibers are found in small mammals and are the most fatiguable but fastest-contracting fiber types. They also are the largest in diameter. They utilize anaerobic glycolysis primarily and contain a large amount of glycogen but relatively few oxidative enzymes. Human laryngeal muscles generally contain a mixture of Types I, IIA, and IIX fibers, with the proportion of each varying from muscle to muscle. The fiber composition of laryngeal muscles differs from that of most larger skeletal muscles. Elsewhere, muscle fiber diameters are fairly constant, ranging between 60 to 80 microns. In laryngeal muscles, there is considerably more variability,[34,35] and fiber diameters vary between 10 microns and 100 microns, with an average diameter of 40 to 50 microns. The TA and lateral CT muscles are designed for rapid contraction. Laryngeal muscles have a higher proportion of Type IIA fibers than most other muscles, which makes them particularly well suited to rapid contraction with fatigue resistance.[36] In addition, many laryngeal motor units have multiple neural innervations. There appear to be approximately 20 to 30 muscle fibers per motor unit in a human CT muscle,[37] suggesting that the motor unit size of this laryngeal muscle is similar to that of extraocular and facial muscles.[38] In the human TA muscle, 70 to 80% of muscle fibers have two or more nerve endplates and some fibers have as many as five nerve endplates.[39] Only 50% of CT and LCA muscle fibers have multiple endplates, and multiple endplates are even less common in the PCA muscle (5%). It is still not known whether one muscle fiber can be part of more than one motor unit (receive endplates from different motor neurons), or whether all of the endplates on each muscle are associated with the same motor neuron.[36]

Recent research has provided additional interesting observations in laryngeal muscles. Wu et al found that human PCA and TA muscles express three types of myosin heavy-chain (MyHC) isoforms, including slow type I, fast type 2A, and fast type 2X.[40] Single-fiber analysis has demonstrated regional differences, and the common occurrence of hybrid fibers.[40] Recent research by Malmgren and coworkers has also demonstrated that laryngeal muscles remain capable of spontaneous regeneration over a lifetime and that the proportion of regenerating fibers (identified immunohistochemically by the presence of the developmental myosin isoforms) increases as the TA muscle ages.[41] Malmgren et al also speculate that the increase in regenerating fibers may be a compensatory response to an age-related increase in muscle fiber injury or death. These new findings are consistent with clinical observations that many "aging changes" of the voice can be reversed through voice therapy.[42]

Larynx: Innervation

The recurrent and superior laryngeal nerves are branches of the tenth cranial nerve, or the vagus nerves, which are the longest of the cranial nerves. The vagus nerves originate from 8 to 10 rootlets in a groove in the brainstem between the olive and inferior cerebellar peduncles, in close association with the origins of the ninth and eleventh cranial nerves. The rootlets attach to the medulla oblongata in the brainstem, and course below the cerebellar flocculus, where they unite to form the tenth cranial nerve, which exits the cranium through the jugular foramen with the spinal accessory nerve, the glossopharyngeal nerve, and the jugular vein. The hypoglossal nerve exits the skull through the hypoglossal canal, which is adjacent to the jugular foramen and separated from it by a septum. The first ganglion of the vagus nerve is the jugular ganglion, which is located in the jugular foramen, and is known also as the superior ganglion of the vagus nerve. The nodose ganglion (inferior ganglion) is the second ganglion of the vagus nerve and is located in the neck, slightly inferior to the jugular foramen. The vagus nerve contains branchial motor fibers, somatic sensory fibers (from the posterior external auditory canal, from skin adjacent to the ear in some people, and from the tympanic membrane and pharynx), special sensory fibers (taste), visceral motor fibers, and visceral afferent fibers (from the upper respiratory tract, esophagus, stomach, pancreas, abdominal viscera, aortic bodies, aortic arch, and heart). Cells for the visceral, special sensory afferent, and somatic sensory afferent fibers originate in the jugular ganglion and the nodose ganglion. Visceral afferent fibers have cell bodies in the inferior vagal ganglion. Their axons ascend to the medulla oblongata, then descend in the tractus solitarius from which they enter the caudal aspect of the nucleus of the tractus solitarius, also called the nucleus solitarius. Sensory afferent fibers from the larynx and pharynx travel with the visceral afferent fibers via the recurrent and superior laryngeal nerves to their cell bodies in the inferior ganglion.

The nucleus ambiguus is the branchial motor nucleus for the external branch of the superior laryngeal nerve, the recurrent laryngeal nerve, and the pharyngeal nerve and its plexus. Bilateral corticobulbar fibers from the motor cortexes descend through the internal capsule to synapse with the nucleus ambiguus. This bilateral innervation is important in maintaining coordinated, voluntary control of the laryngeal muscles. The motor neurons of the CT muscle are situated rostrally in the nucleus ambiguus, just caudal to the nucleus of the facial nerve. More rostrally, the motor neurons of the TA, LCA, and PCA muscles are located in overlapping pools.[43,44] The LCA, TA, and IA motor neurons are located in close association to each other (partially overlapping) and are separate from the CT motor neurons, which are more rostrally co-located with pharyngeal and palatal motor neurons.[45] Davis and Nail[43] have shown that there are larger motor neurons associated with the TA and LCA muscles (fast acting muscles used to constrict and protect the airway) than with the PCA and CT muscle (slower acting muscles that dilate the airway for respiration). Many other neuromotor regions of importance to phonation are beyond the scope of this chapter (mouth, tongue, palate, pharynx, chest, abdomen) but should be considered part of the anatomy of the voice.

Premotor neurons, or interneurons, control motor neurons; and motor neurons with multiple functions may be controlled by more than one premotor neuron. For example, for phonation, the premotor neuron controlling the TA muscle is associated with the nucleus retroambiguus, located caudally in the medulla. However, for swallowing functions, the TA muscle can be driven by premotor neurons elsewhere in the medulla and pons.[46]

The periaqueductal gray (PAG) matter is a central area of particular interest to voice specialists and has been studied elegantly by several investigators, especially Pamela Davis, PhD, in Sydney, Australia. The PAG is a region of gray matter, composed of neuronal cell bodies, surrounding the cerebral aqueduct. It is contiguous with gray matter surrounding the third ventricle in the hypothalamus and thalamus rostrally and with gray matter surrounding the pontine portion of the fourth ventricle caudally. Stimulation of the PAG, or of other regions that stimulate the PAG (such as the hypothalamus),[47] produces vocalization; and destruction of the PAG produces mutism.[48-51] The neurons in the PAG form longitudinal columns and are essential to emotional expression.[52] The lateral column of neurons in the PAG is responsible for vocalization, increases in blood pressure and heart rate associated with the fight-or-flight response, alterations in bodily blood flow, and non-opioid analgesia.[53-56] PAG neurons control vocalization by anastomosing with cells in the nucleus retroambiguus, the

origin of premotor neurons discussed above. In addition to stimulating motor neurons in the nucleus ambiguus associated with the larynx, the nucleus retroambiguus also stimulates motor neurons associated with chewing; movements of the tongue, palate, face, and pharynx; and motor activity in the chest and abdomen.[43] The PAG region receives numerous connections from the cortex;[57] and it may be involved in emotional expression associated with the voice in speech and song. It clearly plays an important role in spontaneous emotional voicing in animals, newborns, and adult humans.[58] The PAG matter is also involved in muscle control during respiration,[53,59,60] a function linked closely with phonation. Interestingly, Davis and coworkers have shown that vocalization activated by the PAG is also associated with laryngeal and vagal afferent input, suggesting that the duration of vocalization is controlled, not just by stimulation of vocalization (including emotional content), but also by the amount of air available in the lungs.[61] Ambalavanar demonstrated that afferents from the internal branch of the superior laryngeal nerve travel to the portions of the PAG involved in vocalization, which may be the pathway associated with coordinating such reflex control.[62] Interestingly, the Lombard effect, which is so important to speakers and singers (the tendency to speak more loudly in the presence of background noise), is also represented in the PAG.[63]

Bandler et al have suggested that the PAG may not activate and deactivate laryngeal, respiratory and orofacial motoneurons directly, but rather may establish "emotional and vocal readiness," with activation actually being dependent on higher brain structures.[56] They suggest that this may explain why damage to the PAG and/or the anterior cingulate cortex produces mutism, even when other components of the voluntary vocal motor system are intact, and why motor cortex injury does not cause mutism when the lateral PAG remains intact to produce emotional vocalization.

Broca's area and the sensory-motor regions of the lateral cerebral cortex are involved in control for vocalization. In 1959, Penfield and Roberts published classic descriptions of the function of the primary motor cortex based on cortical stimulation performed in patients with epilepsy.[64] Vocalization was localized in the lowest portion of the cortical strip. Stimulation of this region produced activity not only in laryngeal muscles, but also in those of the jaw, lips and tongue. The premotor cortex (Brodmann's area 6) is located close to the primary voice motor cortex, as is the supplementary motor region, which is involved in initiation of speech. Adjacent subcortical areas are also important for speech, but their functions are not understood completely. Most axons in the cerebral cortex cross the midline. So, functions such as motor control from the left hemisphere may affect primarily the right side of the body. However, some functions, including those controlled by cranial nerves (ie, facial and laryngeal muscle function), may be ipsilateral and/or contralateral.

Studies utilizing dynamic imaging techniques such as positron-emission tomography (PET) have begun to improve our understanding of function in these areas of the brain. Perry et al used PET to study singing.[65] They found hyperperfusion during singing in various areas associated with the motor cortex, including the anterior cingulate cortex, precentral gyri, anterior insula, supplementary motor area, and the cerebellum. In addition to dynamic imaging (cerebral blood flow) studies, a variety of other methods can be used to study neurophysiology of brain function, including neuropsychological testing, dichotic listening, dichaptic touching, split-field tachistoscopic viewing, electroencephalography with evoked potential testing, and other techniques. Some of these approaches have been used to study cerebral dominance and its relationship to musical faculty. It is popularly believed that music and art are associated with the type of thinking performed primarily in the right brain of a right-handed individual, while language is represented primarily by processes in the left brain. At present, it is unclear whether these traditional models are valid; and it seems probable that complex interactions involving numerous cortical and subcortical areas of both sides of the brain are involved in complicated activities such as emotional expression through speech or song.

The superior laryngeal nerve branches off the vagus nerve high in the neck at the inferior end of the nodose ganglion. It travels between the internal and external carotid arteries, dividing into an internal and external branch near the posterior aspect of the hyoid bone. The external branch courses inferiorly with the superior thyroid artery and vein over the constrictor muscle and through the posterior cricothyroid membrane into the larynx (see Fig 6–8B). The external branch supplies the CT muscle. An extension of the external branch may also supply motor and sensory innervation to the vocal folds. Wu et al have identified this extension of the external branch of the superior laryngeal nerve as the human communicating nerve.[66] This neural connection was found in 12 (44%) of 27 specimens. When present, it exited the medial surface of the cricothyroid muscle and entered the lateral surface of the thyroarytenoid muscle. The communicating nerve was composed of an intramuscular branch, which combined with the recurrent laryngeal nerve or terminated within the thyroarytenoid muscle directly, and

an extramuscular branch that passed through the thyroarytenoid muscle and terminated in the subglottic mucosa in the region of the cricoarytenoid joint. The communicating nerves contain an average of 2,510 myelinated axons, of which 31% were motor neurons. Wu et al believe that when the communicating nerve is present, it supplies a second source of motor innervation to the thyroarytenoid muscle and extensive sensory innervation to the subglottic area and cricoarytenoid joint.

The internal branch of the superior laryngeal nerve is responsible primarily for sensation in the mucosa at and above the level of the vocal fold, but it may be responsible for some motor innervations of laryngeal muscles, as well. The internal branch of the superior laryngeal nerves is divided into three divisions.[67] The superior division supplies the mucosa on the laryngeal surface of the epiglottis. The middle division supplies portions of the true vocal folds, false vocal folds, and the aryepiglottic folds. The inferior division supplies the mucosa of the arytenoids, the portion of the subglottis not supplied by the recurrent laryngeal nerve, the upper esophageal sphincter, and the anterior wall of the hypopharynx. The internal branch of the superior laryngeal nerves also supplies the thyroepiglottic and cricoarytenoid joints.

Terminal sensory nuclei also are involved in reflex pathways associated with the reticular formation. The distributions of the sensory nerves within the larynx in humans remain somewhat speculative, being inferred primarily from research performed in cats.[68] Yoshida and coworkers found that the internal branch at the superior laryngeal nerve supplies the ipsilateral side of the epiglottis, aryepiglottic fold, arytenoid eminence, rostral aspect of the vocal fold, vestibule, and mucosa overlying the PCA muscle. The posterior branch of the recurrent laryngeal nerve divides into two branches, one of which goes to Galen's anastomosis. The other sensory branch provides bilateral supply with ipsilateral dominance to the caudal aspect of the vocal fold and the subglottic region. Some fibers from the internal branch of the superior laryngeal nerve join with fibers from the posterior branch of the recurrent laryngeal nerve to share innervation of the posterior wall of the glottis and the medial aspect of the arytenoids bilaterally with ipsilateral predominance.[69] The cell bodies of the sensory fibers arise primarily in the nodose ganglion and project to the ipsilateral nucleus solitarius. Special sensory fibers for taste from the epiglottis and the larynx course with the vagus nerve to the tractus solitarius and its nucleus.

The recurrent laryngeal nerves branch off the vagus in the chest. On the left, the nerve usually loops around the aortic arch from anterior to posterior and passes lateral to the ligamentum arteriosum behind the arch to enter the tracheoesophageal groove. Occasionally, the nerve is not "recurrent," and does not loop around the aortic arch. Instead it branches directly off the vagus nerve in the neck and courses directly to the larynx. On the right, it usually loops around the brachiocephalic or subclavian artery. This anatomic relationship is usually, but not always, present; and nonrecurrent recurrent nerves occur, probably in less than 1% of people. Nonrecurrent right "recurrent" laryngeal nerves are seen most commonly when the right subclavian artery arises from the descending aorta. In such cases, the "recurrent" nerve arises in the neck and travels directly to the larynx. The recurrent nerves travel superiorly in the tracheoesophageal grooves, entering the larynx between the esophagus and tracheopharyngeus muscle. As they course toward the larynx, the recurrent nerves give off branches to the heart, esophagus, trachea, pharynx, and larynx. The recurrent nerves run perpendicularly between the first two branches of the inferior thyroid artery and are attached closely to the posterior, medial aspect of the thyroid lobe. They enter the larynx coursing just below or under the inferior constrictor muscle and communicate with the ansa Galeni, a connection between the posterior branch of the recurrent laryngeal nerve and the internal branch of the superior laryngeal nerve, which is described in more detail in the next paragraph below. Interestingly, it has been found that the myelinated fibers in the left recurrent laryngeal nerve are larger in diameter than those on the right.[70] This led Malmgren and Gacek to speculate that differences in fiber size may allow the simultaneous activation of laryngeal muscles via faster transmission rates on the left, despite the fact that the right recurrent laryngeal nerve is shorter than the left[71] and thus should otherwise transmit faster causing signal activation sooner. Within the larynx, the recurrent laryngeal nerve crosses from posterior to anterior usually at a level slightly below the cricoarytenoid joint. Usually, the recurrent nerve passes approximately 4 to 5 mm posterior to the cricothyroid joint; but in up to about 15% of adults, the nerve may split around the joint, or it may pass anterior to it. These landmarks may be particularly important during surgical procedures in which identification of the criocothyroid joint is necessary. As the recurrent nerve enters the region of the cricothyroid joint, it divides into branches to each of the intrinsic muscles to which it provides motor innervation. It appears that the first branch usually goes to the PCA muscle. This posterior branch also innervates the IA muscles. An anterior branch courses toward the LCA muscle and supplies the TA muscle, as well. Detailed studies of the courses and

variations on the terminal branches of the recurrent laryngeal nerves have not been published yet. Research is currently underway to address this deficiency in knowledge, which has become relevant clinically because of surgical procedures such as thyroarytenoid neurectomy. Consequently, the thyroarytenoid branch was studied first.[72] In this study, we determined that the median distance from the inferior tubercle of the thyroid cartilage to the thyroarytenoid branch of the recurrent laryngeal nerve was 3.75 mm. Fifty-four percent of the nerves traveled in a horizontal direction within the larynx, but vertical and oblique orientations were observed. The thyroarytenoid division of the recurrent laryngeal nerve branched in approximately 20% of specimens. From this study, we concluded that surgeons performing thyroarytenoid neurectomy can identify the likely position of the thyroarytenoid nerve by measuring approximately 4 mm from the inferior tubercle along a perpendicular line. In most specimens, the nerve was encountered within 1 to 4 mm from the inferior tubercle. In addition to motor innervation, the recurrent laryngeal nerves are also responsible for sensory innervation primarily below the level of the true vocal folds, and of the spindles of the intrinsic muscles,[73] although they may supply portions of the vocal folds as noted above. There are interconnections between the superior and recurrent laryngeal nerves, particularly in the region of the IA muscles. The IA muscles are also the only laryngeal muscles that receive bilateral innervation (both recurrent laryngeal nerves).

Sympathetic innervation of the larynx is from the superior cervical ganglion. Parasympathetic innervation from the dorsal motor nucleus travels to the supraglottic larynx with the internal branch of the superior laryngeal nerves and to the subglottic larynx with the recurrent laryngeal nerves. The larynx also contains other important structures not discussed in detail in this chapter, including chemoreceptors, taste buds, and various mechanoreceptors, Meissner corpuscles, free nerve endings, and Merkel cells. The superior and recurrent laryngeal nerves are also connected through the ramus communicans, also called the ansa Galeni or nerve of Galen, which supplies motor innervation to the tracheal and the esophageal mucosa and the smooth muscle of the trachea. It also supplies the chemoreceptors and baroreceptors of the aortic arch. The laryngeal chemoreflex is an interesting phenomenon that produces cardiovascular changes and central apnea in response to chemical stimulation of the larynx.[74,75] The laryngeal chemoreflex may be triggered by stimuli such as gastric acid and can produce responses including laryngeal adduction, bronchoconstriction, hypotension, bradycardia, apnea, and possibly sudden infant death syndrome.[76] Like sudden infant death syndrome, the laryngeal chemoreflex is seen usually only in infants under the age of one. It differs from the glottic closure reflex in response to swallowing and from laryngospasm, which involves glottic closure without central apnea or cardiovascular changes. There is also a laryngeal reflex that results in glottic closure in response to gentle supraglottic tactile stimulation.

The larynx also contains low-threshold, rapidly adapting proprioceptors and low-threshold slowly adapting proprioceptors. The low-threshold, rapidly adapting proprioceptors are found in laryngeal joint capsules and control laryngeal muscle tone during joint movement (such as during singing or speech). Low-threshold, slowly adapting proprioceptors are found in the laryngeal muscles and help to fine-tune laryngeal muscle tone during activities such as phonation. The laryngeal proprioceptors are associated with two interesting polysynaptic reflex arcs that were identified in 1966.[77] When stimulated, the facilitory reflex arc increases the rate of motor unit firing in the TA and CT muscles. When the inhibitory reflex arch is stimulated, motor unit firing is decreased in the TA, CT, and sternothyroid muscles. Proprioceptors are probably also important in control of laryngeal muscle tone during respiration.[78]

Larynx: Extrinsic Muscles

Extrinsic laryngeal musculature maintains the position of the larynx in the neck. This group of muscles includes primarily the strap muscles. Because raising or lowering the larynx may alter the tension or angle between laryngeal cartilages, thereby changing the resting lengths of the intrinsic muscles, the extrinsic muscles are critical in maintaining a stable laryngeal skeleton that permits effective movement of the delicate intrinsic musculature. In the Western classically trained singer, the extrinsic muscles maintain the larynx in a relatively constant vertical position throughout the pitch range. Such training of the intrinsic musculature results in vibratory symmetry of the vocal folds, producing regular periodicity of vocal fold vibration. This contributes to what the listener perceives as a "trained" voice.

The extrinsic muscles may be divided into those below the hyoid bone (infrahyoid muscles) and those above the hyoid bone (suprahyoid muscles). The infrahyoid muscles include the thyrohyoid, sternothyroid, sternohyoid, and omohyoid muscles (Fig 6–9). As a group, the infrahyoid muscles are laryngeal depressors. The thyrohyoid muscle originates obliquely from the thyroid lamina and inserts into the lower

border of the greater cornu of the hyoid bone. Contraction brings the thyroid cartilage and the hyoid bone closer together, especially anteriorly. The sternothyroid muscle originates from the first costal cartilage and the posterior aspect of the manubrium of the sternum, and it inserts obliquely on the thyroid cartilage. Contraction lowers the thyroid cartilage. The sternohyoid muscle originates from the clavicle and posterior surface of the manubrium of the sternum, inserting into the lower edge of the body of the hyoid bone. Contraction lowers the hyoid bone. The inferior belly of the omohyoid originates from the upper surface of the scapula and inserts into the intermediate tendon of the omohyoid muscle low in the lateral neck. The superior belly originates from the intermediate tendon and inserts into the greater cornu of the hyoid bone. The omohyoid muscle pulls the hyoid bone down, lowering it.

The suprahyoid muscles include the digastric, mylohyoid, geniohyoid, and stylohyoid muscles. As a group, the suprahyoid muscles are laryngeal "elevators." The posterior belly of the digastric muscle originates from the mastoid process of the temporal bone and inserts into the intermediate tendon of the digastric, which connects to the hyoid bone. The anterior belly originates from the inferior aspect of the mandible near the symphysis and inserts into the digastric intermediate tendon. The anterior belly pulls the hyoid bone anteriorly and raises it. The posterior belly pulls the hyoid bone posteriorly and also raises it. The mylohyoid muscle originates from the inner aspect of the body of the mandible (mylohyoid line) and inserts into a midline raphe on the hyoid, connecting with fibers from the opposite side. It raises the hyoid bone and pulls it anteriorly. The geniohyoid muscle originates from the spine at the mental symphysis of the mandible and inserts on the anterior surface of the body of the hyoid bone. It raises the hyoid bone and pulls it anteriorly. The stylohyoid muscle originates from the styloid process and inserts into the body of the hyoid bone. It raises the hyoid bone and pulls it posteriorly. Coordinated interaction among the extrinsic laryngeal muscles is needed to control the vertical position of the larynx, as well as other positions such as laryngeal tilt.

The Supraglottic Vocal Tract

The supraglottic larynx, tongue, lips, palate, pharynx, nasal cavity (see Fig 6–3A), oral cavity, and possibly the sinuses shape the sound quality produced by the vocal folds by acting as resonators. Minor alterations in the configuration of these structures may produce substantial changes in voice quality. The hypernasal

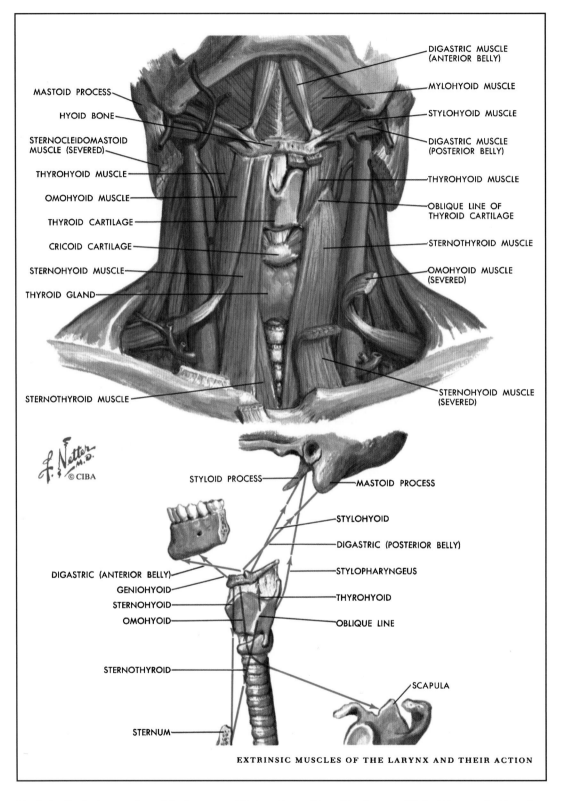

Fig 6–9. Extrinsic muscles of the larynx and their actions. (From *The Larynx. Clinical Symposia.* New Jersey: CIBA Pharmaceutical Company; 1964;16[3]: Plate 4. Copyright 1964. Icon Learning Systems, LLC, a subsidiary of MediMedia USA Inc. Reprinted with permission from Icon Learning Systems, LLC, illustrated by Frank H. Netter, MD. All rights reserved.)

speech typically associated with a cleft palate and/or the hyponasal speech characteristic of severe adenoid hypertrophy are obvious. However, mild edema from an upper respiratory tract infection, pharyngeal scarring, or changes in muscle tension produce less obvious sound alterations. These are immediately recognizable to a trained vocalist or astute critic, but they often elude the laryngologist.

The Tracheobronchial Tree, Lungs, Thorax, Abdomen, and Back

The lungs supply a constant stream of air that passes between the vocal folds and provides power for voice production, which is especially important in singing (Fig 6–10). Singers often are thought of as having "big chests." Actually, the primary respiratory difference between trained and untrained singers is not increased total lung capacity, as popularly assumed. Rather, the trained singer learns to use a higher proportion of the air in his or her lungs, thereby decreasing his or her residual volume and increasing respiratory efficiency.[79]

The abdominal musculature is the so-called "support" of the singing voice, although singers generally refer to their support mechanism as their "diaphragm." The function of the diaphragm muscle in singing is complex, and somewhat variable from singer to singer (or actor to actor). The diaphragm primarily generates inspiratory force. Although the abdomen can also perform this function in some situations,[80] it is primarily an expiratory-force generator. Interestingly, the diaphragm is co-activated by some performers during singing and appears to play an important part in the fine regulation of singing.[81] Actually, the anatomy and physiology of support for phonation are quite complicated and not understood completely, Both the lungs and rib cage generate passive expiratory forces under many common circumstances; however, passive inspiratory forces occur also. The active respiratory muscles working in concert with passive forces include the intercostal, abdominal, back, and diaphragm muscles. The principal muscles of inspiration are the diaphragm and external intercostal muscles. Accessory muscles of inspiration include the pectoralis major; pectoralis minor; serratus anterior; subclavius; sternocleidomastoid; anterior, medial, and posterior scalenus, serratus posterior and superior; latissimus dorsi; and levatores costarum muscles. During quiet respiration, expiration is largely passive. Many of the muscle used for active expiration (forcing air out of the lungs) are also employed in "support" for singing and acting voice tasks, including abdominal, back, and chest muscles.

Muscles of active expiration either raise the intra-abdominal pressure forcing the diaphragm upward or decrease the diameter of the ribs or sternum to decrease the volume dimension of the thorax, or both. They include the internal intercostals, which stiffen the rib interspaces and pull the ribs down; the transversus thoracis, the subcostal muscles, and the serratus posterior inferior muscles, all of which pull the ribs down; and the quadratus lumborum, which depresses the lowest rib. In addition, the latissimus dorsi, which may also act as a muscle of inspiration, is capable of compressing the lower portion of the rib cage and can act as a muscle of expiration as well. The above muscles all participate in active expiration and support. However, the primary muscles of active expiration are the abdominal muscles. They include the external oblique, internal oblique, rectus abdominus, and transversus abdominus muscles. The external oblique is a flat broad muscle located on the side and front of the lower chest and abdomen. Upon contraction, it pulls the lower ribs down and raises the abdominal pressure by displacing abdominal contents inward. It should be noted that this muscle is strengthened by leg lifting and lowering and other exercises but is not developed effectively by traditional trunk curls or sit-ups. Appropriate strengthening exercises of the external oblique muscles are often neglected in voice training. The internal oblique is a flat muscle in the side and front walls of the abdomen. It lies deep to the external oblique. When contracted, the internal oblique drives the abdominal wall inward and lowers the lower ribs. The rectus abdominus runs parallel to the midline of the abdomen, originating from the xiphoid process of the sternum and the fifth, sixth, and seventh costal (rib) cartilages. It inserts into the pubic bone. It is encased in the fibrous abdominal aponeurosis. Contraction of the rectus abdominus also forces the abdominal contents inward and lowers the sternum and ribs. The transversus abdominus is a broad muscle located under the internal oblique on the side and front of the abdomen. Its fibers run horizontally around the abdomen. Contraction of the transverse abdominus compresses the abdominal contents, elevating intra-abdominal pressure. Back (especially lower back) and other muscles (eg, ileocostalis dorsi, ileocostalis lumbarum, longissiumus dorsi) are also extremely important to power source "support" function, and especially to support for projected speech and singing.

The abdominal and back musculature receive considerable attention in vocal training. The purpose of support is to maintain an efficient, constant power source and inspiratory-expiratory mechanism. There is disagreement among voice teachers as to the best mod-

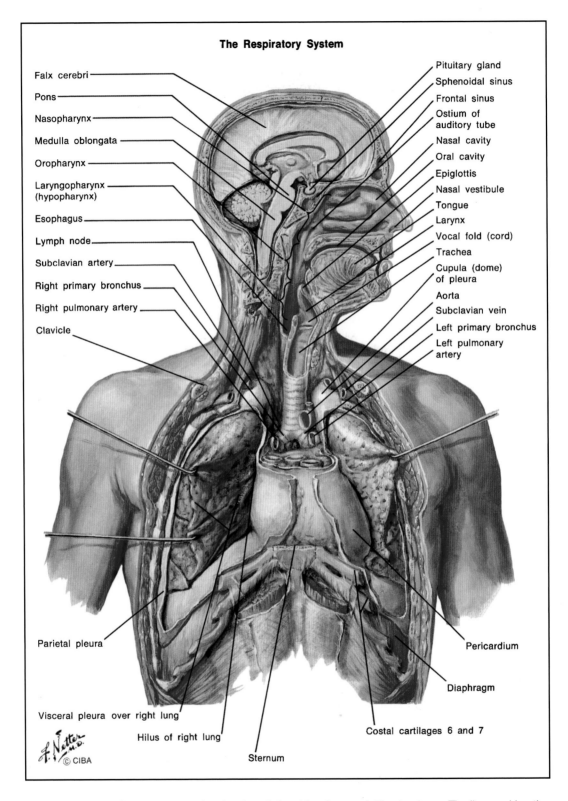

The Respiratory System

Falx cerebri

Pons

Nasopharynx

Medulla oblongata

Oropharynx

Laryngopharynx
(hypopharynx)

Esophagus

Lymph node

Subclavian artery

Right primary bronchus

Right pulmonary artery

Clavicle

Pituitary gland

Sphenoidal sinus

Frontal sinus

Ostium of
auditory tube

Nasal cavity

Oral cavity

Epiglottis

Nasal vestibule

Tongue

Larynx

Vocal fold (cord)

Trachea

Cupula (dome)
of pleura

Aorta

Subclavian vein

Left primary bronchus

Left pulmonary
artery

Parietal pleura

Pericardium

Diaphragm

Visceral pleura over right lung

Hilus of right lung

Costal cartilages 6 and 7

Sternum

Fig 6–10. The respiratory system, showing the relationship of supraglottic structures. The line marking the vocal fold actually stops on the false vocal fold. The level of the true vocal fold is slightly lower. The diaphragm is also visible in relation to the lungs, ribs, and abdomen muscles. (From The Development of the Lower Respiratory System. *Clinical Symposia.* New Jersey: CIBA Pharmaceutical Company; 1975;27[4]: Plate 1. Copyright 1964. Icon Learning Systems, LLC, a subsidiary of MediMedia USA Inc. Reprinted with permission from Icon Learning Systems, LLC, illustrated by Frank H. Netter, MD. All rights reserved.)

el for teaching support technique. Some experts describe positioning the abdominal musculature under the rib cage; others advocate distension of the abdomen. Either method may result in vocal problems if used incorrectly, but distending the abdomen (the inverse pressure approach) is especially dangerous, because it tends to focus the singer's muscular effort in a downward and outward direction, which is ineffective. Thus, the singer may exert considerable effort, believing he or she is practicing good support technique, without obtaining the desired effect. Proper abdominal muscle training is essential to good singing and speaking, and the physician must consider abdominal function when evaluating vocal dysfunction.

The Musculoskeletal System

Musculoskeletal conditioning and position throughout the body (posture) affect the vocal mechanism and may produce tension or impairment of function, resulting in voice dysfunction or injury. Stance deviation, such as from standing to supine, produces obvious changes in respiratory function. However, lesser changes, such as distributing one's weight over the calcaneus rather than forward over the metatarsal heads (a more athletic position), alter the configuration of the abdominal and back muscle function enough to influence the voice. Tensing arm and shoulder muscles promotes cervical muscle strain, which can adversely affect laryngeal function. Careful control of muscle tension is fundamental to good vocal technique. In fact, some teaching methods use musculoskeletal conditioning and relaxation as the primary focus of voice training.

The Psychoneurological System

The psychological constitution of the singer or professional voice user impacts directly on the vocal mechanism. Psychological phenomena are reflected through the autonomic nervous system, which controls mucosal secretions and other functions critical to voice production. The nervous system is also important for its mediation of fine muscle control. This fact is worthy of emphasis, because minimal voice disturbances may occasionally be the first sign of serious neurologic disease.

Physiology

The physiology of voice production is exceedingly complex and will be summarized only briefly in this chapter. Greater detail may be found elsewhere in this

book. For more information, the reader is advised to consult subsequent chapters and other literature, including publications listed in the bibliographies of other chapters and in the Suggested Readings list near the end of this book. Respiratory physiology is included in some detail below.

Overview of Phonatory Physiology

Volitional voice production begins in the cerebral cortex. Complex interactions among the centers for speech, musical, and artistic expression establish the commands for vocalization. The "idea" of the planned vocalization is conveyed to the precentral gyrus in the motor cortex, which transmits another set of instructions to motor nuclei in the brainstem and spinal cord (Fig 6–11). These areas transmit the complicated messages necessary for coordinated activity of the laryngeal, thoracic, and abdominal musculature and of the vocal tract articulators and resonators. Additional refinement of motor activity is provided by the extrapyramidal (cerebral cortex, cerebellum, and basal ganglion) and the autonomic nervous systems. These impulses combine to produce a sound that is transmitted not only to the ears of listeners but also to those of the speaker or singer. Auditory feedback is transmitted from the ear to the cerebral cortex via the brainstem, and adjustments are made to permit the vocalist to match the sound produced with the intended sound. There is also tactile feedback from the throat and other muscles involved in phonation that undoubtedly help in fine-tuning vocal output, although the mechanism and role of tactile feedback are not fully understood. In many trained singers, the ability to use tactile feedback effectively is cultivated as a result of frequent interference with auditory feedback by ancillary noise in the concert environment (eg, an orchestra or band).

The voice requires interactions among the power source, the oscillator, and the resonator. The power source compresses air and forces it toward the larynx. The vocal folds close and open, permitting small bursts of air to escape between them. Numerous factors affect the sound produced at the glottal level, as discussed in greater detail in the next chapter. Several of these factors include the pressure that builds up below the vocal folds (subglottal pressure), the amount of resistance to opening the glottis (glottal impedance), volume velocity of airflow at the glottis, and supraglottal pressure. The vocal folds do not vibrate like the strings on a violin. Rather, they separate and collide somewhat like buzzing lips. The number of times they do so in any given second (ie, their frequency) determines the number of air puffs that escape. The frequency of glottal closing and opening is

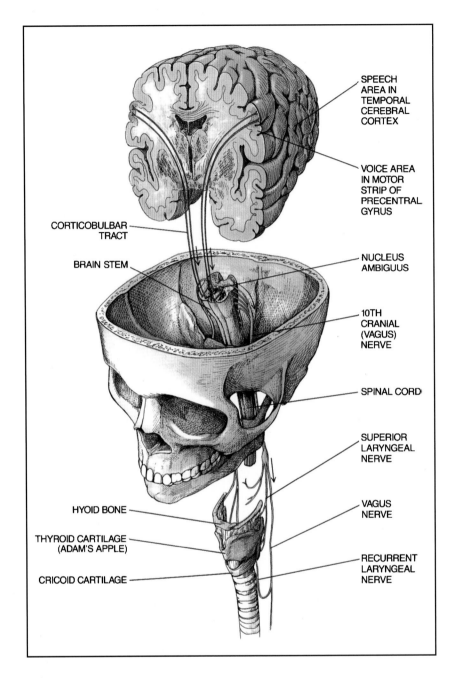

Fig 6–11. How the voice is produced. The production of speech or song, or even just a vocal sound, entails a complex orchestration of mental and physical actions. The idea for making a sound originates in the cerebral cortex of the brain—for example, in the speech area. The movement of the larynx is controlled from the voice area and is transmitted to the larynx by various nerves. As a result, the vocal folds vibrate, generating a buzzing sound. It is the resonation of that sound throughout the area of the vocal tract above the glottis—an area that includes the pharynx, tongue, palate, oral cavity and nose—that gives the sound the qualities perceived by a listener. Auditory feedback and tactile feedback enable the speaker or singer to achieve fine-tuning of the vocal output. (From Sataloff RT. The human voice. *Sci Am.* 1992;267(6):108-115, with permission.)

a factor in pitch determination. Other factors affect loudness, such as subglottal pressure, glottal resistance, and amplitude of vocal fold displacement from the midline during each vibratory cycle. The sound created at the vocal fold level is a buzz, similar to the sound produced when blowing between two blades of grass. This sound contains a complete set of harmonic partials and is responsible in part for the acoustic characteristics of the voice. However, complex and sophisticated interactions in the supraglottic vocal tract may accentuate or attenuate harmonic partials, acting as resonators (Fig 6–12). This portion of the vocal tract is largely responsible for the beauty and variety of the sound produced. Because of its complexity and importance, vocal tract resonance is explained in chapter 13 by Sundberg.

Interactions among the various components of the vocal tract ultimately are responsible for all the vocal characteristics produced. Many aspects of the voice still lack complete understanding and classification. Vocal range is reasonably well understood, and broad categories of voice classifications are generally accepted (Fig 6–13). Other characteristics, such as vocal register, are controversial. Registers are expressed as quality changes within an individual voice. From low to high, they may include vocal fry, chest, middle, head voice, falsetto, and whistle, although not everyone agrees that all categories exist. The term modal register, used most frequently in speech terms, refers to the voice quality generally used by healthy speakers, as opposed to a low, gravelly vocal fry, or high falsetto.

Vibrato is a rhythmic variation in frequency and intensity. Its exact source remains uncertain, and its desirable characteristics depend on voice range and the type of music sung. It appears most likely that the frequency (pitch) modulations are controlled primarily by intrinsic laryngeal muscles, especially the cricothyroid and adductor muscles. However, extrinsic laryngeal muscles and muscles of the supraglottic vocal tract may also play a role. Intensity (loudness) variations may be caused by variations in subglottal pressure, glottal adjustments that affect subglottal pressure, secondary effects of the frequency variation because of changes in the distance between the fundamental frequency and closest formant, or rhythmic changes in vocal tract shape that cause fluctuations in formant frequencies. When evaluating vibrato, it is helpful to consider the waveform of the vibrato signal, its regularity, extent, and rate. The waveform is usually fairly sinusoidal, but considerable variation may occur. The regularity, or similarity of each vibrato event compared to previous and subsequent vibrato events, is greater in trained singers than in untrained voice users. This regularity appears to be one of the characteristics perceived as a "trained sound." Vibratory extent refers to deviation from the standard frequency (not intensity variation) and can be less than ±0.1 semitone in some styles of solo and choral singing, such as some Renaissance music. For most well trained Western operatic singing, the usual vibrato extent at comfortable loudness is ±0.5 to 1 semitone for singers in most voice classifications. Vibrato rate

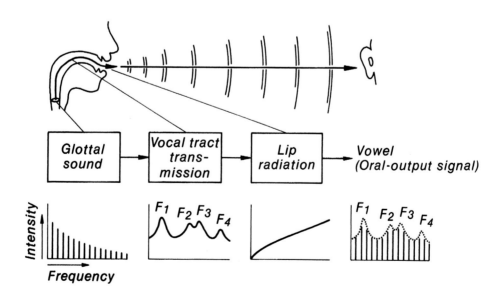

Fig 6–12. Some of the factors determining the spectrum of a vowel. (From Hirano M. *Clinical Examination of Voice.* New York: Springer-Verlag; 1981:67, with permission.)

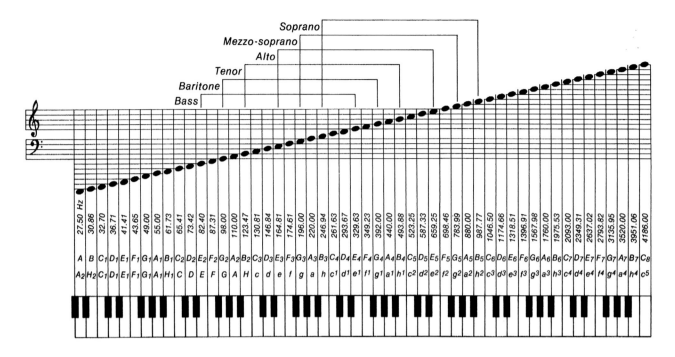

Fig 6–13. Correlation between a piano keyboard, pitch names (the lower in capital letters is used in music and voice research, and in this book), frequency, musical nota- tion, and usual voice range. (From Hirano M. *Clinical Examination of Voice.* New York: Springer-Verlag; 1981:89, with permission.)

(the number of modulations per second) is generally 5 to 7. Rate may also vary greatly from singer to singer and in the same singer. Vibrato rate can increase with increased emotional content of the material, and rate tends to decrease with older age (although the age at which this change occurs is highly variable). When variations from the central frequency become too wide, a "wobble" in the voice is perceived; this is generally referred to as tremolo. It is not generally considered a good musical sound, and it is unclear whether it is produced by the same mechanisms responsible for normal vibrato. Ongoing research should answer many of the remaining questions.

Respiration

Basic functions of the nose, larynx, and elemental concepts of inspiration and expiration are discussed elsewhere in this book. However, a brief review of selected aspects of pulmonary function is included here to assist readers in understanding the processes that underlie "support," as well as in understanding pulmonary disorders and their assessment.

Starting from the mouth, the respiratory system consists of progressively smaller airway structures. The trachea branches at the carina into mainstem

bronchi, which then branch into progressively smaller bronchial passages and terminate in alveoli. Gas exchange (oxygen and carbon dioxide, primarily) between the lungs and the bloodstream occurs at the alveolar level. Air moves in and out of the alveoli in order to permit this exchange of gases. Air is forced out of the alveoli also to creates the air stream through which phonation is produced. Hence, ultimately alveolar pressure is the primary power source for phonation and is responsible for the creation of the subglottal pressure involved in vocal fold opening and closing. Alveolar pressure is actually greater than subglottal pressure during phonation and expiration, because some pressure is lost due to airway resistance between alveoli and the larynx. As the air passes the alveoli, it enters first the bronchioles, which are small, collapsible airways surrounded by smooth muscle but devoid of cartilage. From the bronchioles, air passes to progressively larger components of the bronchial tree and eventually to the trachea. These structures are supported by cartilage and are not fully collapsible, but they are compressible and respond to changes in external pressure during expiration and inspiration. During expiration, the pressure in the respiratory system is greatest in the alveolus (alveolar pressure) and least at the opening of the mouth where pressure is theoretically equal to atmospheric pressure. Thus, theoretically, all pressure is dissipated between the alveolus and the mouth during expiration due to airway resistance between these structures. Expiration pressure is the total of the elastic recoil combined with active forces created by muscular compression of the airway. The active pressure is distributed throughout all the components of the airway, although it may exert greater effect on the alveoli and bronchioles because they are fully collapsible. When the airway is opened, the air pressure in the alveoli (alveolar pressure) is equal to the atmospheric pressure in the room. In order to fill the alveoli, the alveolar pressure must be decreased to less than atmosphere pressure, creating a vacuum, which sucks air into the lungs. In order to breathe out, alveolar pressure must be greater than atmospheric pressure. As discussed above, there are passive and active forces operative during the inspiratory/expiratory process.

To clarify the mechanisms involved, the alveoli may be thought of as tiny balloons. If a balloon is filled with air, and the filling spout is opened, the elastic properties of the balloon will allow most of the air to rush out. This is analogous to passive expiration, which relies on the elastic properties of the respiratory system. Alternatively, we may wrap our hands around the balloon and squeeze the air out. This may allow us to get the air out faster and more forcefully, and it will allow us to get more of the air out of the balloon than is expelled through the passive process alone. This is analogous to active expiration, which involves the abdominal, chest, and back muscles. If we partially pinch the filling spout of the balloon, air comes out more slowly because the outflow tract is partially blocked. The air also tends to whistle as it exits the balloon. This is analogous to obstructive pulmonary disease, and its commonly associated wheeze. If we try to blow up the balloon while our hands are wrapped around it, the balloon is more difficult to inflate and cannot be inflated fully; because it is restricted physically by our hands. This is somewhat analogous to restrictive lung disease. Under these circumstances, it may also take more pressure to fill the balloon, because the filling process must overcome the restricting forces. Under any of these circumstances, the more we fill the alveolar "balloon," the greater the pressure, as long as the balloon is not ruptured. When the pressure is greater, the increased elastic recoil results in more rapid and forceful air escape when the air is released. The pressure inside the balloon can be increased even above its maximal elastic recoil level simply by squeezing the outside of the balloon. This analogy is helpful in understanding the forces involved in breathing (especially expiration) and in generating support for phonation.

Although inspiration is extremely important, this discussion will concentrate primarily on expiration, which is linked so closely to "support" for speech and singing. The elastic component of expiratory pressure (specifically, alveolar pressure), depends on lung volume and the elastic forces exerted by the chest and the lungs. The lung is never totally deflated. At rest, it is inflated to about 40% of total lung capacity (TLC), as illustrated in chapter 2. The amount of air in the lungs at rest is the functional residual capacity (FRC). At FRC, the thorax is at a volume much less than its rest (or a neutral) posture, which is actually closer to 75% of TLC. Hence, at FRC the thorax has a passive tendency to expand, as happens during inspiration. Conversely, at FRC the lung is greater than its neutral position and would collapse if it were not acted upon by other forces. The collapsing elastic forces of the lung are balanced by the expanding elastic forces of the thorax. The lung and thorax interact closely, and their relative positions of contact vary constantly. This is facilitated by the anatomy of the their boundary zone. The inner surface of the thorax is covered by a membrane called the parietal pleura, and the lung is covered by a similar membrane called the visceral pleura. A thin layer of pleural fluid exists between them. Hydrostatic forces hold these surfaces together while allowing them to slide freely. Under pathologic circumstances (eg, following surgery or radiation) these surfaces may stick together impairing lung function and affecting support for phonation adversely.

Thoracic and lung elastic behavior can be measured. The basic principle for doing so involves applying pressure and noting the volume changes caused by the pressure. This creates a pressure/volume (P/V) curve. The slope with the P/V curve for the thorax reflects its compliance (c_{CW}); and the slope of the P/V curve for the lung represents its compliance (C_L). When pressure is applied to the entire system, a difference P/V curve is created and its slope reflects the compliance of the entire respiratory system (C_{RS}). Starting from FRC, if air is expelled the volume of the system is dropped below FRC, and an expanding force is created. It is increased as the volume decreases. Conversely, during inspiration above FRC, collapsing forces increase with increasing volume.

To phonate, we inspire, increasing volumes well above FRC. If we wish simply to expire, we relax and the passive elastic recoil forces air out of the alveoli, because inflating them has created an alveolar pressure that is greater than atmospheric pressure (and is predictable using the pressure-volume curve). The deeper the inspiration, the greater the elastic recoil, hence the greater the expiratory air pressure. Inspiration from FRC is an active process, primarily. Thoracic muscles elevate the ribs and increase the diameter of the thorax. The external intercostal muscles are important to this process. Inspiration also involves contraction of the diaphragm muscle, which flattens and also increases thoracic volume, and accessory muscles discussed above.

Expiration is created by forces that decrease thoracic volume. If the entire thoracic and pulmonary complex is thought of as a balloon, this process is easy to understand. If one wishes to increase the pressure in a balloon to force the air out, one simply squeezes the balloon. When the container (balloon or thorax) containing a volume of gas (air) is decreased, the pressure in the gas increases. Expiration is achieved by muscles that pull the ribs down or compress the abdominal contents and push them up, making the volume of the thorax smaller. The principle muscles involved are the internal intercostal muscles, which decrease intercostal space and pull the ribs down, abdominal, back, and other muscles, as reviewed earlier in this chapter.

For projected phonations such as singing or acting, support involves (essentially, is) active expiration. After inspiration, elastic recoil and external forces created by expiratory muscles determine alveolar pressure, which is substantially greater than atmospheric pressure. The combination of passive (elastic) and active (muscular) forces pushes air out against airway resistance. As the pressure decreases on the path from alveolar (maximal to mouth atmospheric) pressure, there is a point at which the pressure inside the airway equals the active expiratory pressure (without the elastic recoil component), which is called the equal pressure point (EPP). As expiration continues toward the mouth, pressure drops below the EPP. As airway pressure diminishes below the active expiratory pressure, the airways begin to collapse. This physiologic collapse of the airways increases airway resistance by decreasing the diameter of the airways. The greater the active expiratory forces, the greater the airway compression after the EPP has been passed. Expiratory pressure and airway compression are important to control of expiratory airflow rate and are influenced by EPP.

Under normal circumstances, the EPP is reached in the cartilaginous airways, which do not collapse completely ordinarily, even during very forceful expiration or phonation. This is part of the physiological mechanism that allows us to continue to sing even as we are running out of air. However, under pathologic circumstance, the location of the EPP may be shifted. Asthma is the classic example. During bronchospasm or bronchoconstriction, the diameter of the bronchioles is narrowed by smooth muscle contraction; and airway resistance in the bronchioles is increased.

Hence, as the air moves from the alveoli into the bronchioles, airway pressure diminishes much more quickly than normal; and EPP may be reached closer to the alveoli and bronchioles, in smaller airways that collapse more easily and more completely. In severe circumstances, the distal airways may collapse fully causing hyperinflation of the lungs and trapping air in the alveoli. Expiratory airflow rate is lowered substantially by the increased resistance in the distal airways, resulting in a lower-than-normal subglottic pressure. This can have profoundly adverse effects on phonation.

Other lung dysfunction also can impair subglottal pressure even if airway resistance is normal. The classic example is emphysema, which occurs commonly in smokers. This condition results in damage to the alveoli. Consequently, because elastic recoil pressures are lower, alveolar pressure is decreased compared to normal. Even if the active expiratory forces are normal, if passive (elastic) expiratory forces are decreased, the normal airway resistance acting against diminished alveolar pressure will shift the EPP distally toward or into collapsible airways. Even when active expiratory efforts are increased under these circumstances, they do not help because they collapse the distal airways trapping air in the alveoli, and diminishing subglottal pressure.

Although this overview is oversimplified and highlights only some of the more important components of lower respiratory physiology, it is important for laryngologists to bear these principles in mind in order to understand the importance of diagnosis and treatment of respiratory dysfunction in voice professionals. In patients with Olympic voice demands, even slight changes from optimal physiology may have profound consequences on phonatory function; and they are responsible commonly for compensatory efforts that are diagnosed (correctly) as hyperfunctional voice use (muscle tension dysphonia). If we treat voice hyperfunction as if it were the primary problem, failing to recognize that it is secondary to an underlying, organic, pulmonary disorder, then treatment will not be successful in the long term; and preventable voice dysfunction and vocal fold injury may ensue.

Conclusion

This chapter and those that follow provide only enough information on the terminology, components, and workings of the voice to permit an understanding of practical, everyday clinical problems and their solutions. The otolaryngologist, speech-language pathologist, singing or acting teacher, singer, actor, or other voice professional would benefit greatly from more extensive study of voice science.

Acknowledgment The author is grateful to Mary Hawkshaw and Yolanda Heman-Ackah for their assistance in reviewing this chapter.

References

1. Hatley W, Samuel E, Evison G. The pattern of ossification in the laryngeal cartilages: a radiological study. *Br J Radiol.* 1965;38:585–591.

2. Adams J, Gross N, Riddle S, Andersen P, Cohen JI. An external landmark for the anterior commissure. *Laryngoscope.* 1999;109:1134–1136.

3. Randestad Å, Lindholm CE, Fabian P. Dimensions of the cricoid cartilage and the trachea. *Laryngoscope.* 2000; 110:1957–1961.

4. Thompson AC, Griffin NR. Langerhan cells in normal and pathological vocal cord mucosa. *Acta Otolaryngol* (Stockh). 1995;115:830–832.

5. Hirano M. Structure and vibratory pattern of the vocal folds. In: Sawashima M, Cooper FS, eds. *Dynamic Aspects of the Speech Production.* Tokyo: University of Tokyo Press; 1977:13–27.

6. Gray SD, Pignatari SS, Harding P. Morphologic ultrastructure of anchoring fibers in normal vocal fold basement zone. *J Voice.* 1994;8:48–52.

7. Hammond TH, Zhou R, Hammond EH, Pawlak A, Gray SD. The intermediate layer: a morphologic study of the elastin and hyaluronic acid constituents of normal vocal folds. *J Voice.* 1997;11:59–66.

8. Hammond TH, Gray SD, Butler J, Zhou R, Hamond E. Age- and gender-related elastin distribution changes in human vocal folds. *Otolaryngol Head Neck Surg.* 1998; 119:314–322.

9. Catten M, Gray SD, Hammond TH, Zhou R, Hammond E. Analysis of cellular location and concentration in vocal fold lamina propria. *Otolaryngol Head Neck Surg.* 1998;118:663–667.

10. Gray SD, Hammond E, Hanson DF. Benign pathologic responses of the larynx. *Ann Otol Rhinol Laryngol.* 1995; 104:13–18.

11. Hirano M, Kurita S, Nakashima T. Growth, development of aging of human vocal folds. In: Bless DM, Abbs JH, eds. *Vocal Fold Physiology.* San Diego, Calif: College-Hill Press; 1983: 22–43.

12. Hirano M, Nakashima T. Vascular network of the vocal fold. In: Stevens KN, Hirano M eds. *Vocal Fold Physiology.* Tokyo, Japan: University of Tokyo Press; 1981:45–59.

13. Sato, K. Functional Fine Structures of Human Vocal Fold Mucosa. In: Rubin JS, Sataloff RT, Korovin G, eds. *Diagnosis and Treatment of Voice Disorders.* 2nd ed. Albany, NY: Singular Thomson Learning; 2003:41–48.

14. Kurita S, Nagata K, Hirano M. Comparative histology of mammalian vocal folds. In: Kirchner JA, ed. *Vocal Fold Histopathology: A Symposium.* San Diego, Calif: College-Hill Press; 1986:1–10.

15. Stiblar-Martincic D. Histology of laryngeal mucosa. *Acta Otolaryngol Suppl* (Stockh).1997;527:138–141.

16. Friedrich G, Kainz J, Freidl W. Zur funktionellen Struktur der menschlichen Stimmlippe. *Laryngorhinootologie.* 1993;72(5):215–224.

17. Hirano M, Kurita S, Kiyokawa K, Kiminori S. Posterior glottis. Morphological study in excised human larynges. *Ann Otol Rhinol Laryngol.* 1986;95:576–581.

18. Hirano M. Surgical anatomy and physiology of the vocal folds. In: Gould WJ, Sataloff RT, Spiegel JR, eds. *Voice Surgery.* St. Louis, Mo: Mosby; 1993:135–258.

19. Sato K, Hirano M, Nakashima T, Stellate cells in the human vocal fold. *Ann Otol Rhinol Laryngol.* 2001;110: 319–325.

20. Sato K, Hirano M, Nakashima T. Vitamin A—storing stellate cells in the human vocal fold. *Acta Otolaryngol.* 2003;123:106–110.

21. Sato K, Hirano M, Nakashima T. 3D structure of the macula flava in the human vocal fold. *Acta Otolaryngol.* 2003;123:269–273.

22. Sato K, Hirano M, Nakashima T. Age-related changes of collagenous fibers in the human vocal fold mucosa. *Ann Otol Rhinol Laryngol.* 2003;111:15–20.

23. Sato K, Hirano M. Age-related changes of elastic fibers in the superficial layer of the lamina propria of the vocal folds. *Ann Otol Rhinol Laryngol.* 1997;106:44–48.

24. Hirano M, Kurita S, Sakaguchi S. Ageing of the vibratory tissue of the human vocal folds. *Acta Otolaryngol* (Stockh). 1989;107:428–433.

25. Sato K, Sakaguchi S, Kurita S, Hirano M. A morphological study of aged larynges. *Larynx Jpn.* 1992;4:84–94.

26. Hirano M. Yoshida T, Kurita S, et al. Anatomy and behavior of the vocal process. In: Baer T, Sasaki C, Harris K, eds. *Laryngeal Function in Phonation and Respiration.* Boston, Mass: College-Hill Press; 1987:1–13.

27. Gray S. Basement membrane zone injury in vocal nodules. In: Gauffin J, Hammarberg B, eds. *Vocal Fold Physiology: Acoustic, Perceptual and Physiologic Aspects of Voice Mechanics.* San Diego, Calif: Singular Publishing Group; 1991:21–27.

28. Sundberg J. The acoustics of the singing voice. *Sci Am.* 1977;236(3):82–91.

29. Franz P, Aharinejad S. The microvascular of the larynx: a scanning electron microscopy study. *Scanning Microsc.* 1994;5:257–263.

30. Nakai Y, Masutani H, Moriguchi M, Matsunaga K, Sugita M. Microvascular structure of the larynx. *Acta Otolaryngol Suppl* (Stockh). 1991;486:254–263.

31. Hochman I, Sataloff RT, Hillman RE, Zeitels SM. Ectasias and varices of the vocal fold: clearing the striking zone. *Ann Otol Rhinol Laryngol.* 1999;108:10–16.

32. Frenzel H, Kleinsasser O. Ultrastructural study on the small blood vessels of human vocal cords. *Arch Otorhinolaryngol.* 1982;236:147–160.

33. Sanders I. Microanatomy of the vocal fold musculature. In: Rubin JS, Sataloff RT, Korovin GS, eds. *Diagnosis and Treatment of Voice Disorders.* 2nd ed. Clifton Park, NY: Delmar Thomson Learning; 2003:49–68.

34. Brooke MH, Engle WK. The histographic analysis of human muscle biopsies with regard to fibre types. 1. Adult male and female. *Neurology.* 1969;19:221–233.

35. Sadeh M, Kronenberg J. Gaton E. Histochemistry of human laryngeal muscles. *Cell Mol Biol.* 1981;27:643–648.

36. Lindestad P. *Electromyographic and Laryngoscopic Studies of Normal and Disturbed Vocal Function,* Stockholm, Sweden: Suddinge University;1994:1–12,

37. English DT, Blevins CE. Motor units of laryngeal muscles. *Arch Otolaryngol.* 1969;89:778–784.

38. Faaborg-Andersen K. Electromyographic investigation of intrinsic laryngeal muscles in humans. *Acta Physiol Scand Suppl.* 1957;41(suppl 140):1–149.

39. Rossi G, Cortesina G. Morphological study of the laryngeal muscles in man: insertions and courses of the muscle fibers, motor end-plates and proprioceptors. *Acta Otolaryngol* (Stockh). 1965;59:575–592.

40. Wu YZ, Crumley RL, Armstrong WB, Caiozzzo VJ. New perspectives about human laryngeal muscle: single-fiber analyses and interspecies comparisons. *Arch Otolaryngol Head Neck Surg.* 2000;126:857–864.

41. Malmgren LT, Lovice DB, Kaufman MR. Age-related changes in muscle fiber regeneration in the human thyroarytenoid muscle. *Arch Otolaryngol Head Neck Surg.* 2000;126:851–856.

42. Sataloff RT. Vocal aging. *Curr Opin Otolaryngol Head Neck Surg.* 1998.6:421–428.

43. Davis PJ, Nail BS. On the location and size of laryngeal motoneurons in the cat and rabbit. *J Comp Neurol.* 1984;230:13–22.

44. Yoshida Y, Miyazaki O, Hirano M, et al. Arrangement of motoneurons innervating the intrinsic laryngeal muscles of cats as demonstrated by horseradish peroxidase. *Acta Otolaryngol.* 1982;94:329–334.

45. Yoshida Y, Miyazaki T, Hirano M, Kanaseki T. Localization of the laryngeal motoneurons in the brain stem and myotopical representation of the motoneurons in the nucleus ambiguus of cats—an HRP study. In: Titze I, Scherer R, eds. *Vocal Fold Physiology: Biomechanics, Acoustics and Phonatory Control.* Denver, Co: The Denver Center for the Performing Arts, Inc; 1983:75–90.

46. Zhang SP, Bandler R, Davis P. Integration of vocalization: the medullary nucleus retroambigualis. *J Neurophysiol.* 1995;74:2500–2512.

47. Bandler R. Induction of "rage" following microinjections of glutamate into midbrain but not hypothalamus of cats. *Neurosci Lett.* 1982;30:183–188.

48. Kelly AH, Beaton LE, Magoun HW. A midbrain mechanism for facio-vocal activity. *J Neurophysiol.* 1946;9:181–189.

49. Adametz J, O'Leary JL. Experimental mutism resulting from periaqueductal lesions in cats. *Neurology.* 1959; 9;636–642.

50. Skultety FM. Experimental mutism in dogs. *Arch Neurol.* 1962;6:235–241.

51. Esposito A, Demeurisse G, Alberti B, Fabbro F. Complete mutism after midbrain periaqueductal gray lesion. *Neuroreport.* 1999;10:681–685.

52. Bandler R, Shipley MT. Columnar organization in the midbrain periaqueductal gray: modules for emotional expression? *Trends Neurosci.* 1994;17:379–389.

53. Zhang SP, Davis PJ, Bandler R, Carrive P. Brain stem integration of vocalization: role of the midbrain periaqueductal gray. *J Neurophysiol.* 1994;72:1337–1356.

54. Bandler R, Carrive P. Integrated defence reaction elicited by excitatory amino acid microinjection in the midbrain periaqueductal grey region of the unrestrained cat. *Brain Res.* 1988;439:95–106.

55. Bandler R, Depaulis A. Midbrain periaqueductal gray control of defensive behavior in the cat and the rat. In: Depaulis A, Bandler R, eds. *The Midbrain Periaqueductal Gray Matter: Functional, Anatomical and Immunohistochemical Organization.* New York, NY: Plenum Press; 1991:175–198.

56. Bandler R, Keay K, Vaughan C, Shipley MT. Columnar organization of PAG neurons regulating emotional and vocal expression. In: Fletcher N, Davis P, eds. *Vocal Fold Physiology: Controlling Complexity and Chaos.* San Diego, Calif: Singular Publishing Group; 1996:137–153.

57. Shipley MT, Ennis M, Rizvi TA, Behbehani MM. Topographical specificity of forebrain inputs to the midbrain periaqueductal gray: evidence for discrete longitudinally organized input columns. In: Depaulis A, Bandler R, eds. *The Midbrain Periaqueductal Gray Matter: Functional, Anatomical and Immunohistochemical Organization.* New York, NY: Plenum Press; 1991:417–448.

58. Davis P, Zhang SP. What is the role of the midbrain periaqueductal gray in respiration and vocalization? In: Depaulis A, Bandler R, eds. *The Midbrain Periaqueductal Gray Matter: Functional, Anatomical and Immunohistochemical Organization.* New York, NY: Plenum Press; 1991:57–66.

59. Davis P, Zhang SP, Winkworth A, Bandler R. The neural control of vocalization: respiratory and emotional influences. *J Voice.* 1996;10:23–38.

60. Davis PJ, Zhang SP, Bandler R. Midbrain and medullary control of respiration and vocalization. *Prog Brain Res.* 1996;107:315–325.

61. Davis PJ, Zhang SP, Bandler R. Pulmonary and upper airway afferent influences on the motor pattern of vocalization evoked by excitation of the midbrain periaqueductal gray of the cat. *Brain Res.* 1993;607:61–80

62 Ambalavanar R, Tanaka Y, Damirjian M, Ludlow CL. Laryngeal afferent stimulation enhances Fos immunoreactivity in periaqueductal gray in the cat. *J Comp Neurol.* 1999;409(3):411–423.

63. Nonaka S, Takahashi R, Enomoto K, Katada A, Unno T. Lombard reflex during PAG-induced vocalization in decrebrate cats. *Neurosci Res.* 1997;29:283–289.

64. Penfield W, Roberts L. *Speech and Brain Mechanisms.* Princeton, NJ: Princeton University Press; 1959.

65. Perry DW, Zatorre RJ, Petrides M, Alivisatos B, Meyer E, Evans AC. Localization of cerebral activity during simple singing. *Neuroreport.* 1999;10:3979–3984.

66. Wu BL, Sanders I, Mu L, Biller HF. The human communicating nerve: an extension of the external superior

laryngeal nerve that innervates the vocal cord. *Arch Otolaryngol.* 1994;120(12):1321–1328.

67. Sanders I, Mu L. Anatomy of human internal superior laryngeal nerve. *Anat Rec.* 1998;252:646–656.

68. Yoshida Y, Tanaka Y, Mitsumasu T, Hirano M, Kanaseki T. Peripheral course and intramucosal distribution of the laryngeal sensory nerve fibers of cats. *Brain Res Bull.* 1986;17(1):95–105.

69. Yoshida Y, Tanaka Y, Hirano M, Nakashima T. Sensory innervation of the pharynx and larynx. *Am J Med.* 2000; 108(suppl 4a):51S–61S.

70. Harrison D. Fibre size frequency in the recurrent laryngeal nerves of men and giraffe. *Acta Otolaryngol.* 1981; 91:383–389.

71. Malmgren L, Gacek R: Peripheral motor innervation of the larynx. In: Blitzer A, Brin MF, Sasaki CT, Fahn S, Harris KS, eds. *Neurologic Disorders of the Larynx.* New York, NY: Thieme Medical Publishers; 1992; 36–44.

72 Scheid SC, Nadeau DP, Friedman O, Sataloff RT. Anatomy of the thyroarytenoid branch of the recurrent laryngeal nerve. *J Voice.* 2004;8(3):279–284.

73. Sato K, Hirano M. Fine three-dimensional structure of pericytes in the vocal fold mucosa. *Ann Otol Rhinol Laryngol.* 1997;106:490–494.

74. Heman-Ackah YD, Goding GS Jr. Laryngeal chemoreflex severity and end-apnea Pa2, and PaCO$_2$. *Otolaryngol Head Neck Surg.* 2000;123(3):157–163.

75. Heman-Ackah YD, Goding GS Jr. The effects of intralaryngeal carbon dioxide and acetazolamide on the laryngeal chemoreflex. *Ann Otol Rhinol Laryngol.* 2000;109(10): 921–928.

76. Heman-Ackah YD, Rimell F. Current progress in understanding sudden infant death syndrome. *Curr Opin Otolaryngol Head Neck Surg.* 1999;7(6):320–327.

77. Abo-el-Enein M. Laryngeal myotactic reflexes. *Nature.* 1966; 209:682–685.

78. Tomori Z, Widdicomb J: Muscular bronchomotor and cardiovascular reflexes elicited by mechanical stimulation of the respiratory tract. *J Physiol.* 1969;200:25–49.

79. Gould WJ, Okamura H. Static lung volumes in singers. *Ann Otol Rhinol Laryngol.* 1973;82:89–95.

80. Hixon TJ, Hoffman C. Chest wall shape during singing. In: Lawrence V, ed. *Transcripts of the Seventh Annual Symposium, Care of the Professional Voice.* New York, NY: The Voice Foundation; 1978;9–10.

81. Sundberg J, Leanderson R, von Euler C. Activity relationship between diaphragm and cricothyroid muscles. *J Voice.* 1989;3(3):225–232.

7

Arytenoid Movement

James A. Letson, Jr., and Renny Tatchell

The Arytenoid Cartilages

The paired *arytenoid cartilages* and the perch upon which they rest, the cricoid (*Cricos*, Greek for ring or circle), form the architectural and anatomical foundation of the larynx (Fig 7–1.). These three cartilages

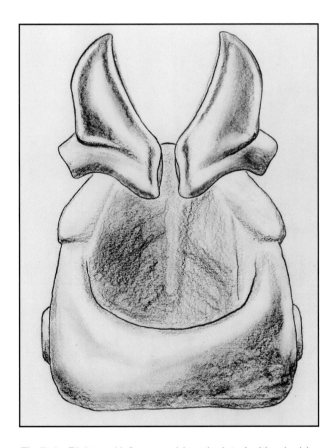

Fig 7–1. Right and left arytenoids articulated with cricoid.

assume even greater significance when the main and one of the secondary functions of the larynx are considered. It is accepted that the primary functions of the larynx are to protect the lower airway, to provide an entranceway to that airway, and to allow the lower and upper airways to be in communication. Although the production of voice is meaningful, it is still considered to be a function of only secondary importance.

Most textbooks describe lower airway protection to be accomplished by a three-layered valvelike system: The first tier is formed by a posterior and inferior infolding of the epiglottis and its approximation to the two aryepiglottic folds, the arytenoid, corniculate, and cuneiform cartilages. The second layer is accomplished by closure of the false vocal folds. Closure of the true vocal folds forms the final third layer. On swallowing a large bolus, the entire larynx comes to rest beneath the base of the tongue. This approximation of the larynx to the base of the tongue serves to vertically compress the three laryngeal valves. When the laryngeal structures responsible for the three valves, the epiglottis, the aryepiglottic folds, the false vocal folds, and the true vocal folds are surgically removed, the provision for and the protection of the airway can still be accomplished, provided that the arytenoid and cricoid cartilages, together with the muscles responsible for arytenoid motion, are preserved.

This is exactly what occurs in an operation designed for extensive laryngeal cancer and known as *supracricoid laryngectomy*. The thyroid cartilage, the majority of the epiglottis, and the true and false vocal folds are surgically removed. Left remaining are the piriform recesses, the hyoid bone, and as stated, the cricoid and arytenoid cartilages, together with their functional musculature. Since the muscles that are used to raise the larynx during swallowing are also removed, the trachea is released from below, which in turn, brings the tongue base and hyoid closer to the arytenoid and cricoid cartilages. The use of cinefluoroscopy during the act of swallowing (a video of the cine study was provided to the author through the courtesy of Dr Gregory S. Weinstein) demonstrates that arytenoid cartilages are brought together in the midline and together revolve over the cricoid, moving inferiorly and anteriorly. The tongue base can still make contact with the arytenoid cartilages and the remaining skeleton of the larynx can be tucked and protected by the backward descending base of the tongue. The combined tongue base and arytenoid mass form a ramp over which and to the sides of which ingested foods and liquids, as well as secretions, can pass safely into the digestive tract, thus preventing them from penetrating the lower airway. In addition, expiratory airflow can set the redundant soft tissue, covering the arytenoids, into a vibration providing a rough but functional voice.

On commenting on the protection of the airway, few texts mention the favorable angle that the trachea and larynx bears to the tongue base. Rather than being vertical (ie, 90° to the horizontal), the axes of the trachea and the larynx form an angle roughly 120° from the horizontal or 30° from the vertical. As such, the larynx is inclined so that it faces the posterior aspect of the tongue. On swallowing, the larynx is drawn upward and forward and the base of the tongue moves downward and backward. The structures of the larynx are carefully tucked beneath the tongue base and the airway is thus protected. Hence, protection of the airway is accomplished by the favorable geometry of the tongue base and larynx, the joining of these two structures, as well as the three tiered laryngeal valve system.

The shape of the arytenoids is unusual. Their name is derived from the resemblance that each arytenoid bears to an ancient water ladle or pitcher. *Arytaina* or *arytaena*, is a Greek word meaning *ladle* or *pitcher*.[1,2] *Eidos* originates also from the Greek, meaning *form*. The composite word, *arytainoeide(s)*, has the meaning of in the form of a ladle or pitcher. If the arytenoids are viewed either from their medial or lateral sides, each arytenoid bears a distinct resemblance to an old-fashioned high-button shoe (Fig 7–2). A resemblance also can be made to the foot (Fig 7–2), ankle, and lower part of the leg which would occupy that shoe. If one uses the latter similarity, the foot is found to be slightly deformed by a bunion located at the metatarsal head of the great toe (Fig 7–3). The bunion creates a malalignment of the great toe (vocal process) from the remaining part of the foot (body of the arytenoid). Rather than being in a linear alignment with the rest of the foot, the long axis of the toe (vocal process) deviates laterally.

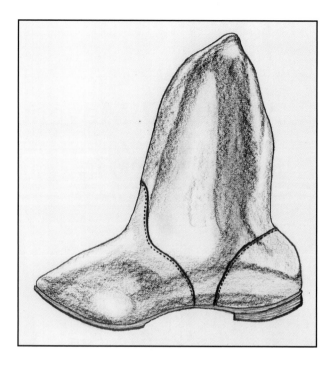

Fig 7–2. Lateral view of right arytenoid depicted as an old-fashioned high button shoe.

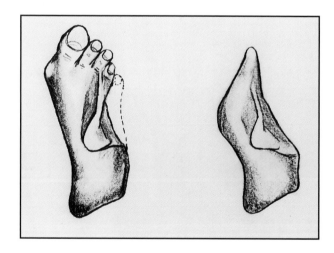

Fig 7–3. Drawing of a right foot. A bunion causing an outward deviation of the big toe and a right arytenoid with the vocal processes representing the outwardly deviated big toe and the foot and ankle representing the body and sides of the arytenoid.

Each arytenoid possesses a base and three sides, which, in turn, meet at an apex. The base is concave and the sides are irregularly shaped and unequal in size. This architectural design has led some investigators to describe the arytenoids as being irregularly shaped pyramids. The faces or sides of the arytenoids are designated as medial, posterior, and antero-lateral (Figs 7–4 and 7–5). From the inferior aspect of the con-

joined medial and antero-lateral faces is found a tapered structure which projects both in an anterior and lateral fashion. This structure is known as the *vocal process*. Projecting posteriorly from the inferior aspect of the posterior face is a broader, blunter, and thicker structure known as the *muscular process*. The antero-lateral face of the arytenoid (Fig 7–6) contains two concavities or foveae. Superiorly lies the largest or *triangular fovea* and inferiorly is the *fovea oblonga* (Fig 7–7). As suggested by its name, this lower concavity is relatively long and narrow (Fig 7–7). The fovea oblonga indents both the muscular and vocal processes. If one

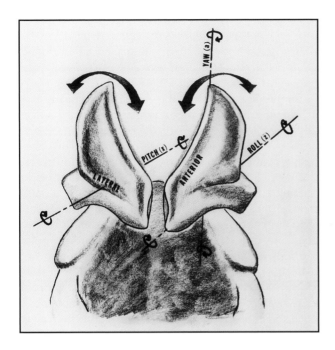

Fig 7–4. Arytenoids perched on the cricoid. The anterior and lateral faces are labeled. Axes *y*, *x*, and *z* are labeled.

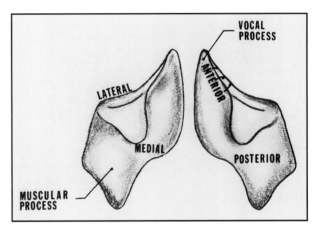

Fig 7–6. Arytenoids and cricoid viewed from above with vocal and muscular processes and these sides labeled.

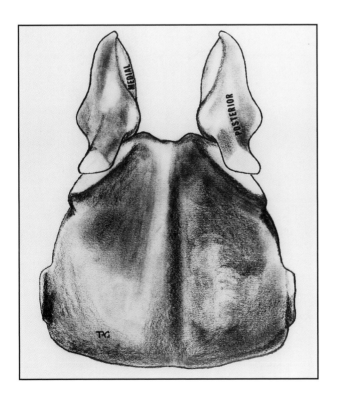

Fig 7–5. Posterior view of arytenoid and cricoid with medial and posterior sides or faces labeled.

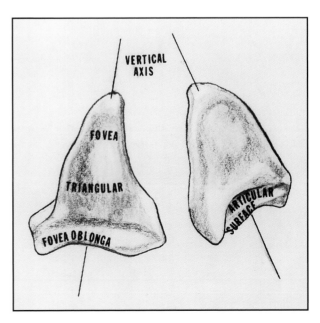

Fig 7–7. Arytenoids, with triangular and oblonga fovea and articulating surfaces or bases labeled.

were to direct a line beginning at the medial and mid-vertical portion of the muscular process and follow the long axis of the muscular process anteriorly, the line would pass through the vocal process. Understanding this fact, together with the concave curvature of the arytenoid's articulating surface, which in turn corresponds to the minor axis of the cricoarytenoid facet[3] is important in understanding the mechanics of arytenoid motion.

Arytenoid Motion

The facet of the cricoid designed to receive the arytenoid is a raised structure, convexly curved and elliptically shaped. An ellipse has a major or longitudinal axis and a minor or horizontal axis. The longitudinal axis of the cricoarytenoid facet runs along the posterior, lateral, and superior margin of the cricoid cartilage (Fig 7–8). With the length of the major axis exceeding the transverse diameter of the articulating surface of the arytenoid, a sliding motion of the arytenoid along the longitudinal axis of the cricoid facet is made possible.[4] This sliding movement may be utilized during forceful closure of the larynx. Although a slide along the major axis of the cricoid facet is possible, the principal motion of the arytenoid is a forward and backward gliding along the minor axis of the cricoid facet. This sliding over a convexly curved surface results in a simultaneous *bidirectional motion*,[4–9] which results in changes not only anteriorly and posteriorly but vertically, as well (Fig 7–9). Bidirectional movement of the arytenoid is poorly described in almost all basic texts and, as a consequence, these key motions remain widely misunderstood.

On moving anteriorly, the vocal process of the arytenoid descends and the muscular process rises. On gliding posteriorly, (Fig 7–10) the vocal process ascends or rises as the muscular process descends.[4] This alternating change in both the vertical and anterior-posterior directions resembles that of a rocking horse or rocking chair.[10] As such, *rocking* has become a common term to describe the motion of the arytenoid. This motion of the arytenoid also bears a distinct resemblance to *rotary movement*. In fact, it is rare to find a textbook or article describing arytenoid motion not using the term *rotation* somewhere in that description. The introduction of the term rotation has created problems, which have significant clinical consequences. With the concept of rotation in mind and the larynx viewed from above (Fig 7–11), changes in verticality are not well appreciated, whereas medial and lateral motions are emphasized (Figs 7–12, 7–13, and 7–14). Vertical displacement of the arytenoid is significant.[11] However, for each unit of vertical displacement that

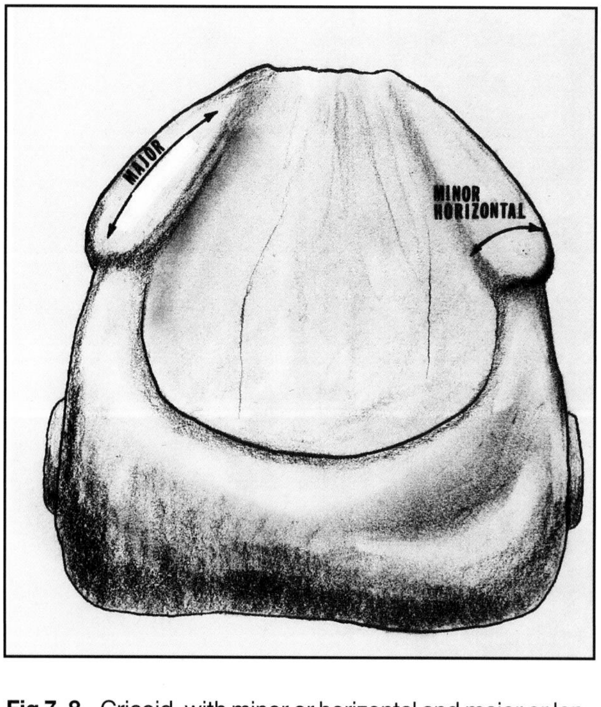

Fig 7–8. Cricoid, with minor or horizontal and major or longitudinal axes of the cricoarytenoid facet labeled. Notice the lateral, anterior, and interior inclinations of the cricoarytenoid facet.

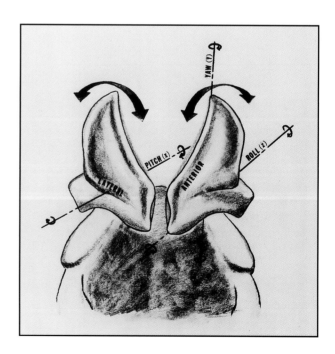

Fig 7–9. Bidirectional movement occurring during revolving of the arytenoid is depicted. The three major axes of rotation (yaw-pitch-roll) are depicted in relationship to the arytenoids.

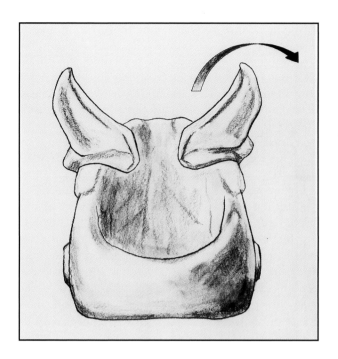

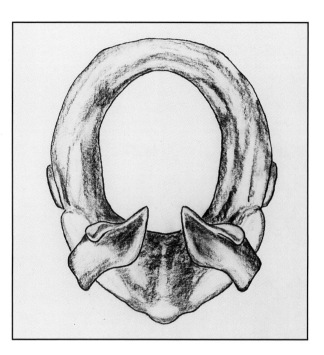

Fig 7–10. Posterior revolving or negative pitchlike rotations. The lateral movement responsible for opening the glottis is due to the positioning of the arytenoid on the cricoarytenoid facet.

Fig 7–12. Superior view of the arytenoids and cricoid, showing forward revolving, gradually approaching almost full adduction. Notice from this perspective the medial and lateral movements are emphasized. Changes in vertical position are hard to discern from this view. Frable[5] states that medial and lateral changes in position occur at twice the magnitude of vertical.

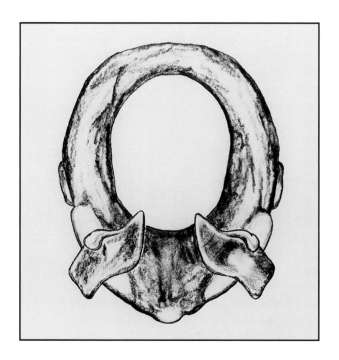

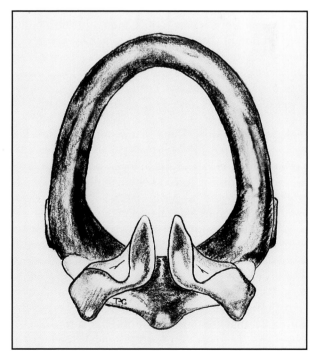

Fig 7–11. Superior view of arytenoids and cricoid with arytenoids revolved posteriorly (abducted).

Fig 7–13. See Fig 7–12 legend.

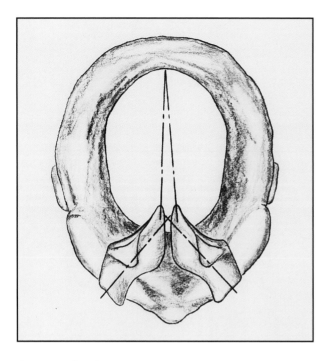

Fig 7–14. See Fig 7–12 legend.

occurs, there are two units of medial-lateral displacement[5]; this gives a false impression that the arytenoids turn on their vertical axes. The *vertical axis* is known as the *y axis*, and motion around this axis is known as *yaw rotation*. The architecture of the cricoarytenoid joint prevents even minimal rotation on the vertical axis.[5, 6, 8]

Unfortunately, many publications, including the 1985 edition of *Gray's Anatomy*, persist in incorrectly describing the arytenoid movement as a rotation about the vertical axis. Arguments countering the concept of yaw rotation have been the subject of several articles. Sonesson[7] and Frable[5] used mathematical models to prove that arytenoid rotation on the vertical axis was impossible. These mathematical models left the impression that rotation was possible on the *transverse (pitch or x)* axis or the anterior-posterior *(roll or z)*[5,7] axis. According to von Leden, if the pivot point is transferred to the posterior cricoid ligament, there may be some minimal rotation allowable on the roll axis.[8] Rotation requires a rotating object to turn on an internal axis. The arytenoid does not turn dynamically on any internal axis. The axis upon which the arytenoids turn is not internal, but rather has its point of origin within the cricoid.

Although the term rocking appears to avoid the difficulty that the term rotation has, it too has its problems. The base of the rocking chair or rocking horse, unlike the arytenoid, is curved not to the concave but rather to the convex. Rocking back and forth

on such a base requires that there be, at every moment, a point of contact with the surface upon which the rocking occurs. The arytenoid as it glides or slides over the cricoid facet has no one point of contact to the cricoid; rather the entire arytenoid base is in contact with the cricoid. Finally, rocking back and forth, whether it be in a rocking chair or on a rocking horse, is actually a rotation on a transverse or pitch axis. In mathematical terms, neither term, rocking or rotating, is considered to be precise.

Over a century ago, Czermak correctly described the gliding of the arytenoid over the facet of the cricoid as, "*the arytenoid processes revolve.*"[10] The gliding movement of the arytenoid over the convexly curved cricoid facet is more properly described as revolving. The difference between a revolving and a rotating object is easily appreciated with the statement "the planets revolve around the sun, while they rotate on their internal axes." Although it is easy to conjure up an image of planets revolving and rotating, it is somewhat difficult for the mind to develop the image of mobile arytenoids revolving on the fixed cricoid. Considering this fact, together with the traditional use of the term rotation and resemblance of motion of a revolving object upon a rounded surface to pitch rotation, a valid argument can be made to accept *pitchlike motion* as an alternative description to *revolving*.

With the arytenoids moving both anteriorly and inferiorly, an additional directional change is also occurring. The arytenoids together with the true vocal folds are observed to move medially, or toward one another *(adduction)*. On moving posteriorly and superiorly, the arytenoids and true vocal folds separate, or move laterally *(abduction)*. Although the arytenoids move medially and laterally during the process of pitchlike motion or revolving, these movements are not due to the pitchlike motion process itself. Rather, the medial and lateral directed movements are due to the alignment of the cricoarytenoid joint. The facets of the cricoid slope laterally, anteriorly, and inferiorly. The arytenoid, on accepting this position, will be inwardly turned on its vertical or yaw axis. This is not a dynamic rotation but rather represents a rotation that is fixed. This subsequent orientation of the arytenoid results in each arytenoid being inclined toward the other and the vocal processes toward the anterior commissure of the true vocal folds (Fig 7–15). This inclination toward one another allows the arytenoids and the true vocal folds to approximate and meet each other during the arytenoid's anterior and inferior pitchlike motion over the cricoid facet. Forward pitch-

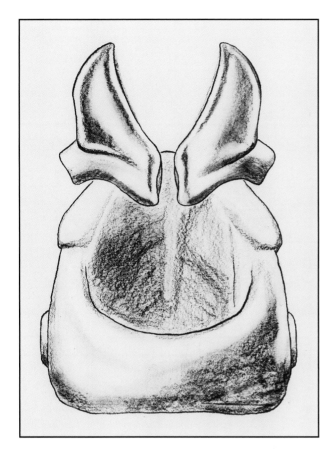

Fig 7–15. The arytenoid, on accepting its position on the cricoid, is inwardly turned on its vertical axis and allows each arytenoid to be inclined toward one another.

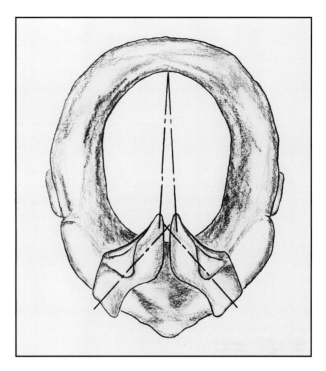

Fig 7–16. Axis drawn through each vocal process demonstrating how this axis diverges from that of the arytenoid body, and in so doing, allows for the convergence of the axes through the vocal processes (vocal ligaments) to meet anteriorly at the midline of the thyroid cartilage.

like motion is known as *positive pitch*. The arytenoids and true vocal folds separate during posterior-superior-directed pitchlike motion of the arytenoids over the cricoid facet (Fig 7–16). This type of pitchlike rotation is known as *negative pitch* (Fig 7–17).

If the vocal processes were not laterally or outwardly angulated from the body of the arytenoid, the anterior and inferior limits of forward movement would never be reached. During positive pitchlike rotation, the vocal processes would prematurely meet. Any further anterior and inferior motion would be arrested. As a result, the position of the posterior one third of the vocal folds during adduction would be higher than the middle third, which in turn would be higher than the vocal fold's anterior third. With the adductory muscles capable of further contraction, the forces generated could conceivably damage the mucosa and perichondrium of the medial edge of each vocal process.

Unfortunately, the detailed measurements of the laryngeal cartilages by Maue and Dickson,[3] as well as

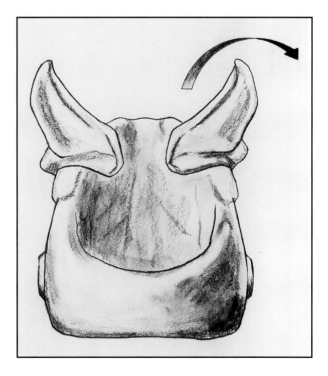

Fig 7–17. Negative pitchlike rotation or posterior or backward revolving.

Hicks (D. Hicks, personal communication), failed to provide the degree of angulation of the vocal processes. If future anatomical studies would demonstrate that the angulation of the arytenoid's vocal process is consistently less in the female than in the male, an explanation would be possible for a posterior glottal chink (Fig 7–18). This is an opening often seen in the female larynx during clinically normal phonation. The tips of each vocal process would meet and prevent contact of the remaining portions of each vocal process and a triangular gap would be created in the posterior glottis.

In summary, arytenoid motion occurs in three directions. Movements involving a change anteriorly and posteriorly, as well as vertically, are due to the revolving or pitchlike motion of the arytenoid along the minor axis of the cricoid's elliptically shaped facet. The medial and lateral movements are due to the orientation of the arytenoid which in turn is determined by the forward, lateral, and inferior inclination of the cricoid-arytenoid facet. During adduction it is the outward angulation of the vocal process from the body of the arytenoid that allows the entire length of the vocal processes to approximate one another and to have this meeting occur at the proper vertical height (Figs 7–19 and 7–20).

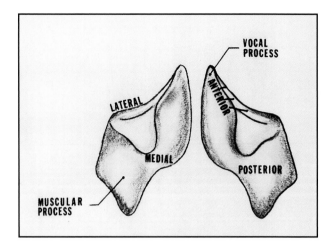

Fig 7–19. Being revolved slightly more forward, the vocal processes will approximate. This meeting is attributed to the outward angulation of the vocal process from the arytenoid body.

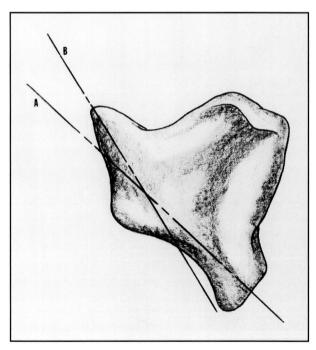

Fig 7–20. Inclination of axis of arytenoid process (B) from the axis of the arytenoid body (A).

Vocal Fold Paralysis

To illustrate the fact that a misconception concerning arytenoid motion still exists in the minds of many experts, one has only to review the procedures designed to treat unilateral vocal fold paralysis. Vocal fold paralysis is a condition generally resulting from a

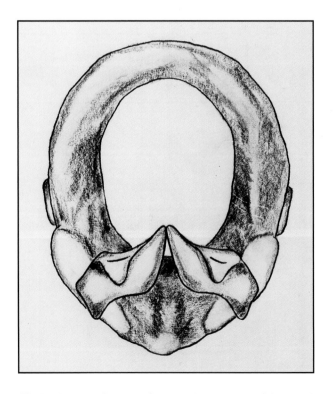

Fig 7–18. Less than usual outward angulation of the vocal processes; on attempted adduction the vocal process tips meet creating a triangular posterior glottal chink.

nonfunctioning recurrent laryngeal nerve. A recently paralyzed vocal fold can have a devastating effect on the individual so afflicted. The basic problem is a continuously opened glottis. With a patent glottis, the lower airway is vulnerable to be penetrated *(aspiration)* by secretions originating in the upper aero-digestive tract, or by ingested food or liquids. Being unable to approximate the true vocal folds, cough strength is appreciably decreased. An inefficient cough can make it difficult to express aspirated material or to raise and clear tracheal-bronchial secretions. In addition, inadequate resistance offered by the vocal folds to expiratory airflow results in a weak and breathy voice, which is difficult to hear at a distance or over background noise and is barely understandable over a telephone. With phonation dramatically reduced from a normal time of 15 to 20 seconds to 4 or fewer seconds, only a few words can be articulated on a single breath, and the rate of respiration during speaking increases some four- to sixfold. So much work and energy are expended during speaking that the individual with a recently paralyzed vocal fold rapidly fatigues and may retreat from all but critical conversations. With time, a poorly understood compensation can occur which reduces the glottal area, thereby diminishing the severity of the problem.

When surgery is considered to treat unilateral vocal fold paralysis, the goal of surgery is to provide a means by which the true vocal folds can be approximated. This goal can be accomplished if a properly positioned medially and inferiorly directed force is applied to the paralyzed true vocal fold. Three common surgical approaches attempt to accomplish this goal:

1. *Foreign material can be injected into the lateral aspect of the membranous true vocal fold.* Materials that have been used include a Teflon-glycerin combination, Gelfoam, collagen, and fat, among others. The concept is that the mass represented by this foreign material will press against the inner aspect of the thyroid cartilage. This rigid structure produces countering medially directed force within the true vocal fold (Newton's third law of motion). Actually, the forces established will be distributed not only medially but also superiorly and inferiorly.

2. *On the side of the paralysis, a rectangular window is created in the ala of the thyroid cartilage.* The upper edge of the window coincides with the superior margin of the true vocal fold. To displace the vocal fold medially, an implant is introduced through the window and fixed into position. This procedure is known as *Thyroplasty Type I* (Figs 7–21, 7–22, and 7–23).

3. *Using a lateral approach, the cricoarytenoid joint is opened and a suture is placed through the muscular process of the arytenoid.* The suture is directed anteriorly and inferiorly then to pass through the ala of the thyroid cartilage (Fig 7–24). This positioning of the suture simulates the pull developed by the contraction of the lateral cricoarytenoid muscle (a major adductor of the larynx). This procedure is known as the *arytenoid adduction procedure.*

One of the first materials to be injected into the vocal folds and to receive widespread use for this procedure was Teflon. The original description of the procedure recommended that Teflon be placed lateral to the vocal process of the arytenoid.[12] When Thyroplasty Type I was a relatively new procedure, several authors described an implant having a posterior extension. The purpose of the posterior extension was to exert a medially directed force on the vocal process. For either procedure to achieve its goal of medialization of the vocal process, the arytenoid would need to be capable of rotating on its vertical or *y* axis. These authors' initial impression of arytenoid motion was in error. Later publications suggest that injections not be made lateral to the arytenoid's vocal process and that implants with a posterior extension not be used. The reasons given were that "they did not work" but an explanation why the procedures performed in this fashion failed was never offered.

The only way that the two arytenoids can be properly approximated for the function of phonation is to move the arytenoid of the paralyzed vocal fold forward and inferiorly (increase the positive pitchlike rotation or anterior revolution of the arytenoid). Such a closure is best accomplished through an arytenoid adduction procedure.

Many experts have also failed to realize that a vertical mismatch exists between the paralyzed and functioning true vocal fold. This vertical malalignment contributes to the open glottis. When viewed from above, the appearance of the paralyzed vocal fold is described as if the arytenoid had previously moved on a cross-sectional plane. Thus, we have the terms *midline, paramedian,* or *lateral.* Motion on a cross-sectional plane would require that arytenoid rotation be on a vertical axis, again a misinterpretation of the facts. By revolving on the cricoid, an arc is created. The posterior-superior and anterior-inferior limits of the arc are defined by the cricoarytenoid joint and the ligamental and muscular attachments to the arytenoid. Summation of the forces acting upon the arytenoid creates motion of the arytenoid over the cricoid, which in turn describes the arc. It is a summation of forces of the paralyzed vocal fold that determines where on that arc the arytenoid will finally rest.

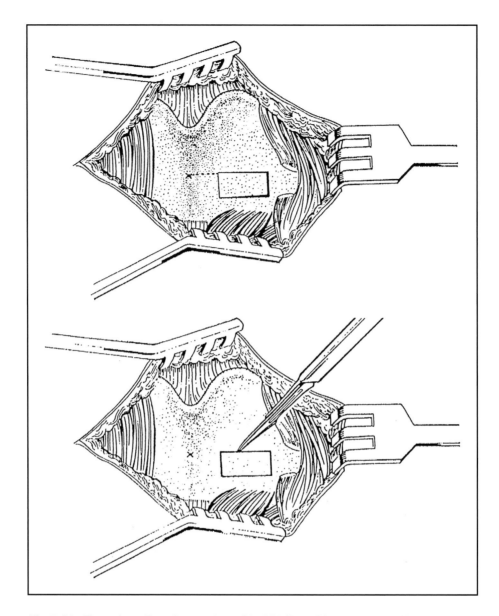

Fig 7–21. Thyroplasty Type I procedure of Isshiki (from *Phonosurgery*, with permission, Isshiki and Springer-Verlag Publishers.)[13] Design of the window. The anterior vertical line of the window is about 5 mm apart from the median line. Direction of the upper transverse line of the window, which corresponds to the upper surface of the vocal fold, must be carefully decided after identifying the line of lower margin of the thyroid ala as shown. Incision is made in the thyroid ala first with BP No. 11 blade.

Important forces to consider are those that result from the contraction of the cricothyroid and interarytenoid muscles. The cricothyroid muscle is the only intrinsic muscle of the larynx not innervated by the recurrent laryngeal nerve. This muscle receives its innervation from the *external branch of the superior laryngeal nerve*. The *interarytenoid muscle* receives bilateral innervation from *the recurrent laryngeal nerve*. The cricothyroid muscle increases longitudinal tension within the vocal fold and with contraction of the upper or anterior fibers (pars recta) allows this pars recta muscle to function as a minor adductor. With further adduction, some additional vertical descent of the vocal process is possible. With contraction of the cricothyroid muscle on the paralyzed side, the arytenoid position is close to, but does not reach the anterior-inferior limit allowable on the arc of revolution. Thus, during inspiration, the recently paralyzed vocal

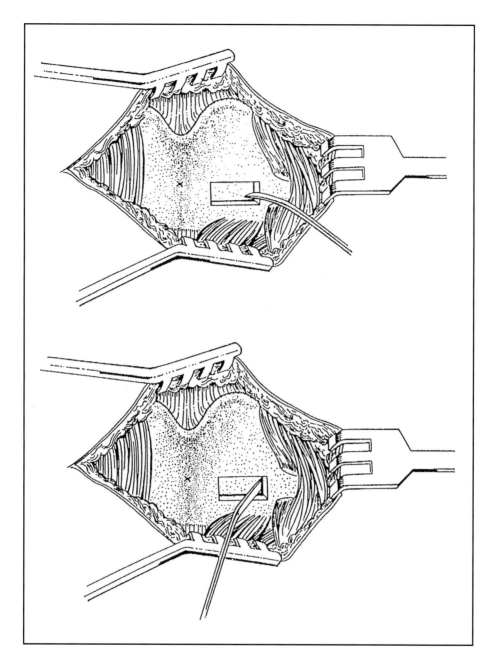

Fig 7–22. See Fig 7–21 legend. After cautious strokes of cutting with the scalpel, or with a burr in old males, a window is pressed inward using an elevator to find where the cut is incomplete.

fold and its vocal process will be in a vertically lower position than the innervated vocal fold. (Fig 7–25). In contrast, during phonation the arytenoid and the paralyzed true vocal fold usually will be in a vertically higher position than the innervated vocal fold (Fig 7–26). In both situations, the functioning arytenoid will revolve past the immobile arytenoid. When asked the question, Does the paralyzed vocal fold ver-

tically lie above or below the innervated vocal fold? the reply should be that the answer depends on the phase of respiration.

During quiet inspiration when the larynx is viewed from above, the prominences created by the arytenoid, corniculate, and cuneiform cartilages on the paralyzed side will be seen to be anterior and medial in comparison to the same prominences of the inner-

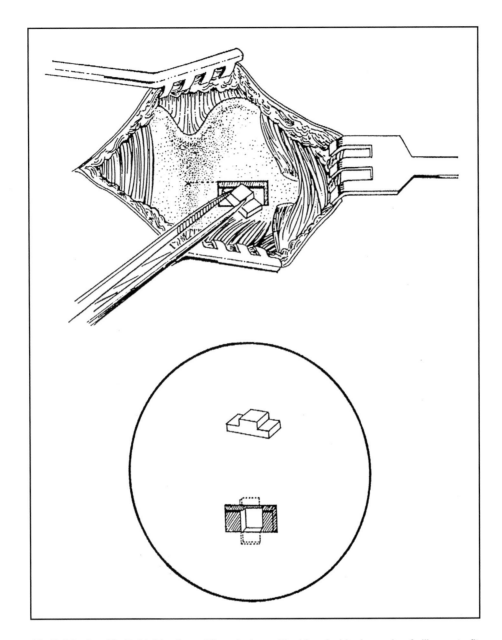

Fig 7–23. See Fig 7–21. Fixation of the window with shim. A shim is made of silicone to fit the size of the window and the desired depth of displacement of the window. This technique, though simple to perform, cannot make fixation of the window so precise as the plug technique can, because the shim tends to bend when inserted.

vated vocal fold. On phonation, the appearance is that these cartilaginous prominences are on the same horizontal plane. Any difference in vertical height is difficult to appreciate.

Conditions in which the cricothyroid fails to activate occur when there is a lesion at the base of the skull or any pathology that results in a high vagal lesion. In this situation, where the cricothyroid muscle is nonfunctional, the arytenoid assumes a position on its arc

near its posterior-superior limits. Hence, the paralyzed vocal fold is not only significantly lateralized, but a considerable vertical gap exists between the two vocal folds, as well. Attempts at medialization of the membranous vocal fold, in this situation, either by vocal fold injection or the Thyroplasty Type I procedure will frequently fail to achieve acceptable vocal strength and quality. The correction of the medial and vertical mismatch between the two vocal folds can be

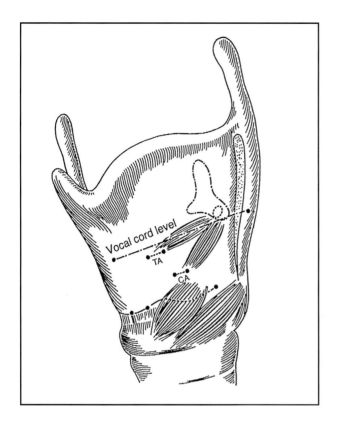

Fig 7–24. Schematic representation of Isshiki's arytenoid adduction procedure. From *Phonosurgery*, with permission of Isshiki and Springer-Verlag Publishers.[13] One of the two sutures is used to pull the muscle process anteriorly: One simulates the thyroarytenoid, the other the cricoarytenoid muscle. When the ala cartilage is calcified, holes must be drilled by a burr at the points indicated as TA and CA.

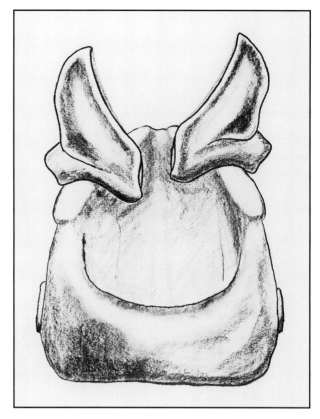

Fig 7–25. Inspiration. Paralyzed right vocal fold (arytenoid) on left of figure. Vocal process of innervated left vocal fold will be vertically higher than right. The innervated vocal fold likewise will be higher and the vertical difference will diminish as the anterior commissure of the true vocal folds are approached.

accomplished by the arytenoid adduction procedure.[13] It is critical for the suture through the muscular process to be placed precisely, and proper tension must be applied to the arytenoid of the paralyzed vocal fold. In this manner, the arytenoid can be moved to a proper forward and inferior position so as to contact the opposite arytenoid during the acts of deglutition and phonation.

When the cricothyroid muscle is functioning, closure of the vertical glottal gap between the membranous vocal folds is frequently accomplished by injection techniques and the Thyroplasty Type I procedure. This is often accomplished more out of serendipity than by thoughtful design. Material injected into the vocal fold, rather than remaining in a distinct cross-sectional plane, will seek an inferior location as well. Injected material will expand the membranous vocal fold vertically, as well as medialize it. Thus, the injection technique can close or approximate the vertical glottal mismatch. However,

injection of most materials into the vocal fold can cause other problems such as a disturbance in phonatory quality. Injections into the vocal fold, rather than lateral to it, are generally considered incorrect. Injection must be lateral to the vocal fold to avoid stiffness and severe dysphonia. Teflon, once placed, cannot be moved and so its placement has to be exact and precise; collagen and fat, once injected, can be maneuvered somewhat into different locations. The ability to reposition these two materials represents a distinct advantage that both collagen and fat have over Teflon.

Despite the concern about injection techniques, when appropriate materials are positioned ideally, it is often possible to plan a procedure so that the vocal process of the arytenoid is brought to or nearly to its appropriate position. Sataloff reports particular success using autologous fat to achieve this goal (RT Sataloff, personal communication). The injected material is positioned lateral to the vocal fold, but no further

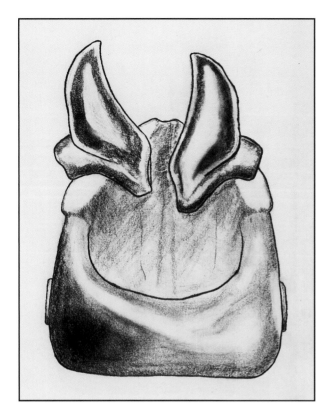

Fig 7–26. Phonation. Paralyzed right vocal fold (arytenoid) on left of figure. The arytenoid of innervated left vocal fold revolves past that of right so it rests vertically lower than the vocal process of the right. The vertical difference between the two vocal folds will be greatest at the level of the vocal processes.

posteriorly than the middle third of the membranous portion.[14] Unlike Teflon, fat allows the safe creation of a slight convexity to the vibratory margin. As the membranous vocal fold is displaced medially, the arytenoid is passively pulled by the attachment of the vocal ligament to the vocal process. Because of the shape of the cricoarytenoid joint, only the desired anterior-inferior motion can occur. If the material is injected too far posteriorly, the injected material elevates the vocal process and mechanically prevents the desired arytenoid repositioning. The thickness of the medial edge of the true vocal folds is about that of a dime. The average width of the implant used in Thyroplasty Type I procedures is several millimeters thicker than this dime-thickness of the free edge of the vocal fold. Thus, when the implant is properly positioned the additional width of the implant will medialize not only the free edge but also several additional millimeters of the subglottal tissue, which should be sufficient to approximate or close the vertical glottal gap.

Ligaments

There are three intralaryngeal ligaments and one elastic membrane that have clinical significance to the student of the larynx. These structures are the following: The *posterior cricoarytenoid ligament*, the *vocal* and *ventricular ligaments*, and the *conus elasticus*.

Running from the medial and inferior portion of the arytenoid body onto the dorsal superior surface of the cricoid is the very dense and strong *posterior cricoarytenoid ligament*. This ligament prevents undue anterior and inferior movement of the arytenoid. Because of its strength, exceptional force is required to dislocate the body of the arytenoid anteriorly.

A physician may have difficulty in distinguishing a recent posterior and lateral dislocated arytenoid from a fresh vocal fold paralysis. Two observations can help distinguish the two entities and hopefully prevent any delay in surgical correction of a dislocated arytenoid. If the larynx is viewed indirectly by a mirror, both the paralyzed vocal fold and the vocal fold with a dislocated arytenoid would appear to be immobilized. Using a flexible or rigid endoscope, some fine movements of the vocal fold with the arytenoid dislocated can generally be perceived at the level of the vocal process and body of the arytenoid during phonation. During inspiration, the arytenoid-corniculate-cuneiform complex (ACCC) of the recently paralyzed vocal fold in most instances would be considerably different than that of a posterior and lateral dislocated arytenoid. During an inspiratory effort, the ACCC of the paralyzed vocal fold will appear to be medial and anterior to that of an innervated vocal fold. In contrast, the ACCC on the side of the posterior and lateral dislocation will appear to have the same anterior-posterior inclination and the same medial orientation of that of the mobile vocal fold. A difference in the vertical position of the two arytenoids would exist but the phenomenon of parallax would make this differentiation difficult to appreciate. The lateral and posterior orientation of the ACCC of the immobile vocal fold on quiet inspiration serves only to suggest the possibility of an arytenoid dislocation. One needs to bear in mind that this same geometric configuration can occur, although rarely, with a vocal fold paralysis. Hence, the observation of low-amplitude coarse movements of the vocal process during phonation should be sought in ruling in or ruling out the possibility of a dislocated arytenoid. If available, an expertly performed EMG of the intrinsic muscles of the larynx is indispensable in distinguishing the two entities.

Running from the tip of each vocal process to the anterior midline of the thyroid cartilage are the vocal ligaments. The two vocal ligaments join at a point on the anterior inferior aspect of the thyroid cartilage. This conjoined attachment of the two vocal ligaments to the thyroid cartilage is known as Broyle's ligament.

A second ligament of importance, the ventricular ligament, also attaches to the arytenoid, but at a locus superior and lateral to the vocal process. The common point of origin for the right and left ventricular ligaments is several millimeters above the attachment of Broyle's ligament. The vocal ligaments approximate the medial boundary of the true vocal fold, and the ventricular ligaments similarly mark the medial boundary of the false vocal fold.

The false or ventricular vocal fold contains little if any musculature and is composed primarily of connective and glandular tissue. What little muscle is present is part of the muscularis portion of the thyroarytenoid muscle. Despite the lack of musculature, the false vocal fold is capable of medial and lateral movement. The mechanisms that control adduction and abduction of the false vocal fold are not fully understood.

The vocal ligament marks not only the medial boundary of the true vocal fold, but also represents the superior margin of a broad expanse of elastic tissue known as the conus elasticus. The conus takes origin from the superior aspect of the cricoid cartilage, and as it ascends to its superior margin, the conus is inclined medially. The conus elasticus is responsible for maintaining the form and shape of the immediate subglottis and the subglottal portion of the true vocal folds.

Arytenoid motion has long been recognized as complex. Misunderstandings about the specifics of arytenoid motion remain prevalent. The resultant misunderstandings have led to erroneous or suboptimal clinical approaches to the treatment of vocal fold immobility. A thorough understanding of the anatomy of the arytenoid and cricoid cartilages, the cricoarytenoid joint, and related ligaments, muscles, and other structures is essential in order to fully understand laryngeal motion disorders. The materials presented in this chapter should be useful not only for diagnostic purposes, but also for designing appropriate non-

surgical and surgical intervention to optimize vocal fold position in three dimensions

Acknowledgment Illustrations in this chapter were provided by Thomas Geyr.

References

1. Abard WR, Howe HA. *Medical Greek and Latin at a Glance*. New York, NY: Harper and Brothers; 1956.
2. *Webster's New World Dictionary*, Second College Edition, Cleveland, Ohio: Collins/World; 1978.
3. Maue W, Dickson DR. Cartilages and ligaments of the adult human larynx. *Arch Otolaryngol*. 1971;94:432–439.
4. Pernkopf E. *Atlas of Topographical and Applied Human Anatomy*. St Louis, Mo: WB Saunders: 1963.
5. Frable MA. Computation of motion at the cricoarytenoid joint, *Arch Otolaryngol*. 1961;73:73–78.
6. Snell C. On the function of the cricoarytenoid joints in the movements of the vocal cords. *Proc. Koninklike Nederlandsche Akad van Wetenschappen*. 1947;50:1370–1381.
7. Sonesson B. Die funktionelle Anatomie des Crico-Arytenoidgelenkes, *Z Anat Entwicklyngsgesch*. 1959;121: 292–303.
8. Von Leden H. The mechanics of the cricoarytenoid joint, *Arch Otolaryngol*. 1961;73:63–72
9. Zemlin WR, *Speech and Hearing Science: Anatomy and Physiology*, 3rd ed. Englewood Cliffs, NJ: Prentice-Hall; 1988:105–109,132–133.
10. Fink BR, *The Human Larynx: A Functional Study*. New York, NY: Raven Press; 1975:122.
11. Baken RJ, Isshiki N. Arytenoid displacement by simulated intrinsic muscle contraction. *Folia Phonatrica*. 1977;29:206–216.
12. Arnold GE. Alleviation of aphonic or dysphonia through intracordal injection of teflon paste. *Ann Otol Rhinol Laryngol*. 1963;72:384–395.
13. Isshiki N. *Phonosurgery: Theory and Practice*. New York NY: Springer-Verlag; 1989:77–129.
14. Mikaelian D, Lowry LD, Sataloff RT. Lipoinjection for unilateral vocal cord paralysis. *Laryngoscope*. 1991;101(5): 465–468.
15. Woodson CE. Configuration of the glottis in laryngeal paralysis, I: clinical study. *Laryngoscope*. 1993;103: 1227–1234.

8

Vocal Fold Injury and Repair

Susan L. Thibeault and Steven D. Gray[†]

Hirano[1,2] was one of the first to recognize the importance of the microstructure of the vocal folds. According to Hirano, the five histological layers of increasing density break down into two biomechanical layers (the body and the cover). The body is composed primarily of muscle, whereas the cover has been described as being composed primarily of collagen and elastin. The shape and tension of the cover determine the vibratory characteristics and subsequent vocal source quality. Its shape and tension may also be modified by lesions that arise from the cover and change the biomechanics and subsequent voice source. Until recently the primary foci of cover descriptions were the thickness of structure and the presence or absence of collagen and elastin. Scientists began to suspect this was not the whole picture after Gray et al[3] described the structure of the basement membrane zone and shearing forces in the vocal fold. Gray and his colleagues[4-7] went on to demonstrate that the normal molecular structure of the lamina propria is constructed of a great deal more than collagen and elastin.

This notion that all of the constituents of the lamina propria and their organization contribute to its biomechanical properties was revolutionary, because it meant there might be other ways to understand and treat laryngeal pathologies than previously known. Furthermore, with the advent of the use of molecular and cell techniques and tools in voice research, there is a field of study that holds considerable promise in providing insights into the cover's characteristics and other aspects of vocal fold biology. One such focus, which will likely provide new vistas for diagnosis and treatment, is an improved understanding of vocal fold injury and the subsequent attempts by the lamina pro-

pria to regulate its repair. The understanding of molecular and cell biology of wound healing is far reaching in other disciplines; whereas, in voice biology, our knowledge is limited. This chapter will introduce the complex processes and the ensuing manifestations of wound healing by the body, as well as evidence of tissue repair in the vocal folds via wound healing pathogenesis.

Wound Healing

Wound healing represents the process of tissue repair with reorganization of the tissue matrix, which produces scar with concomitant loss of tissue function. Generally, scar tissue represents poor reconstitution of epidermal and dermal structures at the site of the healed wound.[8] Specifically, the sequence of repair is comprised of hemostasis, inflammation, mesenchymal cell migration and proliferation, angiogenesis, epithelialization, protein and proteoglycan synthesis, wound contraction, and remodeling. It is beyond the scope of this chapter to discuss all of the intricate factors identified in wound healing; rather the most important known variables and control mechanisms in the normal cascade of biological events of wound healing will be discussed (Table 8–1).

Hemostasis/Coagulation

Blood vessels hemorrhage in all wounds that either damage the epidermal barrier or damage the underlying structures. For the initiation of the wound response, hemorrhage must be truncated by hemostasis. The body generates a clot (made up mainly of

†Deceased.

Table 8–1. Summary of Normal Wound-Healing Mechanisms.

Stage of Wound Healing	Time Course (Approximate)	Principal Molecular and Cellular Events
Hemostasis/Coagulation	Immediately to one day post-injury	Formation of fibrin clot at site of injury.
Inflammation	Immediately to 3 days post-injury	Vasoconstriction and vasodilatation at site of injury.
		Presence of neutrophils followed by macrophages, whose function is to phagocytose bacteria and dead tissue and secrete enzymes for tissue breakdown.
Mesenchymal Cell Migration and Proliferation	2 to 4 days post-injury	Fibroblasts migrate into wound site and become predominant cell type.
		Some fibroblasts phenotypically change into myofibroblasts for tissue repair.
Angiogenesis	2 to 4 days post-injury	Formation of fewer larger blood vessels at site of injury.
Epithelization	Hours to 5 days post-injury	Epithelial cell migration to form epithelium and BMZ.
Protein and Proteoglycan Synthesis	3 to 5 days to 6 weeks post-injury	Formation of ECM through production of proteins, proteoglycans, glycoaminoglycans by fibroblasts.
Wound Contraction and Remodeling	3 days to 12 months post-injury	Myofibroblasts and collagen mediate contraction. Scar remodeling consists of turnover of ECM proteins, proteoglycans, and glycoaminoglycans.
		Apoptosis of myofibroblasts and epithelial cells.

platelets and fibrin) to block the damaged vessels by means of a "coagulation cascade." There are intrinsic and extrinsic pathways to the cascade. The intrinsic pathway of the coagulation cascade is activated when blood is exposed to a negatively charged foreign surface. Factor XII is activated and through a series of further activations enters a common pathway. The extrinsic pathway is initiated when factor VII interacts with tissue factor, an intracellular protein that is expressed in white cells and becomes available when underlying vascular structures are exposed to flowing blood following vessel injury. The extrinsic pathway enters the common pathway directly through activation of factor X. The common pathway results in the production of thrombin, which catalyzes the conversion of fibrinogen to fibrin, and factor XIII, which stabilizes the fibrin polymer in platelet aggregates.

Fibrin becomes the main component of the provisional matrix that provides a scaffold that allows for future migration of inflammatory and mesenchymal cells. The matrix becomes coated with fibronectin and vitronectin from aggregating platelets, serum, and fibroblasts. Fibronectin aids in cellular attachment and modulates the migration of various cell types in the wound. Platelets adhere to fibrin and release adenosine diphosphate (ADP), which in the presence of calcium stimulates further platelet aggregation. Platelet aggregation directs release of multiple cytokines—platelet-derived growth factor (PDGF), TGF-β, TGF-α, bFGF, platelet-derived epidermal growth factor (PDEFG), and platelet-derived endothelial cell growth factor (PDECGF), which contribute to repair at various times of healing.

Inflammation

Inflammation begins very soon after the wound is created and is initiated with intense local vasoconstriction that is replaced by vasodilatation after approximately 10 to 15 minutes.[9] Vasoconstriction contributes to hemostasis and is mediated by circulating catecholamines and the sympathetic nervous system. Vasodilatation generates heat and erythema at the site of injury. Concomitant with vasodilatation, the capillaries develop gaps between the endothelial cells, creating edema. Neutrophils, albumin, and globulin penetrate the fibrin/fibronectin matrix. White cell emigration is controlled, in part, by chemotaxis, which is the unidirectional migration of cells along a chemical gradient.[10] A wide variety of exogenous and endogenous substances have been identified as chemotaxis agents. These include histamine, PDGF, bacterial products, and fibrinopeptides released by thrombin from fibrinogen. In the matrix, large numbers of neutrophils can be found, which serve to engulf foreign material and absorb it using hydrolytic enzymes and oxygen radicals. Forty-eight to eighty-four hours after injury, neutrophils are phagocytosed and destroyed by macrophages.[10] Release of the destructive proteolytic enzymes and free oxygen radical can damage tissue and be held responsible for persistent inflammation and chronic infection in wounds.

Monocytes migrate from the capillaries into the extravascular space via chemotactic factors. Mediated by serum factors and fibronectin, the monocytes are transformed into macrophages. Factors known to stimulate macrophage migration include collagen fragments, fibronectin fragments, and elastin derived from damaged matrices.[10] Macrophages function to phagocytose bacteria and dead tissue and secrete collagenases, elastases, and tissue inhibitors of metalloproteinases (TIMPs). These enzymes aid in the breakdown of the damaged matrix as well as in the breakdown of proteins during remodeling. Macrophages are a primary source of cytokines that stimulate proliferation of fibroblasts and the production of collagen, TGF-β, PDGF, EGF, and fibroblast growth factor. At 48 to 72 hours post-injury, macrophages outnumber neutrophils as the primary cell type. Macrophages stay at the site of injury for several days, after which they are replaced by fibroblasts.

Chronic inflammation can occur if there is foreign material or bacteria at the site of injury. Subsequently, the persistence of inflammation can be deleterious to the healing process. Chronic inflammation can cause tissue damage and infection, because the neurophils release destructive proteolytic enzymes and free oxygen radicals that cause damage.

Mesenchymal Cell Migration and Proliferation

Mesenchymal cell migration and proliferation occur 2 to 4 days after injury, and the fibroblast is the predominant cell implicated in this process. Fibroblasts from surrounding undamaged tissue migrate into the wounded matrix in response to chemotactic signals. Fibroblasts are able to move via their ability to bind and release fibronectin, fibrin, and vitronectin. The direction of movement is guided by the alignment of the fibrils in the matrix. Fibroblasts do not move across matrix fibers. It has been hypothesized that migration is facilitated by the presence of hyaluronic acid.[10] In addition, fibroblasts, which produce proteolytic enzymes such as matrix metalloproteinase 1 (MMP-1), gelatinase (MMP-2), and stromelysin (MMP-3), have been hypothesized as being essential to the migration.

The presence of the fibroblast is important for subsequent synthesis of components of the extracellular matrix (ECM); and fibroblasts are generally considered to be cells of maintenance. Fibroblasts undergo a phenotypic change into myofibrobroblasts that allows them to repair injured tissue. The presence of myofibroblasts is an indication of tissue injury.

Angiogenesis

Angiogenesis restructures new vasculature in the area of injury. This process is mediated by high lactate levels, acidic pH, and decreased oxygen tensions in the tissue. Small capillary sprouts forms on venules at the periphery of the devascularized area. Capillary sprouts grow and proliferate into capillaries, which mature through aggregation of many capillaries into fewer larger vessels.

Epithelialization

Renewal of the epithelial barrier is essential for repair and begins within hours of injury. The earliest sign of epithelialization is thickening of the basal cell layer at the wound edge. Basal cells elongate, detach from the underlying basement membrane, and migrate into the wound. Migration of basal cells along collagen fibers in a leapfrog fashion continues until they reach other cells (contact guidance). If the basement membrane is intact, epithelial cells migrate over it; although the membrane becomes infiltrated with additional fibronectin as the cells move across it.[11] If the basement membrane is not intact, the cells migrate over a provisional matrix.

Once contact inhibition is achieved, cells undergo a phenotypic alteration into more basal-like cells. Compared to normal epithelium, the newly differentiate basal cells are fewer in number and the interface between the dermis and epidermis, the basement membrane zone (BMZ), is atypical. Preserving epithelium and the BMZ improves wound healing.

Protein and Proteoglycan Synthesis

Through phenotypic change, fibroblasts that are in the wound begin to produce proteins. This process begins 3 to 5 days after injury. The major protein synthesized is collagen, which constitutes 50% of the protein found in scar.[12] Collagen synthesis is maximum 2 to 4 weeks after injury and can be altered by several factors (eg, age, stress, and pressure) and various growth factors (eg, FGF, EGF, and TGF-β). A collagen matrix replaces the fibrin scaffold. The presence of the matrix facilitates cellular motility.

Fibroblasts also are responsible for production of the proteoglycans and glycoaminoglycans at the injured site. Hyaluronic acid production is stimulated by PDGF[13] and plays an important role in early wound healing. High levels of hyaluronic acid are found from days 1 through 5, with a decrease between days 5 and 10.[14] Fibronectin is produced throughout all stages of wound healing. Elastin is not synthesized in response to injury. Scar tissue lacks the normal amount of elastin,[15] decreasing the elastic properties of the repaired tissue.

Wound Contraction and Remodeling

Wound contraction is denoted by the centripetal movement of the wound edge towards the center of the wound. The mechanism by which wounds contract is debatable. Myofibroblasts have been described as being responsible for wound contraction.[16] They are present on the third day after injury and remain until 21 days postinjury at the periphery of the wound. Fibroblasts within collagen matrices also have been described as being responsible for wound contraction.[12] The collagen matrices can contract under stress and interact with the matrix around them to mediate contraction.

The final stage of wound healing is scar remodeling. Scar remodeling is characterized by the behavior of collagen at the injured site. It has been found that the net accumulation of collagen becomes stable at approximately 21 days postinjury.[10] Apoptosis of epithelial cells and myofibroblasts occur. Scar remodeling can continue up to 12 months with turnover of collagen in a denser, more organized fashion along lines of stress. Eighty percent breaking strength is achieved in the new scar tissue via an increase in the number of intra- and intermolecular cross-links between collagen fibers. Because of the remodeling, metalloproteinases, tissue inhibitors of metalloproteinases, and enzymes are necessary and are found throughout the injured site. Overall, type I collagen increases and type III decreases, with a decrease in glycoaminoglycans (GAG) and water in the matrix.[12] Early immature scar is present during the first 1 to 3 months following injury.[12] This type of scar is stiff and thick. Mature scar, because of the remodeling of collagen, is generally thinner and more pliable. The differences are attributed to changes in structural proteoglycans.[17]

Vocal Fold Manifestations of Injury and Repair

Vocal fold injury has a variety of etiologies, including excessive vocal use or phonotrauma (resulting from increased mechanical forces on the tissue), intubation, intentional or incidental resection of laryngeal tissue, inflammation caused from infection or physical irritants, and laryngeal injury secondary to acute or blunt accident. The body's attempts to repair the injured tissue can cause alterations in the production of select proteins that subsequently modify normal vocal fold lamina propria viscosity and oscillatory motion. Recent work incorporating genomic methodologies (discussed in chapter 4) into the study of vocal fold injury and repair has provided innovative insight into the etiological wound healing paradigms and their effect on tissue viscosity, in benign lesions.

Wound Healing Paradigms in Benign Vocal Fold Lesions

The most extreme response of injury and repair in the vocal folds is scarring, a response that represents the final stage of wound healing–wound contraction and remodeling, which is characterized by poor reconstitution of the epidermal/dermal tissue. Vocal fold scarring causes significant changes in the physical properties of vocal fold tissue, altering the body-cover relationship and inhibiting propagation of normal mucosal wave. These changes produce hoarseness, loss of vocal control, and fatigue and present significant treatment challenges. The relationship between the ultrastructural alterations of the ECM and their effect on the viscoelastic properties (stiffness and viscosity) of the tissue is an important association that will likely shed significant light on possible treatment avenues. Measurement of the viscoelastic properties and histological characterization of fibrous and interstitial proteins of the lamina propria in vocal fold scarring in the rabbit model[18,19] paralleled the clinical picture seen in vocal fold scarring—loss of mucosal wave and increased stiffness. Rheologically, when compared to the normal lamina propria, scarred vocal fold lamina propria was found to have significantly increased levels of viscosity and stiffness. Scarred lamina propria demonstrated new, unorganized collagen, most likely representing an early stage of remodeling and less elastin distributed in scattered networks, which may be partially responsible for loss of normal tissue elasticity. Decreased decorin levels in scar, whose role is to promote the lateral association of collagen fibrils to form fibers and fiber bundles in the ECM, corresponded to the authors' finding of unorganized collagen. Levels of increased procollagen I (a collagen precursor) appear to correlate with the significantly less fibromodulin measured in the scarred vocal fold. Through fibromodulin's capability to inhibit TGF-β, which upregulates the synthesis of collagen,[20] an increase in collagen production would be expected concomitantly with a decrease in fibromodulin. Lastly, high fibronectin levels in vocal fold scar support the hypothesis that fibronectin induces cell migration and ECM synthesis and suggest that its persistence may be involved in the development of fibrosis.

Vocal fold polyp and Reinke's edema are two benign vocal fold lesions thought to represent wound-healing paradigms. Decreased fibronectin, less basement zone injury and increased vascular injury[21,22] characterize polyps, whereas increased fibrin, hemorrhage and thickening of the basement membrane zone have been described in Reinke's edema.[23] The wound healing stages of inflammation and hemostasis/coagulation are analogous to Reinke's edema and polyps, respectively. Measurement of gene expression levels for procollagen I, collagenase, elastase, fibronectin, fibromodulin, decorin, hyaluronan synthase 2, and hyaluronidase demonstrated similar transcription profiles between the two lesions with the exception of fibromodulin and fibronectin. These differences may provide insight into differences in mucosal wave characteristics. Fibronectin transcription levels were clearly down regulated for Reinke's edema compared to those of polyps. Again, the ability of fibronectin to induce cell migration and ECM synthesis suggests that its persistence might be involved in the development of fibrosis, which might be related directly to viscoelastic parameters of the mucosal wave. The decreased levels of fibronectin in Reinke's edema suggest that there is activity towards a state of less stiffness. Fibromodulin plays a role in collagen fibrillogenesis; fibromodulin-null animals have collagen fiber bundles that are disorganized and have abnormal ECM morphology. Down regulation of fibromodulin, as found in the polyps, suggests a disorganized ECM regulation, which may be moving towards a stiffer environment. Both increases in fibronectin and decreases in fibromodulin support a stiffer phenotype in polyps. The transcriptional levels for fibromodulin and fibronectin predicted mucosal wave scores, rated from preoperative videostroboscopy. Interestingly, transcription levels were confirmed with measurement of protein translation levels for collagen and fibronectin for the polyp group. The changes in the protein levels parallel those found for mRNA and stroboscopy analysis. Low collagen levels appear to be related to a stiffer phenotype, consistent with that reported for vocal fold scar, which has less collagen and increased stiffness. High fibronectin protein levels were associated with stiffer mucosal wave scores.

Protein's Role in Modulating Vocal Fold Tissue Viscosity

The relationship between increased tissue stiffness, viscosity, and changes in the fibrous and interstitial proteins does not seem to be straightforward. The relationship between the biomechanical properties of the vocal fold and the constituents of the lamina propria is related directly and necessitates further discussion. Increased stiffness, increased viscosity, or decreased mucosal wave, which have been documented for vocal fold scar, vocal fold polyp, and Reinke's edema, have lamina propria ECM that is characterized by decreased collagen, increased fibronectin, decreased fibromodulin, and decreased decorin. The finding of decreased collagen levels differs from dermal literature that has shown increased collagen with increased stiffness. Differences may be related to the nature of vocal fold tissue and the vibratory forces that provide an environment that results in constant regulation secondary to mechanical forces. It has been shown that mechanical forces can affect ECM gene expression, upregulate dermal procollagen synthesis, and stimulate collagen turnover.[24] Interstitial proteins play an important role in the organization and regulation of the fibrous proteins; hence, it may be the levels of the interstitial proteins that are directly related to the viscoelastic properties of vocal fold tissue, resultant to their interface with fibrous proteins. Decreases in decorin and/or fibromodulin have a direct effect on collagen organization producing abnormal architecture. The abnormal architecture is associated with altered tissue dynamics. Furthermore, increased fibronectin levels, along with low collagen levels, have been associated with stiffer mucosal wave states in vocal fold polyps, implicating a fibronectin role in effecting tissue stiffness. High fibronectin protein levels allied with stiffer mucosal wave scores corroborate the hypothesis of fibronectin-inducing ECM synthesis,[12] which can produce an unorganized matrix. Fibronectin has an adhesive character that attracts cells and macromolecules.[12] The ensuing altered molecular configuration might affect mucosal wave stiffness directly.

The role of the interstitial proteins in contributing to the fibrous protein architecture is enhanced when considering TGF-β. TGF-β. has been found in chronic wounds that heal with scar formation, but not in fetal wounds that heal without scar formation.[12] Although it is responsible for upregulation of fibronectin and new collagen synthesis, it down-regulates the synthesis of decorin, in vitro.[26] Furthermore, it is inhibited by fibromodulin. These interactions suggest that TGF-β levels would also be expected to be high in vocal fold scar tissue, because the decreased fibromodulin levels would increase TGF-β, with subsequent effects of increased fibronectin, collagen production, and decreased decorin. Thibeault et al[19] demonstrated evidence of increased fibronectin and decreased decorin and fibromodulin in vocal fold scar. Levels of TGF-β in vocal fold lamina propria and disease can only be hypothesized, because it has not been measured to date. However, TGF-β might be the growth factor that interacts with all of the interstitial proteins and is responsible for their modifications in pathology.

Microarray Analysis of Benign Vocal Fold Lesions

To analyze global patterns of gene expression in benign laryngeal disease, DNA microarray (MA), a new high throughput genomic technology, has been utilized to study two benign lesions, polyps and granulomas.[27] Polyps transpire as a sequela of vocal abuse and have been characterized by a hemorrhagic event or increased vascular permeability.[28] Vocal fold granulomas result from injury and histologically have been characterized by focal ulceration, desquamating epithelium, and edematous lamina propria with infiltration by chronic inflammatory cells and neutrophils.[29] MA improves understanding of disease gene profiles and of pathway regulation of such profiles; and this technology may provide essential etiological information that will advance diagnosis and treatment. Overall expression results obtained from MA suggest that vocal fold granuloma and vocal fold polyp have two different levels of cellular activity taking place. Upregulated wounding healing, inflammation and matrix remodeling genes differentiate vocal fold granuloma. This corroborates previous research by Shin et al[29] who describe vocal fold granuloma as an inflammatory lesion. Ylitalo[30] has proposed that the initial inflammatory response to trauma is maintained by variables such as extraesophageal reflux and throat clearing. Because of the spectrum of wound-healing genes present in the granuloma, it has been speculated that a continuous repair response is present for vocal granulomas with an emphasis on the inflammation stage.

Differentiated vocal fold polyp genes did not include inflammatory, wound-healing, or matrix-remodeling genes; rather, immune system response to injury genes were upregulated. This is significant in light of the prevailing notion in the literature suggesting that vocal polyps are a result of vocal trauma and that their histology shows evidence of regeneration and repair.[23] Down-regulated membrane receptor genes for vocal polyps might imply anomalies in normal cellular activity, indicating a system that is in inhibition rather than overexpression of ECM. Moreover, the cluster of epithelial regulated genes highly expressed in vocal fold polyp specifies greater activity in the epithelium compared to normal true vocal fold. Differing reports regarding alterations in the epithelium of vocal fold polyp have been described in the literature. Loire et al[31] report atrophy of the epithelium of vocal fold polyp with a thin basement membrane zone, whereas Kotby et al[32] describe an intact basement membrane zone in their histological samples. The overexpressed genes of the epithelial cluster in this study are already known to be active participants in altering epithelial structure and the basement membrane zone at the level of the anchoring fibers, suggesting anomalies of the epithelium in vocal fold polyp that are related directly to gene expression. It appears as if there is anomalous epithelization wound healing for vocal fold polyps.

Repetitive vocal trauma, as is seen in vocal fold nodules, can represent changes in the BMZ, demonstrating a separation of the epithelium from the underlying dermis. It has been proposed that this area represents an area of stress when the tissue is put into vibration.[33] Electron microscopy studies[13] have demonstrated thickening of the BMZ and increased fibronectin,[21] which may represent tearing forces in the subepithelium. Kotby et al[34] described nodular lesions with gaps at the intercellular junctions, disruption and duplication of the BMZ, and collagen fiber dispositions. The presence of increased fibronectin corresponds to all stages of wound healing; fibronectin is ubiquitous throughout the process. Gray et al[33] proposed that the disorganized BMZ (particularly injury to the anchoring fibers) may leave the vocal fold in a state predisposed for repetitive injury, and fibronectin deposition may lead to increased stiffening of that part of the membranous fold.

In the voice biology literature, relatively few proteins, proteoglycans, glycoproteins, and GAG have been investigated in normal or injured lamina propria. Technology has limited the analysis. Traditionally, the substances considered have been limited to those identified to be present in true vocal folds only (ie, collagen, elastin, decorin, fibronectin, fibromodulin, and hyaluronic acid) (Table 8–2). MA provides large-scale definition of gene patterns at the level of the whole genome. This provides a great deal of information in a shorter amount of time. Interestingly, differentially expressed gene lists ascertained for vocal fold polyps and vocal fold granulomas demonstrate genes that are not those traditionally investigated and listed above. Rather, genes not previously examined appear to be playing major roles in the characterization of these two lesions. Investigations into these gene lists may

Table 8–2. Characteristics of ECM Players in Normal and Injured Lamina Propria.

ECM Player	Function	Localization in Normal Lamina Propria	Localization in Injured Lamina Propria
Collagen	Provide strength to lamina lamina propria.[35]	Density increases across superficial layer of lamina propria to deep layer of lamina propria.[35]	Disorganized and decreased in scarred lamina propria[18] Decreased in vocal fold polyps with stiffer mucosal waves[36]
Elastin	Provide stretch and recoil of the lamina propria[35]	Highest density in middle layer of lamina propria.[35]	Decreased in scar tissue[18]
Procollagen Type I	Precursor to collagen.[37]	Unknown in normal lamina propria.	Increased in scarred lamina propria[18]
Decorin	Promote lateral association of collagen fibrils to form fibers and fiber bundles in the ECM. Binds to fibronectin and TGF-β.[38]	Found throughout lamina propria. Highest density is in superficial layer of the the lamina propria.[6]	Decreased in scarred lamina propria[19]
Fibronectin	Induces cell migration and ECM synthesis. May be involved in the development of fibrosis.[12]	Found throughout the lamina propria including the BMZ (specialized lamina propria).[6]	Increased in scarred lamina propria[19] Increased in vocal fold polyps. Higher levels of fibronectin associated with stiffer mucosal waves in vocal fold polyps.[36] MRNA levels decreased in Reinke's edema.[36] Increased levels in BMZ of nodules.[3]
Fibromodulin	Inhibits TGF-β, which upregulates collagen synthesis. Plays role in collagen fibrillogenesis.[20]	Found in the intermediate and deep layers of the lamina propria.[6]	Decreased in scar lamina propria.[19] MRNA levels decreased in vocal fold polyps and increased in Reinke's edema.[36]
TGF-β	Upregulated fibronectin and collagen synthesis.[26] Downregulates synthesis of decorin.[26] Inhibited by fibromodulin.[20]	Has not been measured in normal lamina propria.	Has not been measured in injured lamina propria.

provide important insights into future treatments for vocal fold disease distinguished by mucosal wave stiffness.

Future Directions

Vocal fold injury and repair are of concern not only because of the resultant lesion but also because of its effect on the vibratory mechanism. Consequently, to appreciate fully the biological manifestations of the complexity of wound healing in the vocal fold lamina propria, a better understanding of the alterations in tissue viscosity and elasticity is needed. Preliminary research in vocal fold biology has demonstrated that the interactions between the ECM components in vocal fold disease states is complicated. The viscoelastic properties of vocal fold tissue appear to be related to relationships between the fibrous and interstitial proteins, rather than to alterations of a single protein as originally considered. Regardless of etiology, all vocal fold lesions do not appear to follow a typical wound-healing paradigm. As we begin to identify these the structural and viscoelastic differences better, there is potential for improved clinical diagnosis and treatment.

References

1. Hirano M. Morphological structure of the vocal cord as a vibrator and its variations. *Folia Phoniatr* (Basel). 1974; 26:89-94.

2. Hirano M. *Clinical Examination of Voice.* New York, NY: Springer-Verlag; 1981.

3. Gray SD, Pignatari S, Harding P. Morphologic ultrastructure of anchoring fibers in normal vocal fold basement membrane zone. *J Voice.* 1994;8(1):48-52.

4. Hammond TH, Zhou R, Hammond EH, Pawlak A, Gray SD. The intermediate layer: a morphologic study of the elastin and hyaluronic acid constituents of normal human vocal folds. *J Voice.* 1997;11(1):59-66.

5. Hammond TH, Gray SD, Butler J, Zhou R, Hammond E. Age- and gender-related elastin distribution changes in human vocal folds. *Otolaryngol Head Neck Surg.* 1998;119(4): 314-322.

6. Gray SD, Titze IR, Chan R, Hammond TH. Vocal fold proteoglycans and their influence on biomechanics. *Laryngoscope.* 1999;109(6):845-854.

7. Hammond TH, Gray SD, Butler J. Age and gender related collagen distribution in human vocal folds. *Ann Otol Rhinol Laryngol.* 2000;109(10):913-920.

8. Nodder S, Martin P. Wound healing in embryos: a review. *Anat Embryol.* 1997;195(3):215-228.

9. Jacobson K, O'Dell D, Holifield B, et al. Redistribution of a major cell surface glycoprotein during cell movement. *J Cell Biol.* 1984;99(5):1613-1623.

10. Lawrence WT. Physiology of the acute wound. *Clin Plast Surg.*1998;25(3):321-340.

11. Fujikawa LS, Foster CS, Gipson IK, Colvin RB. Basement membrane components in healing rabbit corneal epithlial wounds: Immunofluoresence and ultrastructural studies. *J Cell Biol.* 1984;98(1):128-138.

12. Ehrlich HP. Collagen considerations in scarring and regenerative repair. In: Garg HG, Longaker MT, eds. *Scarless Wound Healing.* New York, NY: Marcel Dekker; 2000:99-113.

13. Heldin P, Laurent TC, Heldin CH. Effect of growth factors on hyaluronan synthesis in cultured human fibroblasts. *Biochem J.* 1989;258(3):919-922.

14. Weigel PH, Fuller, GM, LeBouef RD. A model for the role of hyaluronic acid and fibrin in the early events during the inflammatory response and wound healing. *J Theor Biol.* 1986;119:219-234.

15. Martins-Green M. The dynamics of cell-ECM interactions with implications for tissue engineering. In: Chick W, ed. *Principles of Tissue Engineering.* New York, NY: RG Landes Company; 1997.

16. McGrath MH, Hundahl SA The spatial and temporal quantification of myofibroblasts. *Plast Reconstr Surg.* 1982;69:975-985.

17. Garg HG, Warren CD, Siebert JW. Chemistry of scarring. In: Garg HG, Longacre MT, eds. *Scarless Wound Healing.* New York, NY: Marcel Dekker; 2000:1-22.

18. Thibeault SL, Gray SD, Bless DM, Chan R, Ford C. Rheologic and histologic analysis of vocal fold scarring. *J Voice.* 2002;16(1):96-104.

19. Thibeault SL, Bless DM, Gray SD. Interstitial protein alterations in rabbit vocal fold with scar. *J Voice.* 2003; 17(3):377-383.

20. Ignotz RA., Massague J. Transforming growth factor-B stimulates the expression of fibronectin and collagen and their incorporation into the extracellular matrix. *J Biol Chem.* 1986;261(9):4337-4345.

21. Courey M, Shohet J, Scott M, Ossoff R. Immunohistochemical characterization of laryngeal benign lesions. *Ann Otol Rhinol Laryngol.* 1996;105(7):525-531.

22. Gray SD, Hirano M, Sato K. Molecular and cellular structure of vocal fold tissue. In: Titze IR, ed. *Vocal Fold Physiology: Frontiers of Basic Science.* San Diego, Calif.: Singular Publishing Group; 1993:1-34.

23. Dikkers F, Nikkels P. Benign lesions of the vocal folds: histopathology and phonotrauma. *Ann Otol Rhinol Laryngol.* 1995;104(9 Pt1):698-703.

24. Parsons M, Kessler E, Laurent GJ, Brown RA, Bishop JE. Mechanical load enhances procollagen processing in dermal fibroblasts by regulating levels of procollagen C-proteinase. *Exp Cell Res.* 1999;252(2):319-331.

25. Whitby DJ, Ferguson MW. Immunohistochemical localization of growth factors in fetal wound healing. *Dev Biol.* 1991;147(1):207-215.

26. Scott PG, Dodd CM, Ghahary A, Shen Y J, Tredget EE. Fibroblasts from post-burn hypertrophic scar tissue synthesize less decorin than normal dermal fibroblasts. *Clin Sci.* 1998;94(15):541-547.

27. Thibeault SL, Hirschi S, Gray SD. Gene expression patterns of vocal fold polyp and granuloma revealed by DNA microarray analysis. *J Speech Lang Hear Res.* 2003;46(2):491-502.

28. Frenzel H. Fine structural and immunohistochemical studies on polyps of human vocal folds. In: Kirchner JA, ed. *Vocal Fold Histopathology.* San Diego, Calif: College-Hill Press; 1986:39-50.

29. Shin T, Watanabe H, Oda M, Umezaki T, Nahm I. Contact granulomas of the larynx. *Eur Arch Otorhinolaryngol.* 1994;251(2):67-71.

30. Ylitalo R. *Clinical Studies of Contact Granuloma and Posterior Laryngitis with Special Regard to Esophagopharyngeal Reflux* [dissertation]. Stockholm, Sweden: Department of Logopedics and Phoniatrics and Department of Surgery, Karolinska Institute; 2000:54.

31. Loire R, Bouchayer R, Cornut G, Bastian R. Pathology of benign vocal fold lesions. *Ear Nose Throat J.* 1988;67:357-362.

32. Kotby MN, Nassar A, Seif EI, Helal EH, Saleh MM. Ultrastructural changes of the basement membrane zone in benign lesions of the vocal folds. *Acta Otolaryngol.* 1988;113:98-101.

33. Gray SD, Hammond E, Hanson DF. Benign pathologic responses of the larynx. *Ann Otol Rhinol Laryngol.* 1995; 104(1):13-18.

34. Kotby MN, Nassar A, Seif EI, Helal EH, Saleh MM. Ultrastructural features of vocal fold nodules and polyps. *Acta Otolaryngol.* 1988;105:477-482.

35. Gray SD, Titze IR, Alipour F, Hammond TH. Biomechanical and histologic observations of vocal fold fibrous proteins. *Ann Otol Rhinol Laryngol.* 2000;109(1): 77-85.

36. Thibeault SL, Gray SD, Li W, Ford CN, Smith ME, Davis RK. Genotypic and phenotypic expression of vocal fold polyps and Reinke's edema: a preliminary study. *Ann Otol Rhinol Laryngol.* 2003;111(4):302-309.

37. Alberts B, ed. *Molecular Biology of the Cell.* New York, NY: Garland Publishing; 1999.

38. Iozzo RV. The family of small leucine-rich proteoglycans: key regulators of matrix assembly and cellular growth. *Crit Rev Biochem Mol Biol.* 1997;32(2):141-174.

9

Cellular and Molecular Mechanisms of Aging of the Vocal Fold

Leslie T. Malmgren

The vocal folds have a layered structure that consists of the epithelium, the lamina propria, and the thyroarytenoid muscle.[1] Studies concerning the basic cellular and molecular mechanisms underlying vocal fold atrophy and bowing have been carried out primarily in relation to the aging process. The mechanisms underlying vocal fold aging differ between layers and involve not only atrophy and cell death, but also a complex age-related remodeling of the tissue in the lamina propria as well as in the thyroarytenoid muscle.

Remodeling of the Vocal Fold Mucosa

A number of studies have suggested that age-related remodeling of the layered structure of the lamina propria may contribute to an age-related change in the voice. According to the cover-body theory of phonation, the epithelium, superficial layer of the lamina propria, and much of the intermediate layer of the lamina propria vibrate as a "cover" on a relatively stationary "body," which consists of the remainder of the intermediate layer, the deep layer, and the thyroarytenoid muscle.[1] An age-related decrease in the depth of the superficial and intermediate layers of the lamina propria of the vocal fold has been reported,[2] and it has been suggested that this may result in vocal fold bowing.[3] Because elastin likely plays a key role in the biomechanics of the lamina propria,[4] age-related changes in the density of elastin staining have also been examined. These studies are in disagreement. A

qualitative study reported an age-related loss of elastin.[5] However, a more recent quantitative study demonstrated an 879% increase in the density of elastin staining in geriatric subjects with no significant gender-related difference.[6] In addition, there was an age-related increase in the thickness of the intermediate layer of the lamina propria in geriatric subjects and a decrease in the superficial layer of the lamina propria.[6] This decrease in the relative thickness of the superficial layer indicates an age-related change in the cover-to-body ratio, and it was suggested that this remodeling process contributes to the formation of sulcus or to bowed vocal folds.[4] In contrast to the results obtained for age-related changes in vocal fold elastin, there was no significant age-related difference in the density of collagen staining in the lamina propria.[7] However, both female adult and geriatric vocal folds had substantially less (59%) collagen staining than males.[7]

Remodeling of the Thyroarytenoid Muscle

Age-related Fiber Loss and Atrophy

Because laryngeal motor units differ from those of limb muscles with respect to their pattern of innervation, ultrastructure, and contractile proteins,[8-14] it cannot be assumed that the aging process in the thyroarytenoid muscle (TA) is identical to that in the limb muscles. Recent studies concerning age-related changes in the muscle fiber type content of the thyroarytenoid muscle (Fig 11–1) have demonstrated a complex remodeling process, which includes a pattern of muscle fiber loss and atrophy that differs from most other aging skeletal muscles.[15-17] Age-related losses of motor neurons and muscle fibers as well as muscle fiber atrophy are known to contribute to decreased contraction speed, strength, and endurance in limb muscles in the elderly.[18-25] In limb muscles, this process is characterized by a selective loss and atrophy of type 2 (fast-twitch) muscle fibers.[25-27] However, stereological studies on the human thyroarytenoid muscle have demonstrated a preferential 27% loss in the length density (Lv fiber type, muscle) of type 1 (slow-twitch) muscle fibers, which indicates an age-related loss in the number of type 1 fibers.[15] In contrast, there is not a significant age-related decrease in the length density of type 2 fibers in the TA or an overall decrease in the mean diameters of type 2 fibers.[15] However, there is a significant age-related decrease in the surface density of type 2 fibers, as well as an increase in the atrophy factor, which is an index of the content of very small, atrophic fibers.[15] These findings indicate that, although there is not a significant age-related overall atrophy of type 2 fibers as in limb muscles, there is selective atrophy of a small part of the type 2 fiber population in the TA.

Age-related Changes in Muscle Fiber Regeneration

An age-related change in the balance between the frequency of cell death or injury and the rate and viability of nerve fiber and muscle fiber regeneration contributes to the loss and atrophy of muscle fibers in the TA. Studies on limb muscles have suggested that a reduced capacity for muscle fiber regeneration may contribute to age-related losses in fiber numbers, muscle mass, and a decline in strength.[28,29] In spite of the importance of muscle fiber regeneration to the maintenance of muscle mass and strength, the technical challenge of obtaining quantitative estimates of this infrequent process has discouraged relevant studies. However, quantitative estimates of the content of regenerating muscle fibers in the entire volume of the human TA have recently been obtained using stereological techniques.[16] Because the developmental myosin heavy chain isoform is expressed only in regenerating muscle fibers in adults,[30] these studies detected regenerating fibers using immunocytochemical techniques to image this contractile protein (Fig 11–2). It was demonstrated that muscle fiber regeneration plays an important role in compensating for muscle fiber injury and cell death in the TA.[16] Although regenerating muscle fibers comprise only a very small proportion of the total fiber population at

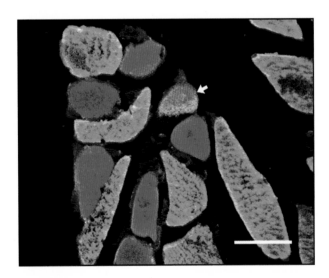

Fig 11–1. Confocal laser scanning micrograph of human TA. Immunocytochemical staining detects slow twitch (type 1) muscle fibers using a CY 3 fluorochrome label (*red*) for the slow myosin heavy chain isoform, and fast twitch (type 2) fibers are imaged using a FITC label (*green*) for the fast myosin heavy chain isoform. Note the red/green fiber (*arrow*) with colocalization of both the fast and slow isoform. Calibration bar = 50 μm. (Reproduced with permission from *Otolaryngology–Head and Neck Surgery*. 1999;121:4414-4451.[15])

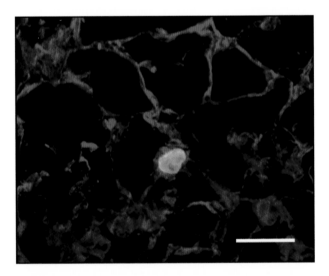

Fig 11–2 Confocal laser scanning micrographs of human thyroarytenoid muscle. Concanavalin A (*red fluorochrome*) images the extracellular matrix and surface of unstained muscle fibers. Small regenerating muscle fibers express the developmental myosin heavy chain isoform (*green fluorochrome*) in isolated regenerating fiber (*arrow*). Calibration bar = 50 μm. (Reproduced with permission from *Archives of Otolaryngology—Head and Neck Surgery*. 2000;126:851-856.[16])

any one time, regeneration replaces almost twice the original muscle fiber population in the human TA by age 70.[16] Muscle fiber regeneration may involve either the entire muscle fiber or only an injured segment of the fiber.[31] Therefore, the contribution of regeneration to the maintenance of the muscle mass and strength is most clearly indicated by the total regenerated muscle fiber length rather than the number of regenerated fibers. These stereological studies demonstrated a 610% age-related increase in the ratio of the length of regenerating muscle fibers to the total muscle fiber length in the entire volume of the human TA.[16] This increase in the relative length of regenerating fibers likely represents a compensatory response to an age-related increase in muscle fiber cell death and injury rather than an increase in regenerative capacity, because there is an age-related decrease in type 1 fibers[15,16] as well as an age-related increase in the frequency of programmed cell death (apoptosis) in type 1 fibers[17] (discussed later).

The demonstrated age-related increase in muscle fiber death and regeneration in the human TA is paralleled by an age-related increase in cycles of denervation and reinnervation in laryngeal motor neurons.[32-35] Age-related changes in the interaction of these processes likely contribute to the observed age-related loss of muscle fibers in the TA as well as to an age-related increase in the remodeling of TA motor units. With advancing age, there is a loss of motor neurons,[18-20] and the capacity for both nerve[36-38] and muscle fiber regeneration is diminished.[39-42] Each cycle of muscle fiber death and regeneration requires successful reinnervation for functional recovery. Consequently, the demonstrated age-related increase in cycles of muscle fiber injury and regeneration increase the demand for reinnervation of regenerated muscle fibers. Because the capacity for reinnervation decreases with age, this increase in the frequency of muscle fiber regeneration contributes to an age-related increase in muscle fiber denervation and atrophy.[43,44]

Myonuclei and Muscle Fiber Diameter

The prevention and treatment of age-related muscle fiber loss and atrophy in the thyroarytenoid muscle requires an understanding of the underlying cellular and molecular mechanisms. A number of recent studies have suggested that muscle fiber atrophy is generally the result of a decrease in the number of nuclei in the muscle fiber and, conversely, that fiber hypertrophy is the result of an increase in the number of myonuclei.[45] Most cells have a single nucleus with a volume of cytoplasm that is relatively constant and specific to the cell type, which suggests that some

unknown mechanism regulates the amount of cytoplasm that can be supported by a nucleus in a particular cell type.[46] Muscle fibers differ from other cell types in that muscle fibers in that they generate force over long distances, which requires a relatively high cellular volume. Because the transcriptional capacity of a single nucleus is spatially limited, muscle fibers have evolved specialized regulatory mechanisms that are based on a syncytium (multiple nuclei in a single cell) in which the cytoplasmic volume maintained by an individual myonucleus can be regulated by changes in the number of myonuclei in the muscle fiber (Fig 11–3). This makes it possible for a single muscle fiber to be very long and to vary in diameter yet maintain a constant amount of cytoplasm controlled by each myonucleus (nuclear domain). Therefore, the diameter of the muscle fiber is a function of the nuclear domain and the number of myonuclei. These relationships have recently been examined in the human thyroarytenoid muscle based on stereological estimates of the numerical densities of myonuclei in muscle fiber types that were identified using immunocytochemical

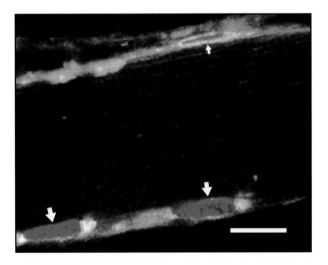

Fig 11–3. Muscle fiber in human thyroarytenoid muscle. Note FITC concanavalin A fluorescence at the interface between the surface of the muscle fiber and the satellite cell (*small arrows*). This interface is seen as a gradation from green fluorescence where there is no overprojection from the red fluorescence of the nuclear stain to a yellow fluorescence where overprojection combines the red ethidium homodimer emission with the green FITC emission. Note that this green/yellow fluorescent interface is not present on the inner surface of myonuclei (*large arrows*). This staining difference was used to distinguish satellite cells from myonuclei. Calibration bar = 20 μm. (Reproduced with permission from *Otolaryngology—Head and Neck Surgery*. 2000;123:377-384.[15])

techniques.[47] The numerical density of myonuclei was demonstrated to be relatively high for both type 1 (71,303/mm^3 of fiber volume) and type 2 fibers (66,072/mm^3 of fiber volume) in the TA with no significant difference between the fiber types. Such high numerical densities of myonuclei are found in fatigue-resistant muscle fiber types that are specialized for oxidative metabolism by having a small diameter and a high mitochondrial content.[48] A high numerical density of myonuclei is thought to provide an increased transcriptional capacity to support a relatively high requirement for mitochondrial gene expression,[48] which compensates for the very limited coding capacity of the mitochondrial genome.[49] The human TA is composed almost entirely of type 1 and type 2a fiber types,[50,51] both of which have a high mitochondrial content,[52] consistent with this relationship. Furthermore, muscle fiber diameters in the TA are substantially smaller than in most other human muscles.[15] This is an adaptation for a high capacity for oxidative metabolism, because smaller fiber diameters facilitate the diffusion of oxygen and nutrients from capillaries.[53] In addition, it was demonstrated that the numerical density of myonuclei increased with decreasing fiber diameter in the human TA in both type 1 and type 2 fibers,[47] which is also likely an adaptation to support an increase in mitochondrial transcriptional requirements with decreasing fiber diameter.[48,53]

Relationship of Satellite Cells to Injury and Myonuclei

Because the mass and strength of a muscle are largely a function of the number of myonuclei, muscle atrophy or hypertrophy results from changes in the relative rates of loss and replacement of myonuclei.[45] Because muscle fibers are postmitotic, the number of myonuclei are determined by the numerical density and proliferative capacity of satellite cells (see Fig 11–3), which are the source of myonuclei.[54] Stereological studies have demonstrated relatively high numerical densities of satellite cells in the human TA.[47] This is consistent with reports indicating that satellite cells are more numerous in oxidative, fatigue-resistant muscles.[54] In addition, it was found that the numerical density of satellite cells was significantly higher for type 1 fibers than for type 2 fibers and that this difference increased with increasing total satellite numerical density.[47] Because the number of satellite cells has been demonstrated to increase in response to challenges such as injury, overwork, denervation, exercise, or stretch[45,54] the relatively high numerical density demonstrated for type 1 fiber satellite cells may be a

response to some form of cellular injury or to some change in trophic interactions. This would be consistent with a hypothesis that the type 1 fibers in the TA are more frequently exposed to injury and that the number of satellite cells on this fiber type increases selectively as the extent of the challenge increases.

Age-related Change in Satellite Cell Numbers

It has been suggested that decreases in satellite cell numerical densities or in their proliferative capacity may contribute to age-related limb muscle atrophy.[55] Design-based stereological techniques have been used to assess age-related changes in the numerical densities of satellite cells and myonuclei in the human thyroarytenoid muscle. It was demonstrated that there is an overall significant age-related decrease in the ratio of satellite cells to myonuclei in the TA.[47] This decrease must be considered in relation to an age-related increase in the demand for satellite cell proliferation as evidenced by an increase in muscle fiber regeneration[16] as well as an age-related increase in muscle fiber programmed cell death in the TA[17] (discussed later). This suggests an age-related decrease in the response of satellite cell proliferation to the demonstrated age-related increase in muscle fiber injury and cell death in the human TA.

Age-related Changes in Apoptosis

Programmed cell death (apoptosis) appears to play a major role in the mechanisms underlying the demonstrated age-related increase in muscle fiber injury and cell death in the human TA. Apoptosis is a complex program of cell suicide, which can be influenced by a variety of regulatory stimuli.[56] This process is characterized by DNA fragmentation, which can be detected in tissue sections using in situ labeling of fragmented nuclear DNA.[57,58] Using these techniques, studies on nonlaryngeal skeletal muscles have demonstrated that apoptosis of myonuclei and satellite cells contributes to a wide variety of pathological conditions in skeletal muscle. These include hindlimb unloading-induced muscle atrophy,[59] exercise-induced muscle fiber damage,[60-62] and denervation atrophy.[63,64] In addition, it has been also shown that diminished supplies of trophic factors[65] and oxidative stress[66] also result in apoptosis of myonuclei and satellite cell nuclei. Qualitative studies have shown that apoptosis of myonuclei accounts for an age-related loss of muscle fibers in the rhabdosphincter.[67] Recent stereological studies have shown that there is a significant age-related increase in the numerical density of apoptotic myonuclei and apoptotic satellite cell nuclei in type 1 but not in type 2 fibers in the entire volume of the human TA.[17] This suggests that an increased frequency of some form of cellular injury contributes to the demonstrated selective loss of type 1 fibers in the human TA. However, as indicated, apoptosis plays a role in a variety of pathological conditions, and the cellular and molecular mechanisms underlying this increase in apoptosis are presently unknown.

Remodeling of Motor Units

In addition to the demonstrated loss and atrophy of muscle fibers, there is also an age-related increase in the remodeling of the motor units in the TA. A number of studies indicate that this results from an ongoing cycle of denervation and reinnervation. Consistent with this mechanism, there is an age-related increase in the numbers of degenerating and regenerating myelinated nerve fibers in the recurrent laryngeal nerve.[32] In addition, there is an increase in extremely small, atrophic type 2 fibers in the human TA with no significant loss in the total number of type 2 fibers.[15] There is also an age-related increase in the content of muscle fibers in the human TA having a coexistence of both slow and fast myosin heavy chain isoforms,[15] which is consistent with results obtained in aging limb muscles.[68] Changes in myosin heavy chain isoform expression occur with altered motor unit activity patterns and a number of other factors.[69] However, these transitions between muscle fiber types also result from age-related remodeling of motor units as a result of cycles of denervation and reinnervation that occur with age-related loss of motor neurons.[70] In this process, denervated muscle fibers are reinnervated by local sprouting of axons; and muscle fiber type conversions can occur consistent with the type of the new motor unit. Because this process occurs locally, the normally random topographical distribution of muscle fiber types can progress to clusters of fibers of the same type (muscle fiber "type grouping").[71] This process probably contributes to the observed increase of transitional fiber types in the aging human TA. More direct evidence for this mechanism is the finding that there is also an increase in muscle fiber "type grouping" in the human TA.[35] Muscle fiber type grouping is a well-established indicator of partial denervation followed by reinnervation. The process of motor unit remodeling that results in muscle fiber "type grouping" can also be detected using electromyography. Consistent with these findings is a recent report that demonstrates a significant age-related increase in motor unit duration in the human thyroarytenoid muscle.[33]

Effect of Muscle Use and Misuse

A better understanding of the relationship of muscle use and misuse to age-related changes in the laryngeal muscles may provide a basis for improved forms of intervention. In limb muscles, age-related muscle atrophy and loss of strength can be slowed or even reversed by exercise.[72,73] Changes in muscle use, such as exercise, stretch, or immobilization, cause changes in the mitotic activity and numerical density of satellite cells.[74-77] The resulting change in the number of myonuclei leads to a corresponding increase or decrease in the muscle fiber diameter and in the mass and strength of the muscle.[78] Although it has been demonstrated that intensive voice and respiration training can improve vocal fold adduction in patients with Parkinson's disease,[79,80] strength or endurance training techniques have not been systematically studied in relation to the prevention or reversal of age-related changes in the laryngeal muscles.

The relationship between specific types of muscle use and contraction-induced muscle fiber injuries also requires clarification, because they may contribute to the observed cycles of muscle and nerve fiber degeneration and regeneration and muscle fiber loss in the aging human TA.[15-17] In limb muscles, eccentric (lengthening) contractions are known to be common and particularly damaging in muscles that have not been adequately conditioned.[81-88] This type of contraction-induced, muscle fiber injury results in an activation of stretch-activated ion channels and prolonged depolarization of muscle fibers[89] followed by ultrastructural lesions, including muscle fiber A-band lesions,[90] and ultimately muscle fiber degeneration. It has also been reported that the muscles of old animals are more vulnerable to eccentric contraction-induced injury and that free radicals contribute to a delayed decrease in maximum isometric tetanic force and morphological fiber damage.[91] Although these degenerated fibers regenerate completely in young adult animals, regeneration is incomplete in old animals.[28,92,93] Furthermore, because this process of muscle fiber regeneration requires reinnervation for recovery of function, contraction-induced fiber injury places an increased demand on an already diminished capacity for nerve regeneration in aging muscle.[94]

Gene Therapy

Because apoptosis plays a role in age-related muscle fiber loss and atrophy in the human TA,[15,47] it may be possible to use gene therapy to prevent or reverse age-related changes in the mass and strength of the TA[56] by targeting one of the many complex pathways that regulate apoptosis.[56] For example, an age-related decrease in insulin-like growth factor I (IGF-1)[95] likely contributes to the demonstrated age-related increase in apoptotic satellite cells in the human TA[17], because withdrawal of IGF-1 results in satellite cell apoptosis.[65] Consistent with these findings, it has been demonstrated that gene therapy based on viral-mediated overexpression of IGF-1 prevents an age-related decrease in rat limb muscle mass and strength[96] as well as denervation atrophy in the rat TA,[97-99] which is likely due to myonuclear apoptosis.[64] These findings suggest that it may be possible to prevent or reverse the demonstrated age-related increase in satellite cell and myonuclear apoptosis[17] in the human TA by using gene therapy or pharmacological intervention to block apoptosis. However, the design of effective therapeutic strategies will require a more complete understanding of the mechanisms underlying myonuclear and satellite cell apoptosis in this highly specialized muscle. Furthermore, it will be necessary to use animal models to clarify the role and interactions of gene therapy with other growth factors[100,101] and with variables such as muscle use[72,73] and age-related changes in blood flow.[102]

References

1. Hirano M. Structure and vibratory behavior of the vocal folds. In: Sawashima M, Cooper FS, eds. *Dynamic Aspects of Speech Production.* Tokyo: University of Tokyo Press; 1977:13–30.
2. Hirano M, Kurita S, Sakaguchi S. Ageing of the vibratory tissue of human vocal folds. *Acta Otolaryngol.* 1989;107:428–433.
3. Tanaka S, Hirano M, Chijiwa K. Some aspects of vocal fold bowing. *Ann Otol Rhinol Laryngol.* 1994;103:357–362.
4. Gray SD, Titze IR, Alipour F, Hammond TH. Biomechanical and histologic observations of vocal fold fibrous proteins. *Ann Otol Rhinol Laryngol.* 2000;109:77–85.
5. Sato K, Hirano M. Age-related changes of elastic fibers in the superficial layer of the lamina propria of vocal folds. *Ann Otol Rhinol Laryngol.* 1997;106:44–48.
6. Hammond TH, Gray SD, Butler J, Zhou R, Hammond E. Age- and gender-related elastin distribution changes in human vocal folds. *Otolaryngol Head Neck Surg.* 1998;119:314–322.
7. Hammond TH, Gray SD, Butler JE. Age- and gender-related collagen distribution in human vocal folds. *Ann Otol Rhinol Laryngol.* 2000;109:913–920.
8. Merati AL, Bodine SC, Bennett T, et al. Identification of a novel myosin heavy chain gene expressed in the rat larynx. *Biochim Biophys Acta.* 1996;1306:153–159.
9. Briggs MM, Schachat F. Early specialization of the superfast myosin in extraocular and laryngeal muscles. *J Exp Biol.* 2000;203:2485–2494.
10. Bendiksen FS, Dahl HA, Teig E. Innervation pattern of different types of muscle fibres in the human thyroarytenoid muscle. *Acta Otolaryngol* (Stockh). 1981;91:391–397.
11. Perie S, St. Guily JL, Callard P, Sebille A. Innervation of adult human laryngeal muscle fibers. *J Neurol Sci.* 1997;149:81–86.
12. Malmgren LT, Gacek RR, Etzler CA. Muscle fiber types in the human posterior cricoarytenoid muscle: A correlated histochemical and ultrastructural morphometric study. In: Titze I, Scherer R, eds. *Conference on Physiology and Biophysics of Voice.* Denver, Colo: Denver Center for Performing Arts; 1983:41–56.
13. Malmgren LT, Gacek RR. Histochemical characteristics of muscle fiber types in the posterior cricoarytenoid muscle. *Ann Otol Rhinol Laryngol.* 1981;90:423–429.
14. Lucas CA, Rughani A, Hoh JF. Expression of extraocular myosin heavy chain in rabbit laryngeal muscle. *J Muscle Res Cell Motil.* 1995;16:368–378.
15. Malmgren LT, Fisher PJ, Bookman LM, Uno T. Age-related changes in muscle fiber types in the human thyroarytenoid muscle: an immunohistochemical and stereological study using confocal laser scanning microscopy. *Otolaryngol Head Neck Surg.* 1999;121:441–451.
16. Malmgren LT, Lovice DB, Kaufman MR. Age-related changes in muscle fiber regeneration in the human thyroarytenoid muscle. *Arch Otolaryngol Head Neck Surg.* 2000;126:851–856.
17. Malmgren LT, Jones CE, Bookman LM. Muscle fiber and satellite cell apoptosis in the aging human thyroarytenoid muscle: a stereological study using confocal laser scanning microscopy. *Otolaryngol Head Neck Surg.* 2001;125:34–39.
18. Wang FC, de Pasqua V, Delwaide PJ. Age-related changes in fastest and slowest conducting axons of thenar motor units. *Muscle Nerve.* 1999;22:1022–1029.
19. Brown WF, Strong MJ, Snow R. Methods for estimating numbers of motor units in biceps-brachialis muscles and losses of motor units with aging. *Muscle Nerve.* 1988;11:423–432.
20. Doherty TJ, Vandervoort AA, Taylor AW, Brown WF. Effects of motor unit losses on strength in older men and women. *J Appl Physiol.* 1993;74:868–874.
21. Jennekens FG, Tomlinson BE, Walton JN. Histochemical aspects of five limb muscles in old age. An autopsy study. *J Neurol Sci.* 1971;14:259–276.
22. Tomonaga M. Histochemical and ultrastructural changes in senile human skeletal muscle. *J Am Geriatr Soc.* 1977;25:125–131.
23. Larsson L. Morphological and functional characteristics of the ageing skeletal muscle in man. A cross-sectional study. *Acta Physiol Scand Suppl.* 1978;457:1–36.
24. Lexell J, Henriksson-Larsen K, Winblad B, Sjostrom M. Distribution of different fiber types in human skeletal muscles: effects of aging studied in whole muscle cross sections. *Muscle Nerve.* 1983;6:588–595.
25. Grimby G. Muscle performance and structure in the elderly as studied cross-sectionally and longitudinally. *J Gerontol A Biol Sci Med Sci.* 1995;50A:17–22.

26. Larsson L, Edstrom L. Effects of age on enzyme-histochemical fibre spectra and contractile properties of fast- and slow-twitch skeletal muscle. *J Neurol Sci.* 1986;76:69–89.

27. Lexell J. Human aging, muscle mass, and fiber type composition. *J Gerontol A Biol Sci Med Sci.* 1995;50A:11–16.

28. Brooks SV, Faulkner JA. Skeletal muscle weakness in old age: underlying mechanisms. *Med Sci Sports Exerc.* 1994;26:432–439.

29. Carlson BM. Factors influencing the repair and adaptation of muscles in aged individuals: satellite cells and innervation. *J Gerontol A Biol Sci Med Sci.* 1995;50A:96–100.

30. d'Albis A, Couteaux R, Janmot C, et al. Regeneration after cardiotoxin injury of innervated and denervated slow and fast muscles of mammals. Myosin isoform analysis. *Eur J Biochem.* 1988;174:103–110.

31. Hall-Craggs EC. The regeneration of skeletal muscle fibres per continuum. *J Anat.* 1974;117:171–178.

32. Malmgren LT, Ringwood MA. Aging of the recurrent laryngeal nerve: an ultrastructural morphometric study. In: Fujimura O, ed. *Vocal Physiology: Voice Production, Mechanisms and Function.* New York, NY: Raven Press; 1988:159–180.

33. Takeda N, Thomas GR, Ludlow CL. Aging effects on motor units in the human thyroarytenoid muscle. *Laryngoscope.* 2000;110:1018–1025.

34. Malmgren LT. Aging-related changes in peripheral nerves in the head and neck. In: Goldstein MA, Kashima HK, Koopman CF, eds. *Geriatric Otorhinolaryngology.* Toronto: BC Decker, Inc; 1989:138–143.

35. Malmgren LT, Fisher PJ, Brandes M. Age-related increase in muscle fiber "type grouping" in the human thyroarytenoid muscle. Presented at the Association for Research in Otolaryngology Twentieth Midwinter Meeting; 1997; St Petersburg, Fla. Available at: http://www.aro.org/abstracts/1997/T597.html

36. Choi SJ, Harii K, Lee MJ, et al. Electrophysiological, morphological, and morphometric effects of aging on nerve regeneration in rats. *Scand J Plast Reconstr Surg Hand Surg.* 1995;29:133–140.

37. Kawabuchi M, Chongjian Z, Islam AT, et al. The effect of aging on the morphological nerve changes during muscle reinnervation after nerve crush. *Restor Neurol Neurosci.* 1998;13:117–127.

38. Verdú E, Butí M, Navarro X. The effect of aging on efferent nerve fibers regeneration in mice. *Brain Res.* 1995;696:76–82.

39. Carlson BM, Faulkner JA. Muscle regeneration in young and old rats: effects of motor nerve transection with and without marcaine treatment. *J Gerontol A Biol Sci Med Sci.* 1998;53:B52–B57.

40. Sadeh M. Effects of aging on skeletal muscle regeneration. *J Neurol Sci.* 1988;87:67–74.

41. Cannon JG. Intrinsic and extrinsic factors in muscle aging. *Ann N Y Acad Sci.* 1998;854:72–77.

42. Marsh DR, Criswell DS, Hamilton MT, Booth FW. Association of insulin-like growth factor mRNA expressions with muscle regeneration in young, adult, and old rats. *Am J Physiol.* 1997;273:R353–R358.

43. Carlson BM, Faulkner JA. The regeneration of noninnervated muscle grafts and marcaine-treated muscles in young and old rats. *J Gerontol A Biol Sci Med Sci.* 1996;51:B43–B49.

44. Carlson BM, Faulkner JA. Muscle regeneration in young and old rats: effects of motor nerve transection with and without marcaine treatment. *J Gerontol A Biol Sci Med Sci.* 1998;53:B52–B57.

45. Allen DL, Roy RR, Edgerton VR. Myonuclear domains in muscle adaptation and disease. *Muscle Nerve.* 1999;22:1350–1360.

46. Hughes SM, Schiaffino S. Control of muscle fibre size: a crucial factor in ageing. *Acta Physiol Scand.* 1999;167:307–312.

47. Malmgren LT, Fisher PJ, Jones CE, et al. Numerical densities of myonuclei and satellite cells in muscle fiber types in the aging human thyroarytenoid muscle: an immunohistochemical and stereological study using confocal laser scanning microscopy. *Otolaryngol Head Neck Surg.* 2000;123:377–384.

48. Tseng BS, Kasper CE, Edgerton VR. Cytoplasm-to-myonucleus ratios and succinate dehydrogenase activities in adult rat slow and fast muscle fibers. *Cell Tissue Res.* 1994;275:39–49.

49. Scarpulla RC. Nuclear control of respiratory chain expression in mammalian cells. *J Bioenerg Biomembr.* 1997;29:109–119.

50. Claassen H, Werner JA. Fiber differentiation of the human laryngeal muscles using the inhibition reactivation myofibrillar ATPase technique. *Anat Embryol (Berlin).* 1992;186:341–346.

51. Guida HL, Zorzetto NL. Morphometric and histochemical study of the human vocal muscle. *Ann Otol Rhinol Laryngol.* 2000;109:67–71.

52. Rivero JL, Talmadge RJ, Edgerton VR. Fibre size and metabolic properties of myosin heavy chain-based fibre types in rat skeletal muscle. *J Muscle Res Cell Motil.* 1998;19:733–742.

53. Sieck GC, Zhan WZ, Prakash YS, et al. SDH and actomyosin ATPase activities of different fiber types in rat diaphragm muscle. *J Appl Physiol.* 1995;79:1629–1639.

54. Bischoff R. The satellite cell and muscle regeneration. In: Engel AG, Franzini-Armstrong C, eds. *Myology.* New York, NY: McGraw-Hill; 1999:97–118.

55. Mezzogiorno A, Coletta M, Zani BM, et al. Paracrine stimulation of senescent satellite cell proliferation by factors released by muscle or myotubes from young mice. *Mech Ageing Dev.* 1993;70:35–44.

56. Thompson CB. Apoptosis in the pathogenesis and treatment of disease. *Science.* 1995;267:1456–1462.

57. Tidball JG, Albrecht DE, Lokensgard BE, Spencer MJ. Apoptosis precedes necrosis of dystrophin-deficient muscle. *J Cell Sci.* 1995;108:2197–2204.

58. Gavrieli Y, Sherman Y, Ben-Sasson SA. Identification of programmed cell death in situ via specific labeling of nuclear DNA fragmentation. *J Cell Biol.* 1992;119:493–501.

59. Allen DL, Linderman JK, Roy RR, et al. Apoptosis: a mechanism contributing to remodeling of skeletal muscle in response to hindlimb unweighting. *Am J Physiol.* 1997;273:C579–C587.

60. Podhorska-Okolov M, Sandri M, Zanada F, et al. Apoptosis of myofibres and satellite cells: exercise-induced damage in skeletal muscle of the mouse. *Neuropathol Appl Neurobiol.* 1999;24:518–531.

61. Sandri M, Carraro U, Podhorska-Okolov M, et al. Apoptosis, DNA damage and ubiquitin expression in normal and mdx muscle fibers after exercise. *FEBS Lett.* 1995;373: 291–295.

62. Sandri M, Podhorska-Okolow M, Geromel V, et al. Exercise induces myonuclear ubiquitination and apoptosis in dystrophin-deficient muscle of mice. *J Neuropathol Exp Neurol.* 1997;56:45–57.

63. Tews DS, Goebel HH, Schneider I, et al. DNA-fragmentation and expression of apoptosis-related proteins in experimentally denervated and reinnervated rat facial muscle. *Neuropathol Appl Neurobiol.* 1997;23:141–149.

64. Yoshimura K, Harii K. A regenerative change during muscle adaptation to denervation in rats. *J Surg Res.* 1999; 81:139–146.

65. Mampuru LJ, Chen SJ, Kalenik JL, et al. Analysis of events associated with serum deprivation-induced apoptosis in C3H/Sol8 muscle satellite cells. *Exp Cell Res.* 1996;226:372–380.

66. Stangel M, Zettl UK, Mix E, et al. H_2O_2 and nitric oxide-mediated oxidative stress induce apoptosis in rat skeletal muscle myoblasts. *J Neuropathol Exp Neurol.* 1996; 55:36–43.

67. Strasser H, Tiefenthaler M, Steinlechner M, et al. Urinary incontinence in the elderly and age-dependent apoptosis of rhabdosphincter cells [letter]. *Lancet.* 1999;354: 918–919.

68. Klitgaard H, Zhou M, Schiaffino S, et al. Ageing alters the myosin heavy chain composition of single fibres from human skeletal muscle. *Acta Physiol Scand.* 1990; 140:55–62.

69. Pette D, Staron RS. Mammalian skeletal muscle fiber type transitions. *Int Rev Cytol.* 1997;170:143–223.

70. Larsson L. Motor units: remodeling in aged animals. *J Gerontol A Biol Sci Med Sci.* 1995;50A:91–95.

71. Ansved T, Wallner P, Larsson L. Spatial distribution of motor unit fibres in fast- and slow-twitch rat muscles with special reference to age. *Acta Physiol Scand.* 1991; 143:345–354.

72. Frischknecht R. Effect of training on muscle strength and motor function in the elderly. *Reprod Nutr Dev.* 1998;38:167–174.

73. Singh MA, Ding W, Manfredi TJ, et al. Insulin-like growth factor I in skeletal muscle after weight-lifting exercise in frail elders. *Am J Physiol.* 1999;277:E135–E143.

74. Darr KC, Schultz E. Hindlimb suspension suppresses muscle growth and satellite cell proliferation. *J Appl Physiol.* 1989;67:1827–1834.

75. Snow MH. Satellite cell response in rat soleus muscle undergoing hypertrophy due to surgical ablation of synergists. *Anat Rec.* 1990;227:437–446.

76. Delp MD, Pette D. Morphological changes during fiber type transitions in low-frequency-stimulated rat fast-twitch muscle. *Cell Tissue Res.* 1994;277:363–371.

77. Kadi F, Eriksson A, Holmner S, et al. Cellular adaptation of the trapezius muscle in strength-trained athletes. *Histochem Cell Biol.* 1999;111:189–195.

78. Allen DL, Yasui W, Tanaka T, et al. Myonuclear number and myosin heavy chain expression in rat soleus single muscle fibers after spaceflight. *J Appl Physiol.* 1996;81: 145–151.

79. Ramig LO, Countryman S, O'Brien C, et al. Intensive speech treatment for patients with Parkinson's disease: short-and long-term comparison of two techniques. *Neurology.* 1996;47:1496–1504.

80. Ramig LO, Dromey C. Aerodynamic mechanisms underlying treatment-related changes in vocal intensity in patients with Parkinson disease. *J Speech Hear Res.* 1996;39:798–807.

81. McCully KK, Faulkner JA. Characteristics of lengthening contractions associated with injury to skeletal muscle fibers. *J Appl Physiol.* 1986;61:293–299.

82. Armstrong RB, Warren GL, Warren JA. Mechanisms of exercise-induced muscle fibre injury. *Sports Med.* 1991; 12:184–207.

83. Hunter KD, Faulkner JA. Pliometric contraction-induced injury of mouse skeletal muscle: effect of initial length. *J Appl Physiol.* 1997;82:278–283.

84. Macpherson PC, Dennis RG, Faulkner JA. Sarcomere dynamics and contraction-induced injury to maximally activated single muscle fibres from soleus muscles of rats. *J Physiol.* 1997;500(Pt 2):523–533.

85. Mair J, Mayr M, Muller E, et al. Rapid adaptation to eccentric exercise-induced muscle damage. *Int J Sports Med.* 1995;16:352–356.

86. Brown SJ, Child RB, Day SH, Donnelly AE. Exercise-induced skeletal muscle damage and adaptation following repeated bouts of eccentric muscle contractions. *J Sports Sci.* 1997;15:215–222.

87. Brown SJ, Child RB, Day SH, Donnelly AE. Indices of skeletal muscle damage and connective tissue breakdown following eccentric muscle contractions. *Eur J Appl Physiol Occup Physiol.* 1997;75:369–374.

88. Faulkner JA, Brooks SV, Opiteck JA. Injury to skeletal muscle fibers during contractions: conditions of occurrence and prevention. [review]. *Phys Ther.* 1993;73:911–921.

89. McBride TA, Stockert BW, Gorin FA, Carlsen RC. Stretch-activated ion channels contribute to membrane depolarization after eccentric contractions. *J Appl Physiol.* 2000;88:91–101.

90. Ogilvie RW, Armstrong RB, Baird KE, Bottoms CL. Lesions in the rat soleus muscle following eccentrically biased exercise. *Am J Anat.* 1988;182:335–346.

91. Zerba E Komorowski TE, Faulkner JA. Free radical injury to skeletal muscles of young, adult, and old mice. *Am J Physiol.* 1990;258(3 Pt 1):C429–C435.

92. Faulkner JA, Jones DA, Round JM. Injury to skeletal muscles of mice by forced lengthening during contractions. *Q J Exp Physiol.* 1989;74:661–670.

93. Brooks SV, Faulkner JA. Contraction-induced injury: recovery of skeletal muscles in young and old mice. *Am J Physiol.* 1990;258(3 Pt 1):C436–C442.

94. Faulkner JA, Brooks SV, Zerba E. Muscle atrophy and weakness with aging: contraction-induced injury as an

underlying mechanism. *J Gerontol A Biol Sci Med Sci.* 1995;50A:24–129.

95. Benbassat CA, Maki KC, Unterman TG. Circulating levels of insulin-like growth factor (IGF) binding protein-1 and -3 in aging men: relationships to insulin, glucose, IGF, and dehydroepiandrosterone sulfate levels and anthropometric measures. *J Clin Endocrinol Metab.* 1997; 82:1484–1491.

96. Barton-Davis ER, Shoturma DI, Musaro A, et al. Viral mediated expression of insulin-like growth factor I blocks the aging-related loss of skeletal muscle function. *Proc Natl Acad Sci U S A.* 1998;95:15603–15607.

97. Shiotani A, O'Malley BWJ, et al. Human insulinlike growth factor 1 gene transfer into paralyzed rat larynx: single vs multiple injection. *Arch Otolaryngol Head Neck Surg.* 1999;125:555–560.

98. Shiotani A, O'Malley BWJ, Coleman ME, et al. Reinnervation of motor endplates and increased muscle fiber size after human insulin-like growth factor I gene transfer into the paralyzed larynx. *Hum Gene Ther.* 1998;9:2039–2047.

99. Flint PW, Shiotani A, O'Malley BWJ. IGF-1 gene transfer into denervated rat laryngeal muscle. *Arch Otolaryngol Head Neck Surg.* 1999;125:274–279.

100. Menetrey J, Kasemkijwattana C, Day CS, et al. Growth factors improve muscle healing in vivo. *J Bone Joint Surg Br.* 2000;82:131–137.

101. Cannon JG. Cytokines in aging and muscle homeostasis. *J Gerontol A Biol Sci Med Sci.* 1995;50A:120–123.

102. Malmgren LT. Age-related changes in blood flow rates in the intrinsic laryngeal muscles of young adult and old rats during quiet respiration. Abstracts of the Fifteenth Midwinter Research Meeting of the Association for Research in Otolaryngology; 1992. Available at: http://www.aro.org/archives/1992/086.html

10

Implications of Nutraceutical Modulation of Glutathione with Cystine and Cysteine in General Health and Voice Medicine

Thomas A. Kwyer, Gustavo Bounous, and Robert Thayer Sataloff

As our understanding of the human voice has progressed, it has become clear that voice preservation and pathology are dependent on the efficient operation of the cellular machinery that maintains the health and optimal function of each organ of the body, including the larynx and lungs. At its most basic level, the source of voice production depends on the availability and absorption of chemical building blocks commonly referred to as nutrients but often overlooked as mediators of cellular function.

Nutritional and metabolic therapies have begun to be researched and applied to clinical conditions with promising results. Therefore, understanding the therapeutic impact of metabolic modulation techniques becomes beneficial to the clinician, as well as the researcher, the patient and the performer. Whether similar research can be applied in humans and expanded to modify clinical outcomes is worthy of evaluation.

Although this chapter is oriented toward recent developments and discoveries in basic science and research, the information is presented to stimulate and accelerate nutritional and metabolic research resulting in the development of clinical strategies to maintain health, enhance performance, and mitigate disease for voice patients and professionals alike.

Of all the potential methods of modifying clinical conditions that affect general health, voice function, and vocal performance that we have scrutinized, glutathione modulation appears particularly promising.

The effects and metabolism of glutathione, cysteine, and to a lesser degree, metallothionein and nitric oxide are reviewed because of the essential and determinant role played by these molecules in the immune system, wound healing, and nitrogen balance. Although the interactions among these molecules are fairly complex, once understood the clinician and patient can utilize this information to influence cellular health, repair, and performance.

The focus of this review is glutathione. It is chosen as a starting point because research documentation on glutathione is plentiful (>64,000 peer-reviewed, scientific publications are already in print); predictable materials for glutathione enhancement have been developed (Immunocal®, IMN-1207) and are clinically available; and of paramount importance to the medical community-at-large, prospective, randomized, double-blind studies are underway (COPD; IMN-1207: Hepatitis C and cancer; John Molson, personal communication, 2004) and a phase I study (Immunocal®; cancer cachexia).

Even though it is still too early to offer definite proof of the effectiveness of glutathione and cysteine enhancement, by the time the fourth edition of this book is published, it would not be surprising to find it has advanced from speculation to routine practice.

Glutathione and the Impact of Glutathione Deficiency in Medicine

Many seemingly unrelated diseases and conditions are unified by the unique properties of cysteine and glutathione (GSH). Glutathione is a tripeptide of L-glutamate, L-cysteine, and glycine. Cysteine is the sulfur-containing amino acid that is the rate-limiting substrate in GSH synthesis. The common features of GSH and cysteine are their ability to donate protons and reduce disulfide bonds.

Metabolic and biochemical reactions involving proton donation affect conditions as diverse as cancer, autoimmune deficiency syndrome (AIDS), sepsis, trauma, burns, Crohn's disease, ulcerative colitis, chronic fatigue syndrome, athletic overtraining, Alzheimer's disease, and Parkinson's disease. Reduction of disulfide bonds is a process that can occur spontaneously with GSH alone or may require GSH dependent enzymes. Essential functions of the immune system (such as antigen presentation), reversal of cataract formation, and repair of denatured enzymes are dependent on the availability of GSH to reduce disulfide bonds.

The impact of these properties of GSH and cysteine has been established by a diverse group of research scientists. Their studies can be assembled into a logical step-wise explanation of how and why GSH and cysteine reproducibly effect fundamental metabolic reactions, enhance immune response, reduce the potential of early apoptotic cell death, and reverse molecular reactions associated with aging (cataract formation).

Glutathione Enzymes

The rate-limiting enzyme of GSH synthesis is γ-glutamylcysteine synthetase (γ-GCS), which joins glutamic acid (glutamate) to cysteine. Glutathione synthetase attaches the glycine to cysteine to complete the synthesis of glutathione. GSH exerts a feedback inhibition on γ-GCS that safeguards against overproduction of intracellular GSH.

Excess GSH also stimulates γ-glutamyl transpeptidase the enzyme that modulates the first step in GSH breakdown back into its component amino acids. This further minimizes any chance of "overdosage" and promotes redistribution of the essential substrate, cysteine, to cells that are deficient in cysteine or GSH.[1]

In this way, glutathione functions as the storage molecule for cysteine. The intracellular GSH level is a good measure of the efficiency of cysteine absorption and availability. However, GSH has functions beyond the storage of cysteine.

Glutathione reductase is the enzyme that renews and reduces oxidized glutathione (GSSG) back to reduced glutathione (GSH). Glutathione peroxidase is directly involved with the removal of excess hydrogen peroxide. The glutathione-S-transferase family of enzymes works in tandem with the P450 cytochrome system of the liver to detoxify many organic toxins, including 12 known cancer-causing toxins. Both require GSH.

GSH is itself an antioxidant. It quenches reactive oxygen compounds (free radicals) directly and is also a master antioxidant that reduces and returns ascorbate (vitamin C) and α-tocopherol (vitamin E) back to their bioactive reduced forms.[2] GSH participates in a number of other well-documented metabolic reactions, including, DNA synthesis and repair, protein synthesis, prostaglandin synthesis, amino acid transport, metabolism of toxins and carcinogens, enzyme activation, and enhancement of immune system function.[1]

Proton Donation, Positive Nitrogen Balance, Cysteine and Cystine

As noted in Figure 10–1, the common underlying characteristic of cysteine to donate protons plays a prominent role in hepatic nitrogen recovery metabolism and appears to have a pivotal role in the determination of nitrogen balance. In this way, proton donation is the key to prevent wasting and negative nitrogen balance seen in conditions as diverse as cancer, AIDS, sepsis, trauma, burns, Crohn's disease, ulcerative colitis, chronic fatigue syndrome, athletic overtraining (Table 10–1), Alzheimer's disease, and Parkinson's disease.[3]

The "low cystine, low glutamine" syndrome described by Dröge and Holm[3] links cachexia and muscle wasting seen in many of these conditions to this common hepatic metabolic pathway, which is controlled by the level of cysteine or cystine, two cysteine molecules connected by a disulfide bond, due to their ability to donate protons that promote positive nitrogen balance. This is the scientific basis for cysteine or cystine supplementation in wasting conditions.

Dröge and Holm document how (1) the cystine level is normally regulated by post-absorptive skeletal muscle protein catabolism; (2) the cystine level is a physiological regulator of nitrogen balance and body cell mass; (3) the cystine-mediated regulatory circuit is compromised in various catabolic conditions, including old age; and (4) cysteine or cystine, the most bioactive form of cysteine, supplementation may be a useful therapy when combined with disease-specific treatments such as antiviral therapy in HIV infection.

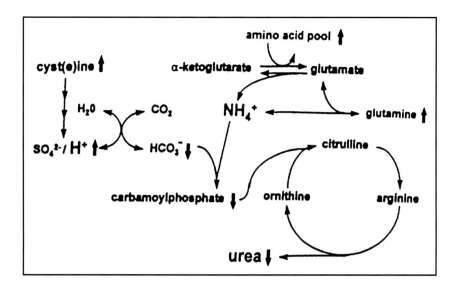

Fig 10–1. Control of nitrogen disposition by hepatic cyst(e)ine catabolism. (Reprinted with permission from Dröge and Holm.[3(p1078)] Copyright © The FASEB Journal.)

Table 10–1. Diseases and Conditions Associated with Abnormally Low Plasma Cystine and Glutamine Levels.

Disease or Condition	Cystine	Glutamine	Glutamate	Urea Production	NK Cell Activity
HIV infection, late asymptomatic stage	↓↓[4]	↓↓[4]	↑	nd	↓↓OI[9,10]
Sepsis, major injury, and trauma	↓↓[5]	↓↓[5]	↑	↑↑[16,18]	↓↓[11,12]
Cancer	↓↓[6]	↓↓[6]	↑	↑↑[16,18]	↓↓[13]
Crohn's disease	↓↓[8]	↓[8]	(↑)	↑↑[17]	↓↓[14,15]
Ulcerative colitis	↓↓[8]	↓[8]	(↑)	↑↑[17]	↓↓[14]
Chronic fatigue syndrome	↓↓[7]	↓↓[7]	nd	nd	↓↓[7]
Overtraining	nd	↓[20]	nd	↑[21]	↓ OI[22]
Starvation	↓↓[23,24]	nd	nd	↓↓[25]	↓ OI

nd = not determined or not detected; OI = opportunistic infections.
Reprinted with permission from Dröge W, Holm E. Role of cysteine and glutathione in HIV infection and other diseases associated with muscle wasting and immunological dysfunction. *FASEB J.* 1997;11(13):1078.[3] Copyright © The FASEB Journal.

According to Dröge and Holm, it appears that the cystine level is the ultimate determinant factor of nitrogen recovery, nitrogen balance, weight loss and body cell mass (see Fig 10–1). Cystine appears to be the optimal source of cysteine. If dietary cystine is insufficient, then muscle catabolism (breakdown) provides cystine, resulting in muscle loss.

Many voice professionals and other fitness-conscious people, especially those in the entertainment industry, pursue physical fitness through dieting and exercise programs. Sometimes, these activities can be pushed to the extreme, especially when diets are deficient in cystine or cysteine, which can lead to muscle breakdown and have deleterious effects on the muscles of respiration (the vocal support system), as well as the delicate muscles of the larynx (the source of sound).

Cysteine supplementation has been shown to enhance strength and endurance significantly in highly trained endurance athletes[26] (long-distance cyclists). This cysteine-enhancing strategy has proven to be critical for maximal physical performance, endurance, and recovery. It has also been shown to improve pulmonary function parameters in a patient with chronic obstructive pulmonary disease (COPD).[27]

These findings have special relevance to voice professionals, because all vocal exercise requires optimal function of the muscles of respiration. Further study is required before definitive statements can be made regarding cysteine or cystine supplementation and pulmonary function improvement in COPD, not to mention its effect in other conditions. However, the athletic endurance study was a prospective, double-blind, randomized, placebo-controlled study showing a 13% increase in peak power performacnce and endurance as well as a 35% increase in white blood cell glutathione level.[26]

Glutathione Is a Determinant Factor of the Type of Immune Response

Antigen presenting cells (APCs) that include macrophages, dendritic cells, and B cells are the first responders of the immune system. They initiate and control the initial event of the immune response: antigen processing. GSH level in APCs determines how antigens are processed and if cytokine (signaling molecule) expression will lead to cellular immunity (adequate GSH associated, T helper 1 [Th1] cytokine response) or humoral immunity (deficient GSH associated, T helper 2 [Th2] cytokine response).[28]

When APCs encounter an antigen, GSH is used to split the antigenic protein-protein disulfide bonds to form protein-GSH disulfide bonds. GSH depletion impedes this process and impairs the APC's ability to form the protein-GSH disulfide bonds required to unfold and disassemble the antigenic protein into fragments that allow for effective processing.[29] Adequate GSH levels lead to effective antigen unfolding followed by the release of Th1-specific cytokines that mediate lymphocyte activation and enhance the cellular immune response.

Adequate Glutathione Level Favors Lymphocyte-Mediated Cellular Immunity

In cell culture, cellular versus humoral immune determination occurs in the first few hours of antigen/APC's interaction.[29] Once expressed, one set of cytokines inhibits expression of the opposite set. Th1 responses develop to battle infections with bacteria, fungi, protozoa, and viruses.[30,31] Th2 responses predominate during helminthic infestations and in response to common environmental allergens.[30] In general, the immune system functions optimally when in the cellular response mode so it can effectively eradicate bacteria, fungi, protozoa, and viruses. GSH is required to maintain this cellular response.

To take full advantage of the immune enhancing effect of GSH, strategies to optimize intracellular GSH levels in APCs and other cells of the immune system need to be developed. Any such strategy must provide the immune system with cysteine or cystine for GSH synthesis. Gmunder et al[32] have noted that different cells of the immune system differ in their preference for cysteine or cystine.

Lymphocytes and Macrophages Differ in Their Preference for Cysteine or Cystine

Lymphocytes are known to preferentially absorb cysteine.[32] Macrophages regulate intracellular GSH levels of lymphocytes by preferentially consuming cystine for intracellular GSH synthesis and then releasing cysteine at a variable and regulated rate for lymphocyte absorption.[32] This has a significant effect on lymphocyte proliferation.[33]

Therefore, macrophages regulate the immunological response by making cysteine available to lymphocytes on an "as needed" basis. For this reason, cystine supplementation feeds all of the cells of the immune system starting with the macrophages and then, through controlled release, to lymphocytes.

On the other hand, cysteine supplementation is not as effective for macrophage GSH production. Because macrophage GSH is the optimal source of the cysteine secreted by macrophages to lymphocytes, providing cysteine instead of cystine reduces the ability of the macrophage to optimally deliver cysteine to the lymphocytes.

Lymphocyte Proliferation and Cytokine Selection

Hamilos also reports that GSH levels play a major role, "Lymphocyte proliferation in response to mitogenic lectins is directly dependent upon glutathione (GSH) availability. Thus, proliferation can be enhanced by providing lymphocytes with excess glutathione, and strongly inhibited by limiting the quantity of intracellular GSH available during the mitogenic stimulation."[33(p223)] Lymphocyte proliferation has been the standard method used to document a material to be immune enhancing.

Cytokines are the cell-signaling molecules that direct the immune differentiation of lymphocytes. The Th1 cytokine pattern is characterized by the production of interleukin 2 (IL-2), IL-12, and interferon-gamma (IFN-γ) and the upregulation of cell-mediated, delayed hypersensitivity, (DTH) responses. The Th2 response pattern is characterized by IL-4 and IL-10 production and upregulation of a variety of antibody responses.[28]

The fundamental biochemical properties of GSH disulfide bond reduction and proton donation underlie the clinically proven benefit of cystine supplementation that provides a reliable, safe and predictable source of GSH for individuals with HIV[34] and probably extend to patients with neurodegenerative diseases.[35]

Many disease states have been associated with GSH deficiency,[1-3,26-28,36-47] but none is more clearly associated with immune deficiency and low GSH than HIV/AIDS. Peterson concludes, "GSH depletion in APC populations may play a key role in exacerbating HIV and other infectious diseases in which Th2 predominance is an important aspect of the disease pathology."[28]

Immune deficiency in AIDS is strongly associated with GSH deficiency. Increasing the intracellular GSH level would be expected to enhance the cellular response of the immune system and have a favorable impact on immune deficiency states, such as in the progression of HIV infection to AIDS. Survival rates in AIDS give insight to the effect of GSH on the progression of HIV to AIDS and the important impact of GSH on survival.

Glutathione Deficiency, HIV/AIDS, and Survival

GSH deficiency is recognized to have a major effect on four important components of the immune response, namely, antigen processing,[28] lymphocyte proliferation,[33] cytokine selection[28,37] and lymphocyte apoptosis[38] (programmed cell death). Clinical observations strongly support the concept that GSH deficiency may be the key to immune deficiency in AIDS and other immune diseases. When GSH levels are maintained or augmented, dramatic improvements in HIV/AIDS clinical outcomes have been documented.[39]

Rodriguez found HIV-infected children to be deficient in GSH compared to controls.[40] Furthermore, "low glutathione concentrations in HIV-infected children are correlated directly with CD4+ T cell counts and correlated inversely with viral loads."[40(p236)] In other words, the lower the GSH, the lower are the CD4+ count and the higher the viral loads.

Herzenberg reported that the GSH level in white blood cells was a *determinant factor* in the survival of AIDS patients.[39] A $p < 0.0001$ level of statistical significance was documented using Kaplan-Meier and logistic regression analyses to evaluate survival data from all HIV-positive patients, as well as from those with a CD4+ cell count greater than $200/\mu l$. The 3-year survival rates in this study were:

Survival in all HIV+:	GSB ≥ 0.91 = 90%.
Survival in all HIV+:	GSB < 0.91 = 32%.
When CD4+ < $200/\mu l$:	GSB ≥ 1.05 = 87%.
When CD4+ < $200/\mu l$:	GSB < 1.05 = 17%.

[GSB = GSH-S-Bimane, a fluorescent form of GSH]

Immune deficiency is associated strongly with GSH deficiency. HIV/AIDS is the prototypic immune deficiency state. Increasing the intracellular GSH level is likely to enhance the cellular response capacity of the immune system, and GSH may prove to be an excellent measure for immune-based therapies. HIV/AIDS survival rates give credence to this conclusion. Close scrutiny of the cellular mechanisms that drive progression of HIV to AIDS and their relationship to immune deficiency is warranted.

Pathogenesis of Immune Deficiency in HIV/AIDS: Cytokine Shift

Clerici has documented that a cytokine shift is associated with progression in AIDS, "a strong type 1/weak type 2 cytokine production profile was observed in HIV-seropositive patients with delayed or absent disease progression, whereas progression of HIV infection was characterized by a weak type 1/strong type 2 cytokine production profile."[37(p185)]

Specifically,

The type 1 to type 2 shift was suggested to be predictive for the following events: (i) rate of decline in the number of CD4+ T lymphocytes; (ii) time to diagnosis of AIDS; and (iii) time to death.[37(p185)]

Progression of HIV infection was suggested to be accompanied by a decline of in vitro production of interleukin-2 (IL-2), IL-12 and interferon gamma (IFN-gamma) (type 1 cytokines) and an increase in the production of IL-4, IL-5, IL-6 and IL-10 (type 2 cytokines) . . . .[37(p185)]

Clerici concluded,

We believe that antiretroviral therapies will not successfully eradicate HIV and that HIV-seropositive patients will not be ultimately cured unless therapies aimed at restoring the immune system are associated with the antiretrovirus drugs currently employed.[37(p187)]

Pathogenesis of Immune Deficiency in HIV/AIDS: Apoptosis

According to Clerici, shifts in cytokines lead to CD4+ cell loss. Antigen stimulation (viral exposure) of lymphocytes of HIV-seropositive individuals in the presence of abnormally low concentrations of IL-2, IL-12 and IFN-γ, and/or of abnormally elevated concentrations of IL-4 and IL-10, would result in the induction of antigen-induced cell death (AICD), also known as apoptosis (programmed cell death), instead of in the induction of T-cell proliferation.[37]

The ultimate cause of cell death in HIV has been debated between a virological or an immunological mechanism.[41] Virological death suggests killing of infected cells by the HIV-1 virus. An immunological mechanism would be more indirect with alteration of CD4+ T-cell function inducing, or associated with increased susceptibility to apoptosis.

Apoptosis is not inherently pathological. Conceptually, programmed cell death represents the reciprocal of monoclonal expansion. As such, it is an integral part of the shutdown mechanism of the immune system. However, T-cells that have been repeatedly stimulated with a specific antigen (such as HIV virus) undergo apoptosis more rapidly than normal, which is why this process is also known as antigen-induced cell death.[42] In AIDS, AICD may account for much the of CD4+ cell loss.

Because HIV infection is associated with persistent or recurrent viral replication throughout the course of the disease, the accelerated apoptosis observed in HIV reflects the intensification of normal AICD occurring in response to the HIV-1 virus as the persistent and recurrent stimulus.[41] Apoptotic susceptibility is affected by the number of antigenic exposures; the more exposures, the more rapidly apoptosis is initiated. The reactions that initiate apoptosis are modulated by cell-signaling molecules such as GSH and Bcl-2.

Apoptosis, Glutathione, and Bcl-2.

B cell lymphoma factor 2 (Bcl-2) is an oncoprotein that is also expressed during times of cellular stress, such as infection, inflammation, and disease. It is one of a large group of cell-signaling proteins that are referred to as heat shock proteins. The Bcl-2 family of proteins regulates the susceptibility of target T-cells to undergo apoptosis.[41]

Under normal circumstances, overexpression of Bcl-2 has been shown to result in the inhibition of some of the common initiators of apoptosis in HIV/ AIDS and other inflammations, including anti-Fas and tumor necrosis factor alpha (TNF-α) mediated apoptosis.[43] One of the determinant factors in this response is the intracellular level of glutathione.

Depletion of GSH caused cells overexpressing Bcl-2 to become sensitized to, and succumb to, apoptotic induction.[38] On the other hand, in cells with adequate levels of GSH, Bcl-2 overexpression led to a relocalization of GSH into the nucleus, thereby altering nuclear redox status and blocking caspase activity, as well as other nuclear initiators of apoptosis.

GSH depletion is also linked to disruption of the mitochondrial transmembrane potential ($\Delta\Psi m$) that is considered to be an early necessary step of apoptosis.[44] A subsequent step is hyperproduction of reactive oxygen species (ROS) with disruption of Ca^{2+} homeostasis.

When there is a sufficient quantity of GSH, Bcl-2 maintains the $\Delta\Psi m$ by enhancing proton efflux from mitochondria, even in the presence of $\Delta\Psi m$-loss-inducing stimuli such as Ca^{2+}, H_2O_2, and tert-butyl hydroperoxide.[45] The proton donor function of GSH, similar to that of cysteine previously described by Dröge in the hepatic cyst(e)ine catabolism cycle, appears to provide the necessary proton for the proton efflux regulating effect of Bcl-2. The action of Bcl-2 prevents apoptotic mitochondrial dysfunction when GSH levels are adequate. This would explain the pivotal role GSH plays in Bcl-2 antiapoptosis.

Mechanism of CD4+ Cell Invasion in HIV/AIDS: Cell Surface Antigen Expression

Sprietsma[46] has reported that the further the AIDS process develops, the more the immune response moves into Th2 phase. Research has shown that HIV multiplies almost exclusively in Th2 cells and rarely, if ever, in Th1 cells.[47,48] The Th2 cytokine, Il-4, promotes the production of the cell surface antigen CXCR4 that allows the more virulent strains of HIV to infect CD4+ cells.[49] BLTR, like CXCR4, is another CD4 cell surface co-receptor that preferentially admits the more aggressive HIV-1 viruses into the cells.[50]

Sufficient intake of the essential nutrients[46] (cysteine; methionine; arginine; vitamins A, B, C and E; zinc; and selenium) maintains the Th1 influence on the immune system, thereby inhibiting the proliferation of viruses such as HIV by inactivating the HIV protease and down-regulating the number of BLTR receptors.

Among essential nutrients that appear to be most commonly deficient in typical diets are the amino acids cysteine, methionine, and arginine. Consequently, supplementation with a source of these amino acids, especially cysteine, is necessary for the production of glutathione, metallothionein, and nitric oxide. Adequate quantities of these three regulatory molecules promote the production of Th1 cytokines and reduce the expression of the cell surface antigens associated with HIV-1 entrance into CD4+ cells and progression to AIDS.

Sprietsma[46] further points out that immune activities under Th1 control can offer protection against a broad range of other clinical conditions that include infectious disease (viral), autoimmune diseases (diabetes and diabetic complications), and other immune conditions (asthma, rheumatoid arthritis and Crohn's disease). Thus, HIV/AIDS is only one of a host of medical condition affected by cytokine selection.

Therefore, it should also be no surprise that HIV/ AIDS is not the only clinical condition favorably affected by cysteine supplementation.[34] Published reports of: (1) a case report of pulmonary function improvement in chronic obstructive pulmonary disease (COPD),[27] (2) a study in Hepatitis B,[51] and (3) a compilation of case reports in urogenital cancer patients[52] expands the knowledge base found in the peer-reviewed medical literature regarding the impact of cysteine supplementation.

The common denominators in these reports appear to be the promise of essential nutrients and the cell-signaling molecules they are synthesized into, especially cysteine and glutathione. Consistent with this view are other reports in the GSH research literature strongly suggesting that many medical conditions are affected, and even controlled, by GSH level linking the actions of GSH to the common underlying mechanism of oxidative stress.

Oxidative stress has been implicated in a number of diseases, but the research literature is particularly convincing in its association with neurodegenerative diseases, especially Parkinson's disease. Significantly, GSH is a powerful antioxidant.[1]

Neurodegenerative Disorders: GSH Prevention of Neuronal Death

During periods of oxidative stress, GSH is an important protector of energy metabolism (mitochondrial function).[53] Dopaminergic neurons are very sensitive to changes in the internal oxidant buffering capacity of the cell caused by reductions in GSH levels that can lead to disruption of calcium homeostasis and cell death.[54] GSH, but not vitamins C or E, protects human neural cells from dopamine-induced apoptosis.[55] Notably, dopamine treatment during GSH depletion is documented to produce defects in psychomotor behavior in a laboratory animal model.[56]

Oxidative stress has been implicated in various neurodegenerative disorders and may be a common mechanism underlying various forms of cell death including excitotoxicity, apoptosis, and necrosis. Bains and Shaw[57] present evidence for a role of oxidative stress and diminished GSH in Lou Gehrig's disease (ALS), Parkinson's disease, and Alzheimer's disease. GSH modulation may prove to be beneficial in spinal cord injury,[58] multiple sclerosis,[59] and stroke.[60,61] Because cysteine supplementation increases GSH it may hold promise as a method to modulate neurodegenerative diseases.

GSH, Dopamine, and Glutamate: Roles in Parkinson's Disease

GSH is utilized by the granular storage system of dopamine in PC12 pheochromocytoma cells, and it is likely that GSH protects susceptible parts of the granular transport system against (possibly dopamine-induced) oxidative damage.[62] In PC12 and C6 glial cell lines, glutamate toxicity causes oxidative stress and GSH depletion by reducing cystine uptake and results in apoptotic cell death.[63,64] These research models of Parkinson's disease suggest a key role for GSH in glutamate excitotoxicity. Strategies designed to maintain GSH levels protect against glutamate toxicity and prevent dopamine-induced cell death, resulting in enhanced neuronal survival.[65,66]

Astrocyte mediation of enhanced neuronal survival is abolished by GSH deficiency.[67] The neuroprotective role of astrocytes involves a number of activities, including expression of antioxidant enzymes, synthesis of GSH, and recycling of vitamin C, as well as transport and metabolism of glucose, which yields reducing equivalents for antioxidant regeneration and lactate for neuronal metabolism.[68] Many of these functions require GSH or cystine.

Astrocytes, like macrophages, prefer cystine and glutamate for GSH synthesis[69,70]; whereas cysteine and glutamine are preferred by neurons. These differential preferences allow astrocytes to regulate neuronal GSH.[67]

Glutathione Deficiency and Wound Healing

Adamson et al[71] were the first to provide evidence that the temporal course of wound healing is related to glutathione metabolism. In animals deficient in GSH, the content of hydroxyproline in wounds accumulated faster by day 4 but was lower by day 6, resulting in reduced wound strength. This finding establishes a cell-signaling role for GSH in wound healing. Post-surgical patients[72] and patients who are critically ill[73] have reduced stores of glutathione in their skeletal muscles. Because muscle functions as a reservoir for glutathione it is not surprising that low levels of intramuscular GSH are associated with immune dysfunction and negative nitrogen balance,[3] both of which are particularly significant for critically ill patients undergoing surgery.

The deficit of GSH, observed in critically ill patients is likely to contribute to the frequently observed increased incidence of wound breakdown and post-operative infection seen in this population that can also result in decubitus ulcers and hypertrophic scarring.

Chronic, nonhealing wounds are a major challenge for the health care industry. These wounds include pressure ulcers (pressure sores, decubitus ulcers, or bedsores), diabetic ulcers, stasis ulcers (those associated with the circulatory problems seen in peripheral vascular disease), and ulcerations at amputation sites. Data from the Medicare website (from nearly all 7,000 nursing homes caring for an estimated 1.5 million patients) indicate an 8% average national incidence. Estimates for pressure ulcers in skilled nursing facilities, extended care/tertiary hospitals, and subacute care facilities such as freestanding ventilator centers are reported in the 20% range.

Providing a supplemental source of cystine (the bioactive form of the key amino acid for glutathione synthesis, cysteine) optimizes the immune response of macrophages and lymphocytes[32] and is the preferred glutathione source for astrocytes.[69] As noted above,

cysteine[46] and glutathione[71] are both essential regulators of the immune response and wound healing.

Immunonutrients and Clinical Outcomes

Supplementation with immune enhancing formulas has been found to improve immune response and efficiency in a number of clinical studies.[74] Immune efficiency has a profound effect on resistance to infection, need for antibiotic therapy and length of stay in the hospital. IMPACT (Novartis Nutrition, Bern, Switzerland) and Immun-Aid (McGraw, Irvine, Calif) were the two materials used in these studies involving critically ill patients.

One study using Immun-Aid in patients with severe abdominal trauma has documented the dramatic benefit of immune-enhancing nutrients on a number of clinical outcomes in seriously ill patients in the ICU setting.[75] This study compares patients fed either an immune enhancing (Immun-Aid) or an isonitrogenous, isocaloric diet with a control of no diet.

As demonstrated by this study (Table 10–2), antibiotic usage is not the only outcome statistic affected. Significant reduction in length of treatment is noted in this study, as well. All of the findings were found to be statistically significant except hospital charges. This is only one of 12 studies compiled in a 1,482 patient meta-analysis.[76]

In the meta-analysis, IMPACT (10 studies) or Immun-Aid (2 studies) was given to critically ill patients.[76] Dramatically improved outcome statistics were documented including a decreased rate of infec-

Table 10–2. How an Immune-Enhancing Diet Affects Outcome Parameters in Severe Abdominal Trauma.

Antibiotic Use and Hospital Stay	Immune-Enhancing Diet (16)	Isonitrogenous, Isocaloric Diet (17)	Statistical Signficance	Control Group (19)
Antibiotic use (days ± SEM)				
Prophylactic	3.8 ± 0.9	2.7 ± 0.5	NS	4.2 ± 0.7
Empiric	1.4 ± 0.8	2.6 ± 1.1	NS	0.7 ± 0.5
Therapeutic	2.8 ± 1.6	7.1 ± 1.7	$p = 0.02$	17.4 ± 4.6
Hospital stay (days ± SEM)				
Total	18.3 ± 2.8	32.6 ± 6.6	$p = 0.03$	34.9 ± 6.0
In ICU	5.8 ± 1.8	9.5 ± 2.3	$p = 0.10$	15.7 ± 4.9
On ventilator	2.4 ± 1.3	5.4 ± 2.0	$p = 0.09$	9.0 ± 4.2
Hospital charges	$80,515 ± 21,528	$110,599 ± 19,132	NS	$141,049 ± 34,396

SEM = standard error of the mean; NS = not significant; ICU = intensive care unit

Adapted from Kudsk KA et al.[75]

tion ($p = 0.005$) and a reduced hospital stay of 2.3 days ($p = 0.007$) in surgical patients and 2.9 days ($p = 0.0002$) in all patients.

Inflammation: Essential Nutrient Deficiency Resulting in Immune Dysfunction

Inflammation is one of the most pervasive causes of disease and disability. Treatment of inflammation is provided by anti-inflammatory medications that fall into two major categories, steroidal and nonsteroidal. Both approaches have significant drawbacks. Steroids suppress the immune system and can increase the occurrence of opportunistic infections. Most nonsteroidal, anti-inflammatory medications are anticoagulants that are associated with irritation of the gastrointestinal tract and bleeding.

According to the research done by Sprietsma,[46] depletion of essential nutrients is associated with immune dysfunction that results in chronic diseases, including inflammatory conditions. This report identifies nitric oxide as a "shut-off" signal for the immune system. Specifically, Th1-cytokine-directed inflammatory cells respond to nitric oxide and stop their activity but Th2-directed cells do not. Th2 cell activity is associated with GSH deficiency and leads to prolonged immune activity and chronic inflammation.

The essential precursor nutrients for these cellular processes include the amino acids cysteine, methionine, and arginine used for production of glutathione, metallothionein, and nitric oxide.[46] Adequate quantities of these three molecules maintain the Th1 influence on the immune system, resulting in optimal function and responsiveness, including nitric-oxide-mediated cessation of immune activity.

However, as the inflammatory process continues, deficiencies in these amino acids are likely to occur resulting in a reduction in the availability of glutathione, metallothionein, and nitric oxide. Inadequate levels of these critical signaling molecules allows Th2 cytokines to predominate, resulting in continuation of the immune response that further exacerbates the deficiency. This correlates with the common clinical findings associated with Th2 cytokine expression seen in chronic inflammation, including eosinophilia and IgE secretion.

Providing supplemental amounts of the essential nutrients appears to be a viable method to restore Th1 influence in the immune system and may well restore its responsiveness to the nitric oxide stop signal. Whether this strategy will result in a reduction in clinical inflammatory damage and cessation of chronic disease requires further investigation.

Summary of the Effects of Glutathione and Cysteine

A great deal of data has been presented that identifies a rapidly growing body of research that has documented how cysteine and glutathione play significant roles in numerous metabolic, immunologic, and cellular reactions. Cysteine, especially in the form of cystine, is the determinate factor of positive nitrogen balance and is the rate limiting substrate for the synthesis of glutathione.[3]

Glutathione maintenance and/or augmentation regulates many basic immune functions:

- optimization of antigen processing,
- maximization of lymphocyte proliferation and antibody synthesis,
- maintenance of Th1 cytokine production (Interferon-γ, IL-2, IL-12)
- reduction of lymphocyte loss due to disease initiated apoptosis, and
- minimization of persistent inflammation by keeping lymphocytes under Th1 cytokine influence, thereby maintaining responsiveness to nitric oxide shut down.

Glutathione is a requirement in a wide array of metabolic reactions that are pivotal to many cellular functions. Table 10–3 summarizes a number of the functions critical to optimal cellular health. These functions are likely to have a significant impact on a number of disease states and health-related conditions.

Glutathione also optimizes wound healing[71] and has a major beneficial effect on clinical outcomes such

Table 10–3. Functions of Glutathione.

Functions as the central reservoir for cysteine

Protects against disease-initiated apoptosis

Optimizes immune function

Maximizes Interferon-γ

Upregulates IL-2

Assists DNA synthesis

Renews enzyme activation

Contributes to protein synthesis

Supports amino acid transport

Prevents oxidative cell damage (antioxidation)

Metabolizes toxins and carcinogens (detoxification)

as AIDS survival rates.[39] Glutathione deficiency erodes the efficiency of the cellular machinery to perform many of these basic tasks and is associated with progressive worsening of clinically significant disease states such as HIV/AIDS.[39,40]

Increasing Intracellular Glutathione with Cysteine and Cysteine Pro-Drugs

A number of strategies have been tried to increase glutathione. Most approaches use pharmacological doses of glutathione or a form of the rate-limiting substrate, cysteine. Administering GSH by oral, intravenous, intratracheal, and intraperitoneal routes has been tried but has no lasting effect.[76,77] Glutathione is digested if taken orally, has a short half-life if delivered intravenously, and does not significantly increase liver or lymphocyte GSH if given intratracheally or intraperitoneally. Esterified GSH compounds have increased GSH in a few tissues[78] but have limited value in human use due to harmful and potentially toxic metabolic products.[79]

Providing cysteine or methionine directly is associated with significant toxicity.[80] Cysteine is readily metabolized,[77] and methionine can be converted to cysteine in the liver but this requires energy. Also, the conversion process could increase an intermediate metabolite, homocysteine. If it is not fully metabolized, increased levels of homocysteine lead to homocysteinuria, which appears to be associated with atherosclerotic vascular disease.

N-acetyl cysteine (NAC) has been used for treatment of AIDS to increase GSH.[3,28,81-86] However, NAC has only 10% bioavailability when given orally and is associated with significant side effects (rashes and severe gastro-intestinal upset) at therapeutic doses of 4 grams or more per day.[39] Anaphylactic reactions also have been reported.[87]

Even at more moderate pharmacological doses, cysteine pro-drugs, such as NAC, are associated with mobilization of heavy metals across the placenta[88-90] and blood brain barrier,[91-95] as well as into liver, kidney,[85] and astrocytes.[96] Although this may prove useful for some interventional techniques, it may also limit its usefulness as a daily source of cysteine for GSH enhancement. Various forms of cysteine, including NAC, cause excitotoxin release in certain areas of the brain such as the hippocampus. The hippocampus is the location of neurodegeneratation in Alzheimer's disease. One of the leading theories advanced to explain the cause of neurodegenerative diseases is excitotoxin release.[97] Excitotoxin release has been documented with various forms of cysteine but does not occur with cystine.[98]

Cystine Is the Optimal Form of Cysteine for Intracellular Glutathione Synthesis

Cystine has been shown to be the cysteine precursor of choice in macrophages[32] and astroglial cells,[69,70] which then feed cysteine to lymphocytes and neurons, respectively, in a highly regulated fashion. The increase in the GSH levels in astrocytes is substantially greater with cystine than with any other cysteine source.[69] Therefore, cystine represents the optimal form of cysteine for GSH production in the antigen presenting macrophage and the neuron protecting astroglial cell.

One way to avoid the multiple drawbacks of using pharmacological doses of cysteine pro-drugs is to use an *undenatured* source of complete amino acids containing a high concentration of cystine, which is now available (Immunocal, Immunotec Research Ltd, Montreal, Quebec, Canada). The effectiveness of this particular approach of GSH production is well documented,[99] and the glutathione produced by this method has been shown to be beneficial in patients suffering from AIDS with wasting syndrome.[100]

The bioactivity and effectiveness of Immunocal appears to be dependent on the *undenature*d quality of this amino acid delivery system, which results in preservation of the disulfide bond that allows a high concentration of cystine to be made available to the liver. This is not a property found in commercial whey proteins.

A full discussion of this topic is beyond the scope of this review, but can be found in a recent text edited by Montagnier, Olivier, and Pasquier.[101]

Nutraceutical Modulation and Cancer Research

One of the earliest examples of nutraceutical modulation of a clinical condition is the treatment of scurvy with vitamin C from citrus fruits. This example is so common and accepted that it may be overlooked as a nutraceutical treatment. On the other hand, nutraceutical modulation of cancer is considered quite controversial and unconventional. However, there are at least three known nutraceutical substances that have anticancer properties reported in peer-reviewed medical journals: lycopenes, isothiocyanates, and an undenatured whey protein concentrate.

Lycopenes are carotenoids, found in red-pigmented foods such as tomatoes and watermelon, and are considered to be powerful antioxidants. An analysis of men who eat tomatoes regularly demonstrated a statistically significant reduction in the rate of prostate cancer.[102] Isothiocyanate is found in cruciferous vegetables such as broccoli and Brussels sprouts and has been identified as having an anticancer effect.[103]

Glutathione[104] and glutathione-S-transferase[105] (GST) are involved in enhancing the intracellular accumulation of isothiocyanates, while intracellular accumulation of isothiocyanates determines their activity in elevating GSH and GST.[106] Antioxidants that are either rejuvenated by GSH (vitamin E) or are integral to glutathione-dependent enzymes (selenium, the cofactor of glutathione peroxidase) appear to play a role in mitigating against carcinogenesis in the prostate.[107]

Two common, fundamental features affecting carcinogenesis of the prostate are the beneficial effect of antioxidation[102] and a defective glutathione-S-transferase pi detoxification system.[107] Glutathione directly conjugates and detoxifies 12 known cancer-causing toxis[108-20] (Table10–4). As noted earlier in this chapter, it is the central antioxidant and GSH is required by GST to detoxify and remove many disease-causing chemicals. Glutathione-S-transferase pi 1 (GSTP1) is one of the four members of the GST family of GSH-dependent, carcinogen-metabolizing, detoxifying enzymes that protects cells from cancer.

The Role of Oxidative Stress in the Moleculopathogenesis of Prostate Cancer

Many, if not all, of the toxins in Table 10–4 are free radical generators that create or become reactive oxygen species (ROS). Generation of ROS creates a pro-oxidant environment that has been demonstrated to be associated with the promotion of prostate cancer.[121] A

Table 10–4. Cancer-Causing Toxins Detoxified by Glutathione.

Aflatoxin B$_1$
N-acetyl-2-aminofluorene
Benz(a)anthracene
Benz(a)pyrene
Benzidine
Dimethylhydrazine
Dimethylnitrosamine
Ethylmethane sulfonate
N-methyl-4-aminoazobenzene
7-methylbenzanthracene
3-methyl-cholanthracene
1-nitropyrene

University of Wisconsin study[121] shows that physiological levels of androgens are capable of decreasing the GSH content of human prostate cells. The reduced antioxidant capability of the cells caused by the reduction of GSH is consistent with the pro-oxidant mechanism for prostate carcinogenesis.

The most common defect described in prostate cancer is inactivation of GSTP1 by hypermethylation. Data on 115 tissue samples found an 87% sensitivity and a 92% specificity for this defect in prostate cancer.[122] The loss of GSPT1 function is directly related to hypermethylation of the CpG island that is the promoter sequence for DNA expression.[123]

"GSTP1 inactivation may render prostate cells susceptible to additional genome alterations, caused by electrophile or oxidant carcinogens…"[124(p1815)] Hypermethylation of the CpG islands is implicated in silencing tumor suppressor genes in cancer.[125] CpG island hypermethylation is an epigenetic lesion[126] and strongly suggests a role for epigenetic changes in carcinogenesis due to inactivation adversely affecting DNA repair, cell cycle function, and apoptosis.[127] It may lead to four specific genetic lesions: microsatellite instability, G to A transitions, steroid-related adducts, and double-strand breaks in DNA.[126]

Hypermethylation of the CpG islands is documented to occur in a number of cancers beside prostate, including ovarian,[128] breast,[129,130] gastric,[131] and colon.[132] "Epigenetic changes, particularly DNA methylation are susceptible to change and are excellent candidates to explain how certain environmental factors may increase the risk of cancer."[127(p1)] Therefore, "aberrant CpG island methylation can also be used as a biomarker of malignant cells and as a predictor of their behavior, and may constitute a good target for future therapies."[127(p1)]

Reversing Epigenetic Lesions: Implications for Prevention and Reversal of Cancer

"Among the many somatic genome alterations present in cancer cells, changes in DNA methylation may represent reversible 'epigenetic' lesions, rather than irreversible 'genetic' alterations."[133(p8611)] "This hypothesized critical role for GSTP1 inactivation in the earliest steps of prostatic carcinogenesis provides several attractive opportunities for prostate cancer prevention strategies, including (1) restoration of GSTP1 function, (2) compensation for inadequate GSTP1 activity (via use of therapeutic inducers of other glutathione-S-transferases (GST), and (3) abrogation of genome-damaging stresses."[134(p39)]

Restoration of GSTP1 function has been reported by Lin et al, "the drug procainamide, a nonnucleoside inhibitor of DNA methyltransferases, reversed GSTP1 CpG island hypermethylation and restored GSTP1 expression in LNCaP human PCA (prostate cancer) cells propagated in vitro or in vivo as xenograft tumors in athymic nude mice."[133(p8611)]

Compensation for inadequate GSTP1 activity is derived from green tea polyphenols (GTP) and curcumin found in the spice turmeric.[135] Curcumin upregulates both glutathione peroxidase (the glutathione-dependent, hydrogen peroxide metabolizing enzyme that requires selenium) and GST in a saturable, dose-dependent manner.[136]

Abrogation of genome-damaging stresses is accomplished through antioxidation, because these stresses in prostate cancer are associated with ROS caused prooxidant shift.[121]

Well-documented, peer-reviewed scientific evidence is published, which establishes that nutraceutical modulation of some malignancies may be possible. Antioxidant dietary supplementation is being evaluated as a chemoprotective strategy in prostate cancer.[107]

Published case reports strongly suggest an anti-tumor effect of a whey protein dietary supplement in some urogenital cancers.[52] Also, Immunocal, the undenatured whey protein used in the urogenital cancer case reports,[52] has been found to modulate the growth characteristics of a dimethylhydrazine-induced malignancy of the colon in animals.[113] These outcomes apparently are due to its ability to increase intracellular glutathione.

Another undenatured whey material, IMN-1207 (Immunotec Research Ltd), is presently being studied in cancer patients as a nutraceutical adjunct for radiation therapy and/or chemotherapy to determine its association with improved quality of life, such as reduced side effects and diminished weight loss (John Molson, personal communication, 2004).

The Glutathione and Cysteine Pathway in Cancer

In the early 1980s, it was found that normal mice fed a whey protein concentrate (WPC) as 20% of a formula diet exhibited marked increase in antibody production in response to T-cell-dependent antigen.[137,138] The relatively high cysteine content of the WPC was found to play a role in the bioactivity of the diet. In fact, optimization of the immune response in animals fed WPC was found to be related to a sustained production of GSH in the lymphocytes through dietary provision of supplementary doses of the GSH precursor cysteine.[99] The enhancing effect of dietary WPC on the immune response was substantially reduced by the administration of S-(n-butyl) homocysteine sulfoximine (BSO), which reduced by half lymphocyte GSH levels,[99] thus confirming the central role of GSH in the immune response. On the other hand, during the days following antigenic challenge in control animals fed a cysteine poor casein diet, a progressive decline of GSH in the challenged lymphocytes correlates with depressed immune response.[99]

Recently, three independent studies showed that whey protein feeding inhibits the development and progression of tumors in laboratory animals.[113-114,139] It is tempting to postulate that the observed effect against small volumes of tumor is somewhat related to potentiation of the immune activity through the GSH pathway facilitated by supplementary cysteine intake as data on the response to SRBC have shown.[99] More specifically with regard to antitumor immunosurveillance, the generation of cytotoxic T-cell activity in mixed lymphocyte cultures was found to be one of several immunological responses that are strongly augmented by thiols.[140] Natural killer cell activity is reduced in cancer patients, but it is restored by additional sources of cysteine.[141] The intriguing role of dietary cysteine and liver GSH in the development of experimental tumors recently reviewed by Parodi[142] clearly indicates an inverse correlation between dietary cysteine, liver GSH and tumor incidence (%), and burden (tumors/group). These observations suggest the concept that protracted anticancer activities by immune cells results in a progressive intracellular depletion of reduced glutathione. Indeed, cancer patients show an accelerated shift to more oxidized conditions.[141]

The overall importance of GSH is emphasized by the drastic attempts to recover all available GSH precursors from GSH catabolism. The degradation of GSH occurs extracellularly through the activity of γ-glutamyl-transpeptidase. Exported GSH and extracellular cystine interact with γ-glutamyl-transpeptidase, leading to the formation of γ-glutamylcystine. The latter is transported into the cell and reduced to form cysteine and γ-glutamylcysteine, which are substrates respectively of γ-glutamylcysteine synthetase and GSH synthetase. This serves as a recovery system for cysteine moieties.[143]

From these observations, it is tempting to speculate that, in the immune cells of the critically ill, the culminating events of cell respiration, electron transport, and oxidative phosphorylation are still functioning and yield energy just as in mouse lymphocytes toward the end of the immune response to SRBC.[99] This assumption is supported by the progressive decline in GSH observed in these cells.

Although oxygen and dietary substrates are still available, what is progressively becoming a limiting factor is the buffering function of the cellular antioxidants, namely, the reduced glutathione system that becomes depleted by the continuous release of oxygen-derived free radicals. For example, the drastic attempt to recover all available essential GSH precursors from the skeletal muscle cells can be viewed as a host survival mechanism.[144]

Finally, cysteine itself may exert a direct antitumor effect in two different ways unrelated to GSH synthesis. It was recently demonstrated that several sulfur-containing antioxidants, such as NAC and OTZ, selectively induce p53-dependent apoptosis in transformed but not in normal cells. In contrast, antioxidants whose action is limited to scavenging radicals do not seem to have this activity.

This activity was found related to a five- to tenfold induction of p53 protein but not to GSH formation. Therefore, a natural cysteine donor such as whey protein concentrate (WPC) could also inhibit tumors by directly increasing cellular thiol levels.[145] A second known effect of a cysteine delivery system is related to the inhibitory effect of cysteine on neoangiogenesis and tumor progression.[146] Locigno and Castronovo recently reviewed the role of the reduced GSH system in cancer development, prevention, and treatment.[147]

GSH-Mediated Reversal of Age-Related Events: Evidence for Biochemical Rejuvenation

Senescent changes lead either to reduced response capacity, such as reduced immunological response, or progressive degeneration, as exemplified by cataract formation. The age-dependent decline in the ability of T-cells to mount a proliferative response is due to an age-related defect in signal transduction.[148] Proliferation of aged T-cells, which is typically 10 to 30% of the level of young controls, was enhanced almost tenfold by increasing GSH and reached levels of young controls.[148]

GSH-dependent reversal of cataract has been reported,[149] and results in improved transparency of the lens. A two-step GSH reduction of disulfide bonds occurs. First, GSH nonenzymatically forms protein-GSH disulfide bonds from lens protein-protein disulfide bonds; then the GSH-dependent enzyme thioltransferase (TTase) reduces the protein-GSH disulfide bond to a protein sulfhydryl bond that unfolds the crystalline protein of the lens.[150] Because TTase is found in the human lens,[151] reversing age-related GSH loss in the lens through GSH enhancement holds great promise for cataract patients.[152] TTase has also been shown to reactivate metabolically important enzymes that have been oxidized such as pyruvate kinase, phosphofructokinase, and glutathione-S-transferase.[150] This may hold promise for patients with diabetes.

Research on life extension has identified endogenous free-radical reactions as a major cause of aging and, "possibly the only one."[153] The higher intracellular glutathione levels found in food-restricted experimental animals has been invoked as the explanation of the life-prolonging effect of food restriction treatment.[154] Because GSH is the major endogenous antioxidant, its preservation and enhancement is central to anti-aging and rejuvenating strategies.

Nutraceutical Modulation and Clinical Outcomes

Although more studies are still needed to move from likelihood to certainty in many specific clinical conditions, the concept of improved outcomes with immune-enhancing nutrients (IMPACT and Immun-Aid) has been fully documented to be safe and effective in many peer-reviewed medical journals, as well as a large (1,482 patients), well controlled, meta-analysis (Table 10–5).[75] The most striking results of this meta-analysis include a 40% reduction of infection ($p = .005$), a nearly 3-day reduction in hospital length of stay ($p =$

Table 10–5. Summary of Meta-Analysis Outcomes of Immunonutrient Enteral Feeds.

Outcomes	Patient Group	Treatment Number	Control Number	Treatment Effect (95% CI)	p-Value
Infection rate	All	437	425	0.60 (0.42, 0.86)	.005
	Surgical	224	223	0.48 (0.28, 0.83)	.01
Length of stay (days)	All	631	642	–2.9 (–4.4, –1.4)	.0002
	Surgical	273	280	–2.3 (–4.0, –0.6)	.007
	Medical	133	125	–9.7 (–17.1, –2.3)	.01
Ventilator days	All	357	369	–2.6 (–5.1, –0.6)	.04
	Trauma	95	101	–4.0, (–7.5, –0.6)	.02

CI = Confidence interval.

.0002) for all patients in the treatment group and for post-surgical patients ($p = .007$).

Nutraceutical Materials

There are a myriad of claims (774,000 on the Google search engine alone) of immune enhancement by many materials, yet there are only three known to the author (TAK) to have been the subject of a significant number of articles published in peer-reviewed, medical journals. Two (IMPACT and Immun-Aid) have demonstrated ability to affect clinical outcomes (Table 10–5). One (Immunocal) is noted to have significant effect on clinical conditions associated with serious disease states—pulmonary functions in COPD,[27] wasting syndrome in HIV/AIDS,[34] and liver function in hepatitis B.[51] Table 10–6 details the usage characteristics of these three medical-grade materials.

The advantage of nutraceuticals is they are natural source materials that the body is able to metabolize with a well-developed and extensive array of enzymes. In the case of the glutathione system, these enzymes synthesize, break down, mobilize, and revitalize glutathione and its precursor amino acids, dramatically reducing the possibility of overdosage and side effects. These features are particularly important, because increasing the concentration and benefit of precursors utilized in glutathione synthesis is central to the mechanism of action of these precursors.

Quantifying and standardizing bioactivity is one of the most challenging aspects of nutraceuticals and functional foods. These products are frequently promoted as good for you, but there is little information on how much isothiocyanate from the broccoli family or lycopene from red fruits is required on a daily basis to be predictably antineoplastic. This has given rise to the "more is better" theory, which has given us any number of food fads that have damaged the credibility of nutraceutical and functional foods in the medical community.

Vitamin C is a good example of the challenges and debates that develop in determining the optimal dosage. High-dose vitamin C was ardently promoted by Dr. Linus Pauling, an early proponent of nutraceutical therapies. Others were particularly concerned about the potential for nutraceutical overdose. Over the years, this debate has waned to obscurity due in large part to the lack of reported side effects. The active ingredients of nutraceuticals and functional foods are likely to demonstrate equivalent safety. It is hard to conceive of overdosing on fruits or vegetables.

Although these materials are safe and effective for promoting health and have shown significant beneficial effect on a variety of conditions associated with disease relevant to clinicians and patients, manufacturers and distributors of nutraceuticals are prohibited from claiming to diagnose, treat, cure, or prevent any disease with their products. This stipulation, enforced by the FDA, has made it difficult to report outcomes of research in plain language, thereby limiting clinicians' and patients' awareness and understanding of the potential benefits of this approach to health care.

Table 10–6. Characteristics of Medical Grade Nutraceuticals.

Characteristics	Immunocal	Immun-Aid	Impact
Amount per unit	10 grams	123 grams	250 ml
Recommended daily dose	40 grams	492 grams	1500 ml
Calories from protein	97.3%	32%	22%
Calories from carbohydrate	2.43%	48%	53%
Calories from fat	0.27%	20%	25%
Fat source	Dairy	Canola oil MCT	Palm kernel, sunflower, and Menhaden oils
Supplemental arginine	No	Yes	Yes
Has immune bioactivity	Yes	Yes	Yes
Mechanism of bioactivity known	Yes	No	No
Proven to increase glutathione	Yes	No	No
Product is in the PDR	Yes	No	No
Cost of recommended daily dose	$8.00	$80.00	$36.00

Another factor limiting wider recognition and broader application of nutraceuticals in health care is the pharmacologic model for developing drugs with specificity of action and target. Emphasis on this model has precluded consideration and focus on development of broad-spectrum, universal agents that mediate a wide array of cellular functions that improve health status and fight disease. As noted by Jeff Donn in his recent article from the Web Site for CBS News, "The quest for broad-spectrum drugs runs against the medical mainstream, which is intent on realizing German researcher Paul Ehrlich's 90-year-old dream of targeting "magic bullets" at specific microbes."[155(p1)]

Strict adherence to this tenet limits the availability of a broad-spectrum approach that offers promising potential solutions for detoxification and protection against a wide variety of threats, including chemical, radiation, and biological agents. Immune enhancement is a good example of the broad-spectrum, universal agent concept.

Immune enhancement techniques can be summarized by a quote from the same article, "Instead of a magic bullet, we are making a better fort," said virologist Roger M. Loria, who researches all-purpose drugs at the Medical College of Virginia in Richmond. The article continues,

Scientists have explored the idea for decades. Often focusing on bolstering the immune system, they hoped to find all-in-one treatments for common ills like cancer, pneumonia or flu, or to mitigate side effects from chemotherapy or radiation treatments. Over the last several years—and especially in recent weeks—worries about terrorism have motivated the search for such drugs. However, they are mostly in early testing and wouldn't be ready for two years, at best.

Although universal drug candidates vary, they tend to work in a common way: by revving up the body's broad, innate defensive shield against foreign germs or their toxins. Unlike antibiotics, most of these new drugs would not directly attack an invader. Unlike vaccines, they would not confine their attack to a narrow group of germs remembered by the immune systems.[155(p1)]

Glutathione and the glutathione family of enzymes represent a common way to rev up the innate defensive shield of the immune system. A nondrug, undenatured whey protein concentrate has been shown to promote and maintain a healthy immune system and to have significant beneficial effect on clinical conditions associated with serious disease states.

Nutraceutical Supplementation in Voice Care

Practical Considerations

So far, no definitive studies have explored application of nutritional and metabolic research to voice patients or voice professionals. However, we believe that such approaches are likely to be beneficial in this population and that these studies are now both practical and feasible to perform.

Immune enhancement, maintenance of body cell mass, and down-regulation of the apoptotic cell death program can be accomplished by increasing intracellular GSH through an orally administered, uniquely formulated, undenatured, whey protein concentrate that provides a novel, nutritional approach to the prevention and reversal of various disease processes.

Recognizing the benefits discussed above, including generalized immune enhancement, as well as beneficial effects on muscle and respiratory function, we hypothesize that manipulation of nutritional substrates affecting synthesis of mediators of cellular metabolism such as glutathione seems likely to help voice professionals and other voice patients in a variety of ways.

General Health and Wellness

If nutritional therapy alters susceptibility to upper respiratory infection or decreases duration of respiratory infection, clearly it would be valuable to singers, actors, and other professional voice users. As noted elsewhere in this book, many voice patients typically lead hectic and irregular lifestyles. The relative malnutrition that accompanies the "fast food" diet so common among performers who travel from hotel to hotel also may be associated with deficits in the optimal function of the immune system.[46] This can result in substantial nutritional deficits that may affect susceptibility to illness, especially respiratory disease, and may contribute to a state of chronic fatigue. Many health-conscious people attempt to avoid colds by boosting their immune function through exercise and vitamin supplements, especially vitamin C. Many use other antioxidants to scavenge free radicals. As discussed above, GSH appears to be an important end-pathway for many of these interventions; and more direct manipulation of this key substrate may prove to be a superior approach. The effectiveness of GSH in enhancing the immune system in patients with HIV/AIDS is particularly impressive. It will be interesting to see whether it has similarly import for use in people with lesser impairment of immune function, such as singers with competent immune systems who are trying to optimize immune response.

Neuromuscular Function

The extensive demands placed on the immune system from recurrent acute illness or chronic disease can adversely affect muscle metabolism,[3] which is the slow recovery following the exercise-induced muscle catabolism that occurs routinely following the exercise of voice performance. Involved muscles include not only laryngeal but also respiratory structures. Maintaining excellent athletic condition in musculature throughout the vocal tract is extremely important to voice performance. Research in other areas suggests that nutritional therapies such as glutathione enhancement should improve these functions in voice patients. Studies of long-distance cyclists appear to be particularly relevant,[26] as does research showing the ability of cysteine supplementation to improve pulmonary function.[27]

Most vocal fold disorders are associated with hyperfunctional compensation, which causes changes in muscle activity that may be associated with voice fatigue, a common complaint among voice patients. Voice misuse may occur in response to muscle functional asymmetries or weakness associated with slow recovery following exercise. This scenario is common among athletes, who are more prone to injury when fatigued than when rested. There is every reason to believe that vocal athletes follow a similar pattern. For actors who perform 8 shows a week, popular singers who present 45-minute sets per night, 6 nights per week, or classical singers who practice daily and perform frequently in large halls without amplification, optimizing muscle function and speed of recovery from exercise are important, often neglected, vocal health issues. Hyperfunctional voice use (muscle tension dysphonia) also occurs commonly in response to even minor neurological abnormalities, such as mild superior laryngeal nerve paresis. Muscle tension dysphonia is recognized as an important cause of vocal injury, including the development of vocal fold masses. Thus, the research reviewed above on the effects of GSH in patients with neurogenic disorders suggests that a similar approach may prove beneficial for neurolaryngologic patients and patients with malignancies involving the vocal tract.

Structural Lesions of the Vocal Fold

Traditionally, structural lesions of the vocal folds have been viewed simplistically. As an example, vocal nodules are believed to be "calluslike" lesions that develop in response to chronic voice abuse or misuse. Since the 1980s, the author (RTS) has hypothesized that voice misuse itself is commonly a response to an unrecognized, underlying organic pathology such as mild paresis. This hypothesis has been borne out in a high percentage of the cases. However, a second long-term question is just beginning to be clarified: Why do some people develop vocal fold nodules (or other structural lesions), while a great many more people who abuse their voices at least as badly fail to develop structural pathology? Research discussed elsewhere in this book (especially in chapters 6 and 10) suggests that various factors at the cellular level determine individual response to trauma, especially materials in the region of the basement membrane. Like all other cells in the body, these cells are dependent on biochemical substrates. These substrates are supplied through an individual's diet. Consequently, it is conceivable that nutritional manipulation may be able to modify some of these important vocal fold cellular functions. This may have implications for prevention of vocal fold nodules and numerous other structural lesions. In addition, the research discussed above (particularly the urological case studies) suggests a beneficial effect from GSH enhancement for patients with neoplastic disease. Similar studies in patients with head and neck malignancies should be considered, including patients with vocal fold cancer and those at high risk to develop laryngeal malignancies.

Voice Surgery

As discussed in chapter 82, vocal fold scarring is one of laryngology's most vexing problems. In large measure, the development of vocal fold scar is a failure of wound healing. Laryngologists traditionally have tried various approaches to optimize healing that include vigorous reflux control, use of antibiotics and steroids to decrease infection and inflammation, postoperative voice rest to minimize stimulation of fibroblast proliferation, and development of minimally traumatic surgical techniques and instruments. Research into genetic and cellular factors that may predict wound healing outcome is ongoing, and further research is planned (Steven Gray, MD, personal communication, 2001). However, as with issues related to the development of structural lesions, it may also be appropriate to investigate not only cellular and genetic issues, but also fundamental biochemical substrates controlled by nutritional intake. The research showing the relationship between glutathione and wound healing is particularly intriguing.[72-74] If increasing GSH levels can improve wound strength and healing in critically ill patients with abdominal wounds, perhaps it can also improve healing characteristics at the opposite extreme of wound healing such as phonomicrosurgical wounds in professional singers. Moreover, if enhancing GSH can promote healing of decubitus ulcers, what might similar metabolic modulation do for recurrent laryngeal granulomas? Although, there is a wide gap between existing research and scientifically validated studies available for application to voice professionals, the potential of this application appears promising. A compelling case for further investigation can be made because GSH augmentation through nutraceutical supplementation is essentially risk free.

Conclusion

Glutathione has been shown to regulate basic immune functions, which may prove beneficial to patients with a broad spectrum of immune-related conditions that include, asthma, rheumatoid arthritis, Crohn's disease, diabetes, and AIDS. It may also play a beneficial role in various neurodegenerative diseases and urological malignancies, as well as improve pulmonary function studies and enhance strength and endurance in athletes.

Although applications for GSH-based metabolic modulation approaches to therapy in voice patients must be considered speculative at present, available information suggests that they are worthy of a concerted research effort. Optimizing cellular functions mediated by GSH appears to be an important approach for preventing disease, improving outcomes in patients who already have pathologic conditions, and possibly for enhancing endurance and optimal performance in healthy voice athletes with Olympic vocal demands.

We look forward to an increasing interest and investigation through rigorous, prospective, controlled studies exploring the potential of GSH modulation, as well as many other nutrition-based approaches for preserving and restoring vocal health.

Acknowledgments The authors (TAK, GB) gratefully acknowledge the contributions made by John Molson to the scientific content of this chapter and to the expanding body of research and medical literature about the impact of glutathione on health and disease. The author (TAK) further acknowledges the valuable contribution made by Jed C. Goldart, MD, MPH, to the refinement of the textual message of this chapter.

References

1. Lomaestro BM., Malone, M. Glutathione in health and disease: pharmacotherapeutic issues. *Ann Pharmacother.* 1995;29:1263–1273.
2. Meister A. The antioxidant effects of glutathione and ascorbic acid, oxidative stress, cell activation and viral infection. In: Pasquier C et al, eds. *Oxidative Stress, Cell Activation and Viral Infection.* Basel, Switzerland: Birkauser Verlag; 1994:101–111.
3. Dröge W, Holm E. Role of cysteine and glutathione in HIV infection and other diseases associated with muscle wasting and immunological dysfunction. *FASEB J.* 1997;11(13):1077–1089.
4. Hack V, Schmid D, Breitkreutz R, et al. Cystine levels, cystine flux, and protein catabolism in cancer cachexia, HIV/SIV infection, and senescence. *FASEB J.* 1997;11(1): 84–92.
5. Roth E, Mühlbacher F, Karner J, et al. Liver amino acids in sepsis. *Surgery.* 1985;97:436–442.
6. Zhang PC, Pang CP. Plasma amino acid patterns in cancer. *Clin Chem.* 1992;38:1198–1199.
7. Aoki T, Miyakoshi H, Usuda Y, Herberman RB. Low NK syndrome and its relationship to chronic fatigue syndrome. *Clin Immunol Immunopathol.* 1993;69:253–265.
8. Erikson LS. Splanchnic exchange of glucose, amino acids and free fatty acids in patients with chronic inflammatory bowel disease. *Gut.* 1983;24:1161–1168.
9. Poli G, Introna M, Zanaboni F, et al. Natural killer cells in intravenous drug abusers with lymphadenopathy syndrome. *Clin Exp Immunol.* 1985;62:128–135.
10. Ullum H, Gotzsche PC, Victor J, et al. Defective natural immunity: an early manifestation of human immunodeficiency virus infection. *J Exp Med.* 1995;182:789–799.
11. Puente J, Miranda D, Gaggero A, et al.[Immunological defects in septic shock. Deficiency of natural killer cells and T-lymphocytes.] *Rev Med Chil.* 1991;119:142–146.
12. Blazar BA, Rodrick ML, O'Mahony JB, et al. Suppression of natural killer cell function in humans following thermal and traumatic injury. *J Clin Immunol.* 1986;6:26–36.
13 Brittenden J, Heys SD, Ross J, Eremin O. Natural killer cells and cancer. *Cancer.* 1996;77:1226–1243.
14. Shanahan F, Leman B, Deem R, et al. Enhanced peripheral blood T cell cytotoxicity in inflammatory bowel disease. *J Clin Immunol.* 1989;9:55–64.
15. Lozano-Polo, J.L., Echevarria-Vierna, S., Casafont-Morencos, F., Ledesma-Castaño, F., Pons-Romero, F. [Natural killer (NK) cells and interleukin-2 (IL-2) in Crohn's disease.] *Rev Esp Enferm Dig.* 1990;78:71–75.
16. Brennan MF. Uncomplicated starvation versus cancer cachexia. *Cancer Res.* 1977;37:2359–2364.
17. Lundsgaard C, Hamberg O, Thomsen OO, et al. Increased hepatic urea synthesis in patients with active inflammatory bowel disease. *J Hepatol.* 1996;24:587–593.
18. Long CL, Crosby F, Geiger JW, Kinney JM. Parenteral nutrition in the septic patient: nitrogen balance, limiting plasma amino acids, and calorie to nitrogen ratios. *Am J Clin Nutr.* 1976;29:380–391.
19. Shaw JH, Wolfe RR. Glucose and urea kinetics in patients with early and advanced gastrointestinal cancer: the response to glucose infusion, parenteral feeding, and surgical resection. *Surgery.* 1987;101:181–191.
20 Parry-Billings M, Blomstrand E, McAndrew N, Newsholme EA. A communicational link between skeletal muscle, brain, and cells of the immune system. *Int J Sports Med.* 1990;11(suppl 2):S122–S128.
21. Janssen GM, van Kranenburg G, and Geurten P. Gender difference in decline of urea concentration during the first 2–3 days postmarathon. *Can J Sport Sci.* 1988;13:18P.
22. Pedersen BK, Kappel M, Klokker M, et al. The immune system during exposure to extreme physiologic conditions. *Int J Sports Med.* 1994;15(suppl 3):S116–S121.

23. Felig P, Owen OE, Wahren J, Cahill GF Jr. Amino acid metabolism during prolonged starvation. *J Clin Invest.* 1969;48:584–594.

24 Smith SR, Pozefsky T, Chhetri MK. Nitrogen and amino acid metabolism in adults with protein-calorie malnutrition. *Metabolism.* 1974;23:603–618.

25. Aoki TT, Müller WA, Cahill GF Jr. Hormonal regulation of glutamine metabolism in fasting man. *Adv Enzyme Regul.* 1972;10:145–151.

26. Lands LC, Grey VI, Smountas AA. Effect of supplementation with a cysteine donor on muscular performance. *J Appl Physiol.* 1999;87(4):1381–1385.

27. Lothian B, Grey V., Kimoff RJ, Lands LC. Treatment of obstructive airway disease with a cysteine donor protein supplement: a case report. *Chest.* 2000;117(3): 914–916.

28. Peterson JD, Herzenberg LA, Vasquez K, Waltenbaugh C. Glutathione levels in antigen-presenting cells modulate Th1 versus Th2 response patterns. *Proc Natl Acad Sci U S A.* 1998;95(6):3071–3076.

29. Short S, Merkel BJ, Caffrey R, McCoy, KL. Defective antigen processing correlates with a low level of intracellular glutathione. *Eur J Immunol.* 1996;26(12):3015–3020.

30. Romagnani S. Lymphokine production by human T cells in disease states. *Annu Rev Immunol.* 1994;12:227–257.

31. Zhang T, Kawakami K, Qureshi MH, et al. Interleukin-12 (IL-12) and IL-18 synergistically induce the fungicidal activity of murine peritoneal exudate cells against Cryptococcus neoformans through production of γ interferon by natural killer cells. *Infect Immunol.* 1997;65:3594–3599.

32. Gmunder H, Eck HP, Benninghoff B, et al. Macrophages regulate intracellular glutathione levels of lymphocytes. Evidence for an immunoregulatory role of cysteine. *Cell Immunol.* 1990;129:32–46.

33. Hamilos D, Zelarny P, Mascali JJ. Lymphocyte proliferation in glutathione-depleted lymphocytes: direct relationship between glutathione availability and the proliferative response. *Immunopharmacology.* 1989;18(3):223–235.

34. Bounous G, Baruchel S, Falutz J, Gold P. Whey protein as a food supplement in HIV-seropositive individuals. *Clin Invest Med.* 1993;16:204–209.

35. Bains JS, Shaw CA. Neurodegenerative disorders in humans: the role of glutathione in oxidative stress-mediated neuronal death. *Brain Res Brain Res Rev.* 1997;25(3):335–358.

36. Short S. Defective antigen processing correlates with a low level of intracellular glutathione. *Eur J Immunol.* 1996;26(12):3015–3020.

37. Clerici M, Fusi ML, Ruzzante S, et al. Type 1 and type 2 cytokines in HIV infection—a possible role in apoptosis and disease progression. *Ann Med.* 1997;29(3):185–188.

38. Voehringer DW, McConkey DJ, McDonnell TJ, et al. Bcl-2 expression causes redistribution of glutathione to the nucleus. *Proc Natl Acad Sci U S A.* 1998;95(6):2956–2960.

39. Herzenberg LA, De Rosa SC, Dubs JG, et al. Glutathione deficiency is associated with impaired survival in HIV disease. *Proc Natl Acad Sci U S A.* 1997;94(5):1967–1972.

40. Rodriguez JF, Cordero J, Chantry C, et al. Plasma glutathione concentrations in children infected with human immunodeficiency virus *Pediatr Infect Dis J.* 1998;17(3): 236–241.

41. Oyaizu N, Pahwa S. Role of apoptosis in HIV disease pathogenesis. *J Clin Immunol.* 1995;15:217–231.

42 Ucker DS, Aswell JD, Nickas G. Activation-driven T cell death. 1: Requirements for de novo transcription and translation and association of genome fragmentation. *J Immunol.* 1989;143:3461–3469.

43. Itoh N, Tsujimoto Y, Nagata S. Effect of bcl-2 on Fas antigen-mediated cell death. *J Immunol.* 1993;151:621–627.

44. Macho A, Hirsch T, Marzo I, et al. Glutathione depletion is an early and calcium elevation is a late event of thymocyte apoptosis. *J Immunol.* 1997;158:4612–4619.

45. Shimizu S, Eguchi Y, Kamiike W, et al. Bcl-2 prevents apoptotic mitochondrial dysfunction by regulating proton flux. *Proc Natl Acad Sci U S A.* 1998;95:1455–1459.

46 Sprietsma JE. Modern diets and diseases: NO-zinc balance. Under Th1, zinc and nitrogen monoxide (NO) collectively protect against viruses, AIDS, autoimmunity, diabetes, allergies, asthma, infectious diseases, atherosclerosis and cancer. *Med Hypotheses.* 1999;53(1):6–16.

47. Mosmann TR. Cytokine patterns during the progression to AIDS. *Science.* 1994;265:193–194.

48. Maggi E, Mazzetti M, Ravina A, al. Ability of HIV to promote a Th1 to Th0 shift and to replicate preferentially in Th2 and Th0 cells. *Science.* 1994;265:244–248.

49. Valentin A, Lu W, Rosati M, et. al. Dual effect of interleukin 4 on HIV-1 expression: implications for viral phenotypic switch and disease progression. *Proc Natl Acad Sci U S A.* 1998;95:11880–11885.

50. Owman C, Garzino-Demo A, Cocchi F, et al. The leukotriene B4 receptor functions as a novel type of coreceptor mediating entry of primary HIV-1 isolates into CD4-positive cells. *Proc Natl Acad Sci U S A.* 1998;95: 9530–9534.

51. Watanabe A, Okada K, Shimizu Y, et al. Nutritional therapy of chronic hepatitis by whey protein (non-heated). *J Med.* 2000;31(5–6):283–302.

52. Bounous G. Whey protein concentrate (WPC) and glutathione modulation in cancer treatment. *Anticancer Res.* 2000;20(6C):4785–4792.

53. Zeevalk, G.D., Bernard, L.P., Nicklas, W.J. Role of oxidative stress and the glutathione system in loss of dopamine neurons due to impairment of energy metabolism. *J Neurochem.* 1998;70(4):1421–1430.

54. Jurma OP, Hom DG, Andersen JK. Decreased glutathione results in calcium-mediated cell death in PC12. *Free Radic Biol Med.* 1997;23(7):1055–1066.

55. Gabby M, Tauber M, Porat S, Simantov R. Selective role of glutathione in protecting human neuronal cells from dopamine-induced apoptosis. *Neuropharmacology.* 1996; 35(5):571–578.

56. Shukitt-Hale B, Denisova NA, Strain JG, Joseph JA. Psychomotor effects of dopamine infusion under decreased glutathione conditions. *Free Radic Biol Med.* 1997;23(3):412–418.

57. Bains JS, Shaw CA. Neurodegenerative disorders in humans: the role of glutathione in oxidative stress-mediat-

ed neuronal death. *Brain Res Brain Res Rev.* 1997;25(3): 335–358.

58. Lucas JH, Wheeler DG, Emery DG, Mallery SR. The endogenous antioxidant glutathione as a factor in the survival of physically injured mammalian spinal cord neurons. *J Neuropathol Exp Neurol.* 1998;57(10):937–954.

59. Singh I, Pahan K, Khan M, Singh AK. Cytokine-mediated induction of ceramide production is redox-sensitive. Implications to proinflammatory cytokine-mediated apoptosis in demyelinating diseases. *J Biol Chem.* 1998; 273(32):20354–20362.

60. Weisbrot-Lefkowitz M, Reuhl K, Perry B, et al. Overexpression of human glutathione peroxidase protects transgenic mice against focal cerebral ischemia/reperfusion damage. *Brain Res Mol Brain Res.* 1998;53(1–2): 333–338.

61. Skaper SD, Ancona B, Facci L, et al. Melatonin prevents the delayed death of hippocampal neurons induced by enhanced excitatory neurotransmission and the nitridergic pathway. *FASEB J.* 1998;12(9):725–731.

62. Drukarch B, Jongenelen CA, Schepens E, et al. Glutathione is involved in the granular storage of dopamine in rat PC12 pheochromocytoma cells: implications for the pathogenesis of Parkinson's disease. *J Neurosci.* 1996; 16(19):6038–6045.

63. Froissard P, Monrocq H, Duval D. Role of glutathione metabolism in the glutamate-induced programmed cell death of neuronal-like PC12 cells. *Eur J Pharmacol.* 1997; 326(1):93–99.

64 Mawatari K, Yasui Y, Sugitani K, et al. Reactive oxygen species involved in the glutamate toxicity of C6 glioma cells via xc antiporter system. *Neuroscience.* 1996;73(1): 201–208.

65. Offen D, Ziv I, Stermin H, et al.. Prevention of dopamine-induced cell death by thiol antioxidants: possible implications for treatment of Parkinson's disease. *Exp Neurol.* 1996;141(1):32–39.

66. Nakamura K, Wang W, Kang UJ. The role of glutathione in dopaminergic neuronal survival. *J Neurochem.* 1997; 69(5):1850–1858.

67. Drukarch B, Schepens E, Jongenelen CA, et al. Astrocyte-mediated enhancement of neuronal survival is abolished by glutathione deficiency. *Brain Res.* 1997; 770(1–2):123–130.

68. Wilson, J.X, Antioxidant defense of the brain: a role for astrocytes. *Can J Physiol Pharmacol.* 1997;75:1149–1163.

69 Kranich O, Dringen R, Sandberg M, Hamprecht B. Utilization of cysteine and cysteine precursors for the synthesis of glutathione in astroglial cultures: preference for cystine. *Glia.* 1998;22(1):11–18.

70. Kranich O, Hamprecht B, Dringen R. Different preferences in the utilization of amino acids for glutathione synthesis in cultured neurons and astroglial cells derived from rat brain. *Neurosci Lett.* 1996;219(3):211–214.

71. Adamson B, Schwarz D, Klugston P, et al. Delayed repair: the role of glutathione in a rat incisional wound model. *J Surg Res.* 1996;62(2):159–164.

72. Luo JL, Hammarqvist F, Andersson K, Wernerman J. Skeletal muscle glutathione after surgical trauma. *Ann Surg.* 1996;223(4):420–427.

73. Hammarqvist F, Luo JL, Cotgreave IA, et al. Skeletal muscle glutathione is depleted in critically ill patients. *Crit Care Med.* 1997;25(1):78–84.

74. Beale RJ, Bryg DJ, Bihari DJ. Immunonutrition in the critically ill: a systematic review of clinical outcome. *Crit Care Med.* 1999;27(12):2799–2805.

75. Kudsk KA, Minard G, Croce MA, et al. A randomized trial of isonitrogenous enteral diets after severe trauma. An immune-enhancing diet reduces septic complications. *Ann Surg.* 1996;224(4):531–543.

76. Witschi A, Reddy S, Stofer B, Lauterburg BH. The systemic availability of oral glutathione. *Eur J Clin Pharmacol.* 1992;43:667–669.

77. Bray TM, Taylor CO. Enhancement of tissue glutathione for antioxidant and immune functions in malnutrition. *Biochem Pharmacol.* 1994;47:2113–2123.

78. Puri RN, Meister A., Transport of glutathione as gamma-glutamylcysteinylglycyl ester, into liver and kidney. *Proc Natl Acad Sci U S A.* 1983;80:5258–5260.

79. Anderson ME, Powric F, Puri RN, Meister A. Glutathione monoethyl ester: preparation, uptake by tissues, and conversion to glutathione. *Arch Biochem Biophys.* 1985;239:538–548.

80. Birnbaum, SM, Winitz, M., Greenstein, J.P. Quantitative nutritional studies with water-soluble, chemically defined diets. III. Individual amino acids as sources of "non-essential" nitrogen. *Arch Biochem Biophys.* 1957;72: 428–436.

81. Dröge W, Gross A, Hack V, et al. Role of cysteine and glutathione in HIV infection and cancer cachexia: therapeutic intervention with N-acetylcysteine. *Adv Pharmacol.* 1997;38:581–600.

82. Gross A, Hack V, Stahl-Hennig C, Dröge W. Elevated hepatic gamma-glutamylcysteine synthetase activity and abnormal sulfate levels in liver and muscle tissue may explain abnormal cysteine and glutathione levels in SIV-infected rhesus macaques. *AIDS Res Hum Retroviruses.* 1996;12(17):1639–1641.

83. Kinscherf R, Fischbach T, Mihm S, et al. Effect of glutathione depletion and oral N-acetyl-cysteine treatment on CD4+ and CD8+ cells. *FASEB J.* 1994;8(6):448–451.

84. Staal FJ, Roederer M, Herzenberg LA, Herzenberg LA. Intracellular thiols regulate activation of nuclear factor kappa-B and transcription of human immunodeficiency virus. *Proc Natl Acad Sci U S A.* 1990;87:9943–9947.

85. Roederer M, Staal FJ, Raju PA, et al. Cytokine-stimulated human immunodeficiency virus replication is inhibited by N-acetyl-L-cysteine. *Proc Natl Acad Sci U S A.* 1990;87:4884–4888.

86. Kalebic T, Kinter A, Poli G, et al. Suppression of human immunodeficiency virus expression in chronically infected monocytic cells by glutathione, glutathione ester, and N-acetylcysteine. *Proc Natl Acad Sci. U S A.* 1991;88: 986–990.

87. Mant TG, Tempowski JH, Volans GN, Talbot JC. Adverse reactions to acetylcysteine and effects of overdose. *Br Med J (Clin Res Ed).* 1984;289:217–219.

88. Kajiwara Y, Yasutake A, Adachi T, Hirayama K. Methylmercury transport across the placenta via neutral amino acid carrier. *Arch Toxicol.* 1996;70:310–314.

89. Aschner M, Clarkson TW. Mercury 203 distribution in pregnant and nonpregnant rats following systemic infusions with thiol-containing amino acids. *Teratology.* 1987;36:321–328.

90. Aschner M, Clarkson TW. Distribution of mercury 203 in pregnant rats and their fetuses following systemic infusions with thiol-containing amino acids and glutathione during late gestation. *Teratology.* 1988;38:145–155.

91. Aschner M, Clarkson TW. Methyl mercury uptake across bovine brain capillary endothelial cells in vitro: the role of amino acids. *Pharmacol Toxicol.* 1989;64: 293–297.

92. Mokrzan EM, Kerper LE., Ballatori N, Clarkson TW. Methylmercury-thiol uptake into cultured brain capillary endothelial cells on amino acid system L. *J Pharmacol Exp Ther.* 1995;272:1277–1284.

93. Aschner M, Clarkson TW. Uptake of methylmercury in the rat brain: effects of amino acids. *Brain Res.* 1988; 462:31–39.

94. Kerper LE, Ballatori N, Clarkson TW. Methylmercury transport across the blood-brain barrier by an amino acid carrier. *Am J Physiol.* 1992;262(5 Pt 2):R761–R765.

95. Aschner M. Brain, kidney and liver 203 Hg-methyl mercury uptakes in the rat: relationship to the neutral amino acid carrier. *Pharmacol Toxicol.* 1989;65:17–20.

96. Aschner M, Eberle NB, Goderie S, Kimelberg HK. Methylmercury uptake in rat primary astrocyte cultures: the role of the neutral amino acid transport system. *Brain Res.* 1990;521: 221–228.

97. Blaylock RL. *Excitotoxins: The Taste that Kills.* Santa Fe, NMex: Health Press; 1997.

98. Abbas AK, Jardemark K, Lehmann A, et al. Bicarbonate-sensitive cysteine induced elevation of extracellular aspartate and glutamate in rat hippocampus in vitro. *Neurochem Int.* 1997;30:253–259.

99. Bounous G, Batist G, Gold P. Immunoenhancing property of dietary whey protein in mice: role of glutathione. *Clin Invest Med.* 1989;12:154–161.

100. Bounous G, Baruchel S, Falutz J, Gold P. Whey protein as a food supplement in HIV-seropositive individuals. *Clin Invest Med.* 1993;16:204–209.

101. Baruchel S, Viau G, Olivier R, et al. Nutriceutical modulation of glutathione with a humanized native milk serum protein isolate, Immunocal™: application in AIDS and cancer. In: Montagnier L, Oliver R, Pasquier C, eds. *Oxidative Stress in Cancer, AIDS, and Neurodegenerative Diseases.* New York, NY: Marcel Dekker; 1997.

102. Chen L, Stacewicz-Sapuntzakis M, Duncan C, et al. Oxidative DNA damage in prostate cancer patients consuming tomato sauce-based entrees as a whole-food intervention. *J Natl Cancer Inst.* 2001;93(24):1872–1879.

103. Smith TJ. Mechanisms of carcinogenesis inhibition by isothiocyanates. *Expert Opin Investig Drugs.* 2001; 10(12):2167–2174.

104. Zhang Y. Role of glutathione in the accumulation of anticarcinogenic isothiocyanates and their glutathione conjugates by murine hepatoma cells. *Carcinogenesis.* 2000;21(6):1175–1182.

105. Zhang Y. Molecular mechanisms of rapid cellular accumulation of anticarcinogenic isothiocyanates. *Carcinogenesis.* 2001;22(3):425–431.

106. Ye L, Zhang Y. Total intracellular accumulation levels of dietary isothiocyanates determine their activity in elevation of cellular glutathione and induction of Phase 2 detoxification enzyme. *Carcinogenesis.* 2001;22(12):1987–1992.

107. Fleshner NE, Kucuk O. Antioxidant dietary supplements: rationale and current status as chemopreventative agents for prostate caner. *Urology.* 2001;57(4 suppl 1):90–94.

108. Newberne PM, Butler WH. Acute and chronic effects of aflatoxins on the liver of domestic and laboratory animals: a review. *Cancer Res.* 1969;29:236–250.

109. Meerman JH, Beland FA, Ketterer B, et al. Identification of glutathione conjugates formed from N-hydroxy-2-actylaminofluorene in the rat. *Chem Biol Interact.* 1982; 39:149–168.

110. Boyland E, Sims P. The metabolism of benz(a)anthracene and dibenz(a,h)anthracene and their 5,6-dihydro derivatives by rat liver homogenates. *Biochem J.* 1965;97:7–16.

111. Waterfall JF, Sims P. Epoxy derivatives of aromatic polycyclic hydrocarbons. The properties and metabolism of epoxides related to benzo(a)pyrene and to 7-, 8-, and 9-dihydrobenzo(a)pyrene. *Biochem J.* 1972;128: 265–277.

112. Yamazoe Y, Roth RW, Kadlubar FF. Reactivity of benzidine diimine with DNA to form N-(deoxyguanosin-9-yl)-benzidine. *Carcinogenesis.* 1986;7:179–182.

113. Bounous G, Papenburg R, Kongshavn PAL. Dietary whey protein inhibits the development of dimethylhydrazine-induced malignancy. *Clin Invest Med.* 1988;11: 213–217.

114. McIntosh GH, Regester GQ, Le Leu RK, Royle PJ. Dairy proteins protect against dimethylhydrazine-induced intestinal cancers in rats. *J Nutr.* 1995;125:809–816.

115. Frei E, Bertram B, Wiessler M. Reduced glutathione inhibits the alkylation by N-nitrosodimethylamine of liver DNA in vivo and microsomal fraction in vitro. *Chem Biol Interact.* 1985;55:123–137.

116. Roberts JJ, Warwick GP. Mode of action of alkylating agents: formation of S-ethyl cysteine from ethyl methanesulphonate in vivo. *Nature.* 1957;179:1181–1182.

117. Coles B, Srai SK, Waynforth HB, Ketterer B. The major role of glutathione in the excretion of N,N-dimethyl-4-amino-azobenzene in the rat. *Chem Biol Interact.* 1983; 47:307–323.

118. Sims P. The metabolism of 3-methylcholanthrene and some related compounds by rat liver homogenates. *Biochem J.* 1966;98:215–228.

119. Sims P. The metabolism of 7- and 12-methylbenz(a)anthracenes and their derivatives. *Biochem J.* 1967;105: 591–598.

120. Djuric Z, Coles B, Fifer EK, et al. In vivo and in vitro formation of glutathione conjugates from the K-region epoxides of 1-nitropyrene. *Carcinogenesis.* 1987;8:1781–1786.

121. Ripple MO, Henry W, Rago RP, Wilding G. Prooxidant-antioxidant shift induced by androgen treatment of human prostate carcinoma cells. *J Natl Cancer Inst.* 1997;89:40–48.

122. Jimenez RE, Fischer AH, Petros JA, Amin MB. Glutathione-S-transferase pi gene methylation: the search for a molecular marker of prostatic adenocarcinoma. *Adv Anat Pathol.* 2000;7(6):382–389.

123. Singal R, van Wert J, Bashambu M. Cytosine methylation represses glutathione S-transferase P1 (GSTP1) gene expression in human prostate cancer cells. *Cancer Res.* 2001;61(12):4280–4286.

124. Lin X, Tascilar M, Lee WH, et al. GSTP1 CpG island hypermethylation is responsible for the absence of GSTP1 expression in human prostate cancer cells. *Am J Pathol.* 2001;59(5):1815–1826.

125. Toyota M, Issa JP. The role of DNA hypermethylation in human neoplasia. *Electrophoresis.* 2000;21(2):329–333.

126. Esteller M. Epigenetic lesions causing genetic lesions in human cancer: promoter hypermethylation of DNA repair genes. *Eur J Cancer.* 2000;36(18):2294–2300.

127. Esteller M, Herman JG. Cancer as an epigenetic disease: DNA methylation and chromatin alterations in human tumours. *J Pathol.* 2002;196(1):1–7.

128. Ahluwalia A, Yan P, Hurteau JA, et al. DNA methylation and ovarian cancer. I. Analysis of CpG island hypermethylation in human ovarian cancer using differential methylation hybridization. *Gynecol Oncol.* 2001; 82(2):261–268.

129. Laux DE, Curran EM, Welshons WV, et al. Hypermethylation of the Wilms' tumor suppressor gene CpG island in human breast carcinomas. *Breast Cancer Res Treat.* 1999;56(1):35–43.

130. Dammann R, Yang G, Pfeifer GP. Hypermethylation of the CpG island of Ras association domain family 1A (RASSF1A), a putative tumor suppressor gene from the 3p21.3 locus, occurs in a large percentage of human breast cancers. *Cancer Res.* 2001;61(7):3105–3109.

131. Kang SH, Choi HH, Kim SG, et al. Transcriptional inactivation of the tissue inhibitor of metalloproteinase-3 gene by DNA hypermethylation of the 5′-CpG island in human gastric cancer cell lines. *Int J Cancer.* 2000; 86(5):632–635.

132. Xiong Z, Wu AH, Bender CM, et al. Mismatch repair deficiency and CpG island hypermethylation in sporadic colon adenocarcinomas. *Cancer Epidemiol Biomarkers Prev.* 2001;10(7):799–803.

133. Lin X, Asgari K, Putzi MJ, et al. Reversal of GSTP1 CpG island hypermethylation and reactivation of pi-class glutathione S-transferase (GSTP1) expression in human prostate cancer cells by treatment with procainamide. *Cancer Res.* 2001;61(24):8611–8616.

134. Nelson WG, De Marzo AM, DeWeese TL. The molecular pathogenesis of prostate cancer: implications for prostate cancer prevention. *Urology.* 2001;57(4 suppl 1):39–45.

135. Stoner GD, Mukhtar H. Polyphenols as cancer chemopreventive agents. *J Cell Biochem Suppl.* 1995;22:169–180.

136. Piper JT, Singhal SS, Salameh MS, et al. Mechanisms of anticarcinogenic properties of curcumin: the effect of curcumin on glutathione linked detoxification enzymes in rat liver. *Int J Biochem Cell Biol.* 1998;30(4):445–456.

137. Bounous G, Stevenson MM, Kongshavn PA. Influence of dietary lactalbumin hydrolysate on the immune system of mice and resistance to salmonellosis. *J Infect Dis.*1981;144:281.

138. Bounous G, Letourneau L, Kongshavn PA. Influence of dietary protein type on the immune system of mice. *J Nutr.* 1983;113:1415–1421.

139. Hakkak R, Korourian S, Shelnutt SR, et al. Diets containing whey proteins or soy protein isolate protect against 7,12-dimethylbenz(a)anthracene-induced mammary tumors in female rats. *Cancer Epidemiol Biomarkers Prev.* 2000;9:113–117.

140. Dröge W, Kinscherf R, Mihm S, et al. Thiols and the immune system: effect of N-acetylcysteine on T-cell system in human subjects. *Methods Enzymol.* 1995;251:255–270.

141. Hack V, Breitkreutz R, Kinscherf R, et al. The redox state as a correlate of senescence and wasting and as a target for therapeutic intervention. *Blood.* 1998;92:59–67.

142. Parodi,P. A role for milk proteins in cancer prevention. *Aust J Dairy Technol.* 1998;53 37–47.

143. Meister A. Glutathione metabolism. *Methods Enzymol.* 1995;251:3–7.

144. Dröge, W., Breitkreutz, R. Glutathione and immune function. *Proc Nutr Soc.* 2000;59:595–600.

145. Liu M, Pelling JG, Ju J, et al. Antioxidant action via p53-mediated apoptosis. *Cancer Res.* 1998;48:1723–1729.

146. Morini M, Cai T, Aluigi MG, et al. The role of the thiol N-acetylcysteine in the prevention of tumor invasion and angiogenesis. *Int J Biol Markers.* 1999;14(4):268–271.

147. Locigno R, Castronovo V. Reduced glutathione system: role in cancer development, prevention, and treatment. *Int J Oncol.* 2001;19:221–236.

148. Weber GF, Mirza NM, Yunis EJ, et al. Localization and treatment of an oxidation-sensitive defect within the TCR-coupled signalling pathway that is associated with normal and premature immunologic aging. *Growth Dev Aging.* 1997;61(3–4):191–207.

149. Wang GM, Raghavachari N, Lou MF. Relationship of protein-glutathione mixed disulfide and thioltransferase in H_2O_2-induced cataract in cultured pig lens. *Exp Eye Res.* 1997;64:693–700.

150. Gravina SA, Mieyal JJ. Thioltransferase is a specific glutathionyl mixed disulfide oxidoreductase. Biochemistry. 1993;32:3368–3376.

151. Raghavachari N, Lou MF. Evidence for the presence of thioltransferase in the lens. *Exp Eye Res.* 1996;63:433–441.

152. Takemoto L. Increase in the intramolecular disulfide bonding of alpha-A crystallin during aging of the human lens. *Exp Eye Res.* 1996;63(5):585–590.

153. Harman D. Extending functional life span. *Exp Gerontol.* 1998;33(1–2):95–112.

154. Armeni T, Pieri C, Marra M, et al. Studies on the life prolonging effect of food restriction: glutathione levels and glyoxalase enzymes in rat liver. *Mech Ageing Dev.* 1998;101(1–2):101–110.

155. Donn J. Search Is on for Universal Drugs. Available at: http://www.cbsnews.com. (Accessed Nov 7, 2001.)

11

An Overview of Laryngeal Function for Voice Production

Ronald J. Baken

It is common to call the larynx the vocal organ, implying that it is the place where the voice is produced. If by "voice" we mean the sound that reaches our ears, then, in the strict sense, nothing could be further from the truth. The larynx generates only the raw material, the basic waveform of voice, that must be modified and shaped by the vocal tract, the highly adjustable tube of the upper airway. The next chapter will consider that crucial shaping process. In this chapter, we shall concentrate on the laryngeal contribution alone. To keep things as clear and distinct as possible, we refer to it as the "vocal source signal."[1]

Some liken the vocal system to a wind instrument. The analogy is useful if it is clear that the instrument in question is brass, and *not* a woodwind. That is, despite the fact that we often (inexactly) speak of "laryngeal vibrations," the vocal folds do not vibrate like a reed at all. Actually they "chop" the airstream into short bursts of airflow. Thus, if the vocal system is analogous to a musical instrument, it is more like a trumpet, and the vocal folds correspond to the trumpeter's lips. The *vocal source signal* is similar to the sound a trumpeter would make with only a mouthpiece. The *voice*, in contrast, is the output from the trumpet's bell.

The Glottal Wave

Before examining the basic mechanisms by which the vocal source signal is produced, it will be worthwhile to take a brief look at the signal itself. In its most fundamental sense, it could be described as a patterned airflow through the glottis (the space between the vocal folds) like the airflow graphed in Fig 11–1. Driven by the pressure of the air in the lungs, the flow increases relatively gradually, reaches a peak, and then decreases suddenly until it stops. After a brief pause, the pattern repeats. This flow pattern is called the "glottal wave."

The sharp cutoff of flow is particularly crucial, because it is this relatively sudden stoppage of the air flow that is truly the raw material of voice. To understand why, think of an experience that you may have had with a poorly designed plumbing system. The faucet is wide open, and the water is running at full force. The tap is then quickly turned off. Water flow stops abruptly and there is a sudden THUMP! from the pipes inside the walls. (Plumbers call this "water hammer.") This happens because, in the simplest terms, the sudden cessation causes moving molecules of water to

---

[1]An effort has been made to keep this chapter as informal as possible in the conviction that what might be lost in rigor will be more than compensated by what is gained in understanding. When basic principles of physics are crucial, however, they are provided for the novice in interruptions of the main flow of the text that are labeled *Intermezzo*. These can be skipped by those already familiar with the concepts in question. Also, the common scholarly practice of citing references in the text has been abandoned so as to improve the flow of information and lessen the intimidation it might engender. The works listed in the Bibliography, however, will buttress the discussion and help satisfy the curiosity of those who may be encouraged to dig deeper.

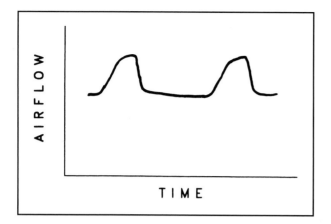

Fig 11–1. Two successive glottal waves. Increasing airflow is vertical.

collide with those ahead of them (like the chain-reaction collision caused when a car suddenly stops on a highway). This generates a kind of "shock wave." When the pipe is jolted by this shock, it moves, creating the vibrations in the air that we hear as a thump. The relatively sudden cutoff of flow that characterizes the glottal wave creates very much the same effect in the vocal tract. An impulse-like shock wave is produced that "excites" the vibration of the air molecules in the vocal tract. That excitation is the voice in its unrefined form.

The rate at which the shocks come is the *fundamental frequency* (F_0) of the voice and is measured in hertz (Hz). (One hertz equals one repetition per second.[2]) The time interval from the start of one cycle to the start of the next is called the *period* and is most conveniently measured in milliseconds. The intensity of phonation is related to the magnitude of the impulses. Now, any complex wave (such as the impulses that the larynx delivers into the vocal tract) is composed of a series of pure tones ("harmonics"), so the glottal source signal provides a palette of frequencies among which the rest of the vocal tract can select for creating the final vocal output.

This palette, or entire family, of frequencies is described as a *spectrum*. The spectrum's lowest tone is called the *fundamental*, and the rest of the tones are called *overtones*. The fundamental plus all of the overtones are called *partials*. Together, their frequencies form a *harmonic series*. The lowest partial is the fundamental. All of the other partials (each of which may be described as partial number N) have frequencies N times the fundamental. For example, the frequency of

the second partial is twice that of the fundamental. The third partial's frequency is three times that of the fundamental, and so on. In other words, the frequencies of the partial are integer multiples of the frequency of the fundamental.

Generating the Source Signal

We are now ready to explore how the glottal source signal is generated. The starring role in that performance definitely belongs to the vocal folds. The rest of the laryngeal structures (reviewed in the previous chapter) are, for our present purposes, essentially only stagehands that we can temporarily ignore.

Seen from the top, the vocal folds appear as whitish bands of tissue that stretch across the airway of the larynx. They join together and are attached to the inside of the thyroid cartilage in front, and each is anchored to an arytenoid cartilage at the rear. The arytenoid cartilages are capable of complex movements that cause the vocal folds to be brought into contact with each other along their length (approximated or adducted), or separated (abducted) to open the air passage for breathing. The space between the vocal folds is called the glottis. Since the vocal folds are movable, the *glottis* can be made quite large or reduced until its size is zero.

If we use special techniques (such as high-speed filming or stroboscopy) to observe vocal fold motion during phonation, we see the movements schematized in Fig 11–2. From an initial condition (Fig 11–2A) in which the vocal folds are in complete contact (and the glottal size is, therefore, zero), they increasingly separate until the glottis attains some maximal size (Fig 11–2D). The vocal folds then snap back to the midline, closing the glottis once again. In an average male voice, this cycle will repeat about 100 times each second. That is, the F_0 will be about 100 Hz. (Females have a higher F_0, on the order of 220 Hz.) Because the air in the lungs is under pressure, air is forced through the glottis during each glottal opening. The result is the patterned air flow of the glottal wave.

What causes this repeated opening and closing of the glottis, and how is its rate controlled? These have been central questions of voice research. Thanks to very rapid and significant advances in the past few years, we now understand quite a bit about what drives the phonatory process. What we know is derived from empirical studies by a large and international array of voice scientists (several of whom are cited in the Bibli-

---

[2]"Fundamental frequency" and "pitch" are related but not the same. F_0 is a physical attribute; pitch is a perception. One does not grow in a lock-step way with the other. The terminological confusion is not helped by the fact that engineers—whose work accounts for a significant fraction of the vocal research literature—typically refer to F_0 as "pitch"!

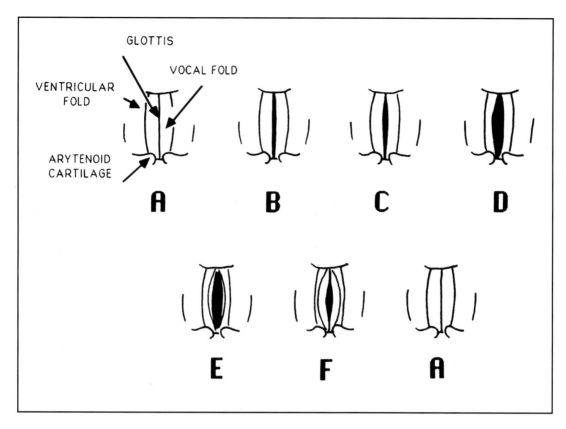

Fig 11–2. The glottal cycle as seen from above. Important anatomical landmarks are indicated.

ography) and from modern mathematical models of the phonatory process, especially those developed by Titze and Ishizaka. As with so much in the natural world, the mechanisms turn out to be both elegant (and simpler than we might have feared) and complex (and hence more complicated than we might have hoped). Although thorough study of the research literature is clearly essential for anyone intending seriously to pursue voice research, and examination of the available models is quite rewarding for those who have the advanced mathematical skills to follow them, we shall only be able to undertake a brief nonmathematical summary of the highlights of the vast store of information that is available. Readers who need to know more or are simply intrigued are urged and implored to delve much deeper.

To understand any of the finer details of the vocal process will require that we view the vocal folds in cross-section (rather than from the traditional viewpoint from above), examine a little bit of their fine structure, and consider a few things about the nature of air flow and pressure.

Structure of the Vocal Folds

The cross-section of a vocal fold in Fig 11–3 shows that it is basically divisible into two zones. Essentially, the vocal fold is built on the supporting mass of the thyroarytenoid muscle that runs along its length. This muscular region, which accounts for most of the bulk of the vocal fold, is referred to as the vocal fold *body*; but it would be a serious mistake to view the body as nothing more than a support for the overlying tissue. Contraction and relaxation of the thyroarytenoid muscle can significantly change its length, thickness, and stiffness. We shall see that these changes play a vital role in determining the characteristics of the vocal source signal.

The body of the vocal fold is wrapped in a layer called the *cover*. Its structure is actually quite complex, but the fine details need not concern us here. It is enough to understand that the cover's outer layer is formed by epithelial tissues (similar to the linings of the rest of the throat and to the upper layers of skin on the surface of the body), and that, under this epithelium, there is a network of fibers that, in some significant ways,

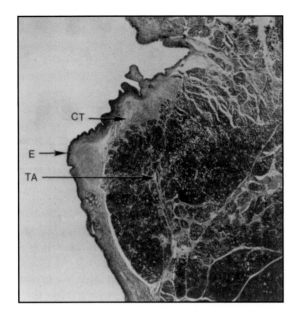

Fig 11–3. Cross-section of the human vocal folds. Courtesy of Dr. Joel C. Kahane, Memphis State University.

resemble rubber bands. The elastic network is particularly well formed near the edge of the upper portion of the vocal fold, where it constitutes the *vocal ligament*. This composite structure has very definite inherent mechanical properties, but, unlike the vocal fold body, those properties cannot normally be altered. The cover is attached relatively loosely. Like the skin on the back of one's hand, it is partially free to slide over the underlying vocal fold body. This mobility is important in phonation.

The Glottal Cycle

We are finally ready to examine the phonatory cycle in more meaningful detail. We shall assume that there is a supply of air in the lungs and that it has been pressurized (as it must be if phonation is to occur) to a level of perhaps 7 cm H_2O (a typical value).[3] The vocal folds are shown schematically in cross-section in Fig 11–4, and we shall consider their changing shape and posture as the vocal cycle progresses.

At the start of the cycle (Fig 11–4A), the vocal folds are approximated. Note their cross-sectional shape: Each is a wedge, with a fairly flat surface on top and a sloping section below. The glottis at this stage is said to be "convergent"—it narrows from a relatively wide

space at the level of the lower surface of the vocal folds to no space at all higher up. The approximation of the vocal folds closes the airway; there is no flow. All the pressure of the air in the lungs acts on the sloping surface of the glottal walls. The pressure tends to push the vocal folds somewhat apart (Fig 11–4B), and the separation grows wider and wider as the pressure continues to act (Fig 11–4C). Finally, the pressure forces separation all the way to the upper surface of the vocal folds, and a glottal space appears (Fig 11–4D). Air flow through the (partially) open glottis begins: the rising part of the glottal flow wave is now under way.

First Intermezzo

At this point, it might be useful to pause briefly to consider some basic facts about the physics of airflow and air pressure. The mathematical values and formulas will not be important to us, but the *concepts* are crucial to understanding the next events in the vocal cycle.

The energy available in the flow of any gas is stored in two forms. Everyday experience tells us that *pressure* represents one kind of energy storage. (Compressed air, for example, is commonly used to power machinery such as jackhammers.) Pressure represents what the physicist calls potential energy, energy waiting to be released to do work. The higher the pressure, the greater the *potential energy* available. Moving gas molecules have momentum, and that momentum also represents energy. So *motion* is the other form of energy storage. (The force against which one must struggle when walking into a very strong wind is produced by the moving air molecules releasing their momentum energy as they collide with you.) The energy of motion is called *kinetic* energy. The faster the gas molecules are moving, the greater is their kinetic energy.

Consider now the flow of air from the lower airway, through the constriction of the glottis, and into the wider space of the upper larynx just above the vocal folds. The diagram in Fig 11–5 represents this flow with the simplifying assumption that the tract has a uniform size except at the glottis, the shape of which has been made geometrically simpler.

Most basic to what will follow is the fact that the rate of air flow must be the same everywhere in the system. If, for example, 100 ml of air is entering the tube each second, then 100 ml/sec must be leaving it. (If not, the tube would soon either blow up and burst or empty itself of all air and generate a potent vacuum!) If the input and

---

[3] cm H_2O (read: centimeters of water) is the standard unit of pressure in vocal physiology. One cm H_2O is enough pressure to hold up a column of water 1 centimeter high.

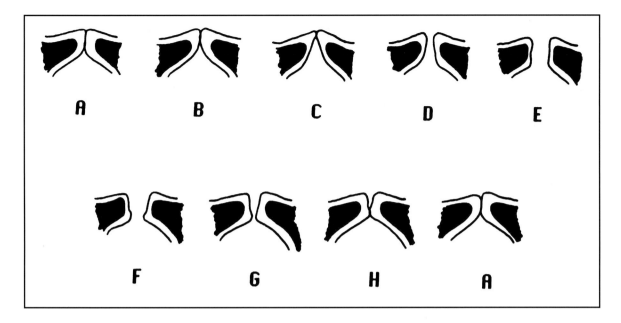

Fig 11–4. Movements of the vocal folds during phonation. The vocal folds are seen in cross-section.

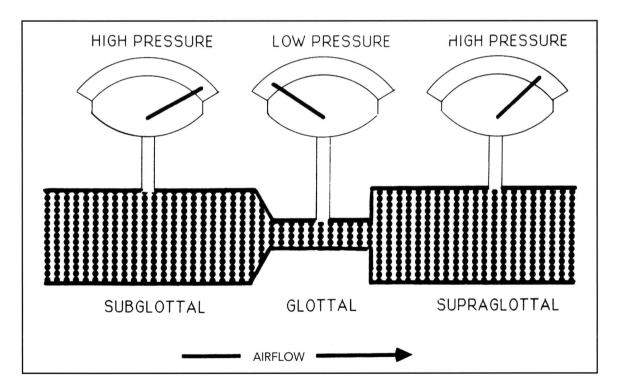

Fig 11–5. Pressure changes in the laryngeal airway, showing the Bernoulli effect. Pressure is sensed by gauges connected to the region below the glottis (subglottal), to the glottal space, and to the area just above the glottis (supraglottal). Air pressure within the glottis is lower than in the spaces above or below it.

output are the same, it must also be true that 100 ml of air moves past *every* point in the tube each second. Let us also remember that (all other things being equal) a given volume of air represents a given number of air molecules. Therefore, we can say that the same number of air molecules passes every point in the system every second.

This does not mean, however, that the *speed* of the air molecules (in meters per second, for example) is the same everywhere. The bottleneck at the glottis poses a special problem. Imagine that the airflow is a parade that fills the street from curb to curb. The marchers are air molecules, arranged in neat rows. Above and below the glottis, the street is quite spacious. In these regions, each row of molecules in the parade is so wide that only a few rows need to pass by every second in order to have a given number of individual marchers pass the spectators, so the rows of molecules do not have to move forward very quickly; just a few rows per second forward movement will do. Now the parade comes to the glottis—a narrowing of the parade route. The rows must become narrower, and fewer marchers can fit in each row, but, every second, the same number of marchers must still pass the parade watchers. (If fewer go by, the marchers to the rear will bunch up on them, creating a major traffic jam.) Since each row holds fewer marchers, and since the same number of marchers must pass every second, there is only one solution: the rows must pass more quickly. All the marchers in the glottal bottleneck have to speed up. When they return to the broader route above the vocal folds, they can all slow down again, but for the moment they must march in quickstep.

The moving air in the lower part of the larynx has a certain amount of energy. It is shared between its potential (pressure) and kinetic (speed of motion) energy, but its energy total is fixed. When the molecules speed up in the constriction, their kinetic energy increases. Such an increase would seem to imply that the total (potential + kinetic) energy would go up, but this cannot be. The total energy cannot increase, because one cannot create energy out of nothing. So, if the total must stay the same, and if the kinetic energy increases, then there is no way around it: The potential energy must decrease, which is another way of saying that the pressure must go down. Of course, when the air molecules reach the wider passage of the laryngeal region above the glottis and slow down again, their kinetic energy will decrease, and so their potential energy will be restored. What all of this means is that, if air is flowing through a narrow glottis, the pressure inside the glottal space will be less than the pressure in the wider spaces above the below it. This phenomenon (which is, of course, true for any constricted tube) is called the Bernoulli effect, and it plays an important role in the closing phase of the vocal cycle.

End of First Intermezzo

Now we can return to the vocal cycle, which we left in Fig 11–4D with the glottis just barely open. In spite of the small opening, the pressure acting on the underside of the vocal folds is still operative, and so the edges of the vocal folds continue to be blown apart. But now there is an airflow through the narrow glottal constriction, which implies that the air pressure inside the glottis must be less than the air pressure above or below it. This relatively negative pressure has the effect of "sucking" the lower margins of the glottis back toward the midline. Also, having been pushed to the side, the lower walls of the glottis have been compressed, almost like foam rubber. The result is that they will tend to spring back, that is, to return to their original position. Therefore, as the cycle proceeds, the lower margins have begun their return to the midline (Fig 11–4E and F), while the upper edges of the vocal folds are still being blown apart.

At this point, a new effect comes into play. Remember that the very edge of the upper portion of the vocal fold contains the highly elastic vocal ligament. As the edge of the vocal fold is pushed farther from the midline, the ligament is stretched more and more. Like a rubber band, the more it is stretched, the stronger is the tendency for it to snap back to its original shape. After a while, this restorative force begins to overcome the outward-pushing force of the air pressure (which, in any case, has been growing weaker as the approximation of lower portions of the folds increasingly pinches off the airflow). The upper portions of the vocal folds, therefore, begin to snap back toward the midline (Fig 11–4 G and H). Ultimately, the glottis will be restored to its original closed shape, and the cycle is ready to repeat.

Let us pause again, this time for a few observations on what has happened. One important consideration is that the motion of the vocal folds has been driven by a combination of *aerodynamic* forces (the lung pressure and the Bernoulli pressure) and the elastic (recoil) properties of the tissues. Hence, the mechanism just described is commonly called the *myoelastic aerodynamic* model of phonation. Another important fact is that the shape of the glottis, and, in particular, its convergence, has played an important role.

Even more interesting is the fact that the upper and lower portions of the vocal folds do not move in synchrony. The lower part is always somewhat ahead of the upper part: It begins to separate earlier, and it begins to return to the midline before the upper portion does. There is, in the more formal language of the vocal physiologists, a *vertical phase difference*. Although the reasons are far beyond the scope of our present discussion, it has been demonstrated that this phase difference is critical in maintaining normal phonation.

Finally, a careful examination of Fig 11–4 shows that a great deal of the vocal fold movement is accounted for by displacement of the mobile vocal fold cover and changes in its shape. (In fact, the rippling of the cover creates a "mucosal wave" that can be seen on the upper surface of the vocal fold during stroboscopic observation.) If there were no vocal fold cover (or its equivalent), normal phonation would not be possible.

Changing Vocal Fundamental Frequency and Amplitude

Several vocal characteristics can be voluntarily altered. The two most significant are F_0 and intensity. Their modification is important in speech and a *sine qua non* of singing.

Control of Vocal Fundamental Frequency

Changing the vocal F_0 means varying the rate at which the glottal wave repeats. The most efficient way of doing this is by modifying the mechanical properties of the vocal folds (although, as we shall see, it is also possible to change F_0 by altering the pressure of the air supply). The structure of the vocal fold, and its relationship to the rest of the larynx makes this fairly easy to accomplish by a number of means. We shall look at the most effective.

A reminder of a few anatomical facts is in order. Recall that the vocal folds stretch from the arytenoid cartilages (which are anchored to the back of the cricoid cartilage) at the rear, to the inside of the thyroid cartilage in front. The thyroid cartilage articulates with the cricoid cartilage in such a way that it can pivot, somewhat like the visor on a helmet. There is a muscle—the cricothyroid—that spans the gap from the thyroid to the cricoid cartilage in front. When it contracts, it pulls the two closer together. Because of the visor-like relationship of the thyroid and cricoid cartilages, contraction of the cricothyroid muscle causes the thyroid cartilage to pivot. Also, the thyroid cartilage will slide forward a bit. The result of these actions is diagrammed in Fig 11–6. Note that the net effect is to increase the distance from the arytenoid cartilages to the inside of the thyroid cartilage. Since the vocal folds must span the arytenoid-to-thyroid space, increasing this distance *stretches* the vocal folds and makes them *longer*.

These changes entail important modifications of the glottal cycle. First, if the vocal folds are longer, then

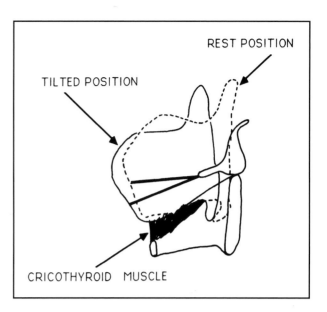

Fig 11–6. Contraction of the cricothyroid muscle causes the thyroid cartilage to rotate about its point of attachment to the cricoid cartilage. It is also pulled slightly forward. The result is to increase the length of the vocal folds, schematized here by *heavy straight lines*.

they present a greater surface area to the pressure in the airway just below them. That, in essence, makes the pressure more effective in separating the vocal folds during the opening phase of the cycle. The vocal folds, therefore, separate more quickly, shortening the cycle. A greater repetition rate, and hence a higher F_0, will be the result. But there is more. Stretching the vocal fold means that the elastic fibers of the vocal fold cover, and in particular the fibers of the vocal ligament, are stretched. The vocal ligament is like a rubber band, and stretching it has the same effect: The resulting increase in stiffness makes it snap back more quickly after being "plucked." Therefore, once the stretched vocal folds have been blown apart, they return more quickly to the midline, so increasing the stiffness of the vocal fold cover (by contracting the cricothyroid muscle) also shortens the cycle (increasing the repetition rate) and thereby contributes to the rise in F_0.

It is also possible to increase the stiffness of the vocal fold body by contracting the thyroarytenoid muscle (which, let us recall, *is* the body of the vocal fold) and having it pull against the stretching influence of the contracting cricothyroid muscle.[4] This increased con-

---

[4]To get a sense of the effect, rest your forearm and elbow on a table, relax your arm, and palpate your biceps muscle. Now (without letting your forearm rise from the table) contract your biceps ("make a muscle") and feel your biceps again. It is now much stiffer.

traction augments the stiffness of the vocal fold cover, and so it, too, helps to shorten the cycle.

Since the phonatory process is governed by aerodynamics as well as by biomechanics, it would be surprising if vocal F_0 could not also be changed by modifying the air pressure driving the cycle. Raising the pressure has the effect of increasing vocal intensity (to be discussed shortly), but, as any vocal artist is no doubt aware, there is a strong tendency for F_0 to increase as well. The exact basis of this effect has not been established for certain, but Titze has proposed a likely hypothesis, which has to do with the distance to which higher pressure drives the edge of the vocal fold from the midline. Several experiments have demonstrated that the vocal F_0 changes by about 4 or 5 Hz for every 1 cm H_2O. For purposes of ordinary conversational speech, this amount of frequency change is not likely to be significant. However, implying as it does that the pitch of the vocal tone will rise as the loudness does, it is clearly of importance to singers, who will have to compensate to deal with it.

Control of Vocal Intensity

Vocal intensity[5] is a function of the amount of excitation that the glottal waves deliver to the air in the vocal tract. It is easy to see that, all other things being equal, the greater the amplitude of the glottal wave, the greater the resulting vocal tract excitation and hence the more intense the vocal signal. Raising the pressure of the air supply effectively increases the amount of air that is pushed through the glottis whenever it is open. That translates to a "taller" glottal flow wave. Hence, increased lung pressure translates to greater vocal intensity.

However, we learned earlier that it is the sudden cessation of the flow that bears the primary responsibility for setting the air of the vocal tract into acoustic vibration. The sharper the flow cutoff, the greater the vocal tract excitation will be and the more intense the resulting vocal signal. Greater vocal intensity is, in fact, associated with a much steeper decreasing phase of the glottal wave. This effect is achieved not only by the higher pressure, but also by voluntary changes in the biomechanics of the vocal folds that tend to resist the increase in airflow that the higher pressure would produce. So intensity increases are produced by a carefully regulated interaction of a higher driving pressure and an increased glottal resistance to flow.

Registers

To an outsider, there is probably no concept in the domain of the vocal arts that seems so contentious as that of vocal registers. Dozens and scores of different terms have been coined to describe subjective voice qualities, and the physiologic reality of almost every one of them as a voice register has been both the victim of vehement denial and the object of passionate defense.

Different registers sound different, to be sure. But variant acoustic impressions derive from changes in the way the vocal source signal is molded by the vocal tract as well as from differences in the vocal source signal itself. Because our concern here is solely with the source signal, we can simplify the problem of registers significantly by looking only at variations in laryngeal function. To keep the matter clear, let us agree to call the results of such differences *laryngeal registers*. We shall also impose the following requirements:

1. A laryngeal register must reflect a specific and distinct mode of laryngeal action. Vocal tract contributions are irrelevant.
2. A laryngeal register is produced across a contiguous range of fundamental frequencies.
3. The F_0 range of any given laryngeal register has little overlap with the F_0 range of any other register.

With these restrictions, only three distinct laryngeal registers have been verified. To avoid problems due to prior—and, frankly, often confused—terminology, and to reduce the influence of connotations commonly associated with older names, Hollien has suggested that we adopt completely new designations for these narrowly defined registers.

1. *Modal register* describes the laryngeal function in the range of fundamental frequencies most commonly used by untrained speakers (from about 75 to about 450 Hz in men; 130 to 520 Hz in women). The name, in fact, derives from the statistical term for "most common value." This register may include the musical "chest," "head," or "low," "mid," and "high" registers, depending on how these are defined.

2. *Pulse register* occurs in the F_0 range at the low end of the frequency scale (25 to 80 Hz in men; 20 to 45 Hz in women). The laryngeal output is perceived as pulsatile in nature. The term is broadly synonymous with "vocal fry," "glottal fry," or the musical term "strohbass."

---

[5]The relationship of vocal intensity and loudness is analogous to that of vocal F_0 and pitch. The former is a physical characteristic, the latter a perception, and the two are not exactly equivalent. We can measure intensity, but only judge loudness, which is influenced by many factors.

3. *Loft register* is employed at the upper end of the vocal continuum (275 to 620 Hz in men; 490 to 1,130 Hz in women). The name is intended to convey a sense of "upper reaches." In general, it corresponds to the older term "falsetto."

Modal register phonation is implicitly accepted as the norm, and, in fact, the glottal cycle we have been considering is that which characterizes it. Pulse and loft differ from modal register in the shape and tension to which the vocal folds are adjusted.

Pulse Register

As diagramed in Fig 11–7, pulse register phonation is accomplished with vocal folds that are rather massive in cross-section, a configuration that is achieved by freeing them of essentially all tension. (Laminagraphic studies by Allen and Hollien have suggested that the relaxation in the glottal region may be so complete that the ventricular folds may actually lie against the upper surface of the vocal folds. If this occurs, the effective mass of the vocal folds would obviously be increased enormously.) These two conditions—increased mass and reduced stretch—account for the very low fundamental frequencies associated with this laryngeal register. It takes longer for the vocal

folds to be blown apart, and, once moving laterally, their increased mass results in greater lateral momentum that sustains the abductory motion longer. The lack of tension implies a reduction of restoring (elastic) recoil, so the abductory motion is not opposed as vigorously, nor does closure, once it is finally under way, proceed as fast.

Pulse register phonation is associated with a very interesting pattern of vocal tract excitations, the results of which are also shown in Fig 11–7. Modal register glottal waves are relatively uniform in duration and amplitude, a fact that is reflected in the great similarity of the acoustic waves that they generate in the vocal tract. Pulse register, however, typically shows a pattern of weaker, shorter glottal waves alternating with larger and longer ones. The exact mechanisms that account for this behavior have yet to be demonstrated, but the phenomenon is so characteristic that some include its presence in the definition of this laryngeal register.

Loft Register

If pulse register represents an extreme in reduction of vocal fold tension, then loft register is just the opposite: Tension is increased to very high levels. The results are diagramed in Fig 11–7. The tension causes the vocal folds to be thinned to such an extent that they take the shape of mere shelves of tissue that may contact each other only over a small vertical distance. (In fact, it is a common observation that loft register phonation may be accomplished with no actual vocal fold contact at all.) A moment's reflection indicates that, under these conditions, vocal fold motion should be rapid but with a small excursion. The increased restorative forces associated with the higher tension cause the opening phase to be terminated early, and the recoil to the midline, driven by greater elasticity, will also be quite fast. On the whole then, loft register adjustment produces high vocal F_0, and the reduction in maximal glottic size generates only weak vocal tract excitations, associated with diminished vocal intensity.

Vocal Source Contributions to Voice Quality

Not all of what we hear in the voice is due to the shaping of the vocal source signal by the resonant and filtering actions of the vocal tract. Any product, after all, is a reflection of the raw material that created it, so some aspects of voice quality are bound to be inherent in the glottal wave itself (and, by inference, in the actions of the vocal folds). The time has now come to

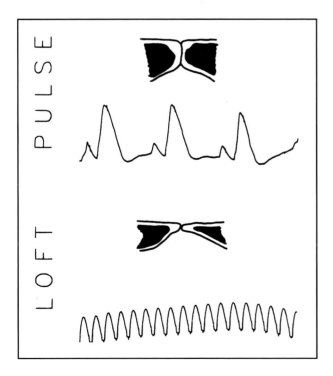

Fig 11–7. Vocal fold configuration and resulting waves in the pulse and loft register. The vocal folds are schematized in cross-section.

examine the vocal source signal in greater detail. To do so, we shall have to consider the *source spectrum*. Some readers may find it useful to pause for the second intermezzo.

Second Intermezzo

We begin with the somewhat startling statement that there really is no separate and distinct physical entity called sound. What we label by that name is simply our perception of changes in air pressure. The pressure changes must occur within a certain range of rates (about 20 to about 20,000 per second) and must be greater than a certain minimal size before we perceive them, but they are physically no different from the air pressure changes measured by a barometer.

The simplest possible way in which any variable—including air pressure—can change is referred to as "simple harmonic motion" and is depicted at the top of Fig 11–8, with pressure on the vertical axis and time on the horizontal axis. The value of the pressure at any given point is proportional to the *sine* of its time location. Hence, this pattern is referred to as a *sine wave*. A sine wave can be almost completely characterized by its F_0 (repetition rate) and by the extent of its pressure change (amplitude).[6]

Very few sounds of the natural world are simple sine waves. Almost all are very much more complex, but a physical law known as the *Fourier theorem* tells us that any complex sound is composed of a series of sine waves of different frequencies and amplitudes. The reality of this statement is demonstrated in Fig 11–9, in which a complex wave is shown with the four sine wave components, which were added together to create it. (Dissecting a complex wave into its sine wave components is known as *Fourier analysis*.) If the repetition rate of the complex wave is perfectly regular, the wave is said to be *periodic*. In that case, all the component sine waves will be integer multiples of the complex wave's F_0. Such components are called *harmonics*. In Fig 11–9, the component sine waves have frequencies of 1,

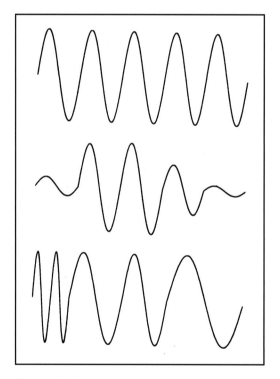

Fig 11–8. Sine waves represent the simplest form of pressure change. **Top:** Five sine wave cycles of equal period and amplitude. **Middle:** Waves of constant period but varying amplitudes. **Bottom:** Constant amplitude and variable period.

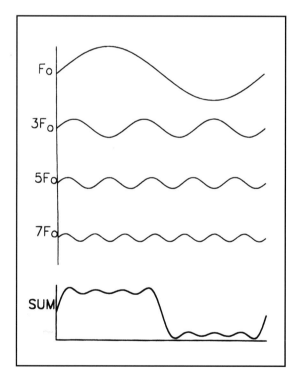

Fig 11–9. Any complex repetitive wave is the sum of a series of sine waves of different frequencies and amplitudes. The wave shown at the **bottom** is the sum of the four "harmonics" shown above it.

---

[6]There is another descriptor, known as the phase angle, that specifies the difference in starting times among two or more waves. When all three parameters—frequency, amplitude, and phase angle—are specified, we know all there is to know about a sine wave. The phase angle is unimportant to the present discussion, however.

3, 5, and 7 times F_0; they are harmonic frequencies. Notice, however, that they have different amplitudes.

So, any complex wave could be expressed as a tabulation of component frequencies with their respective amplitudes, but such a list would hardly be easy to deal with. A better idea is to produce a graph of the information. We can do this by drawing lines along a frequency dimension wherever there is a component sine wave. The height of the line can represent the amplitude of the component. For the wave of Fig 11–10A, such a graph would look like the plot in Fig 11–10B. A plot of this type is known as an *amplitude spectrum*. It is nothing but a graphic summary of the components of a complex periodic wave.

Actually, because of the need to begin with simple cases, we have been a bit dishonest. We have behaved as if the wave that we considered as our example is perfectly periodic, that is, it was assumed to repeat with perfect precision and exactitude, each repetition a precise replica of every other. The spectrum of Fig 11–10B is called a *line spectrum*, because it is composed of lines separated by empty space on the graph. (There are harmonic frequencies, and nothing else.) But a precisely periodic wave is not to be found in nature. There is always some noise, some irregularity of repetition.

Pure noise—a *totally* random wave, such as is shown in Fig 11–10C—has no harmonics. It is composed of sine waves of any and all frequencies (at least within a specifiable range) having unpredictable amplitudes. Its spectrum does not have discrete lines: Since all frequencies are present, the lines fill in all available spaces on the graph, forming a *continuous spectrum*, as in Fig 11–10D. If a signal is essentially periodic, but also has some noise or irregularity, its spectrum will be a combination of a line and a continuous spectrum: There will be some "fill in" between the harmonic lines.

End of Second Intermezzo

The Vocal Source Spectrum

The amplitude spectrum of an ideal (noise free) glottal wave is illustrated in Fig 11–11 (top). The regular spacing of the lines tells us that the components are har-

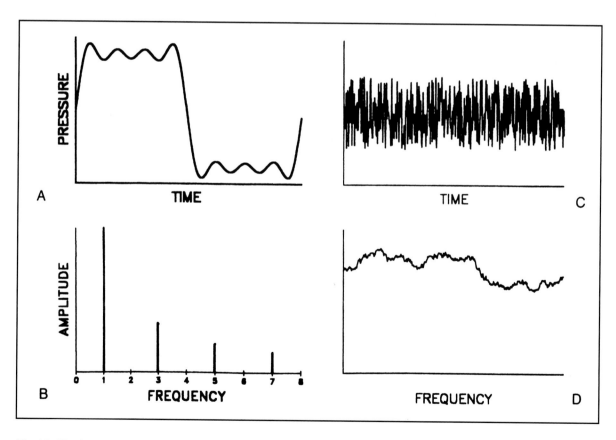

Fig 11–10. Amplitude spectra. The components of the complex wave of Fig 11–9 (redrawn in **A**) can be indicated in the *line spectrum* shown in **B**. Any purely periodic wave has a line spectrum. A random (noise) wave, such as the one shown in **C**, will have a *continuous spectrum*, like that of **D**.

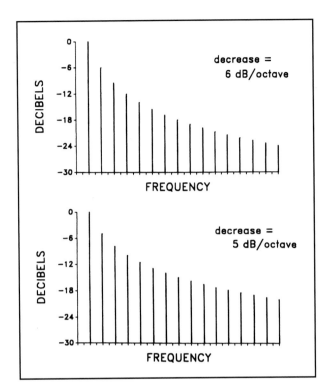

Fig 11–11. Spectra of the glottal wave. In the **upper spectrum**, the "roll-off" (decrease) in the amplitudes of the harmonic lines is at the rate of 6 dB/octave. This is typical of the voice at conversational intensity. Increasing intensity (or voluntary adjustment of the vocal folds) can strengthen the higher harmonics, resulting in a roll-off that is less steep, as in the **lower spectrum**.

monic frequencies. The orderly decrease in their amplitude with increasing frequency is referred to as the spectrum's *roll-off*. For a typical healthy voice, it amounts to an attenuation of approximately 6 dB per octave of frequency increase.

Let us take a moment and explore where the high-frequency harmonics come from. Consider the waveform we have used as an example (Fig 11–9 or 11–10A). It has a sudden shift at its midpoint. Such a sharp movement represents a fairly rapid rate of change in the acoustic pressure. To generate such a quick change, there must be some among the sine wave components of the waveform that also have rapid change. The higher the frequency of a wave, the faster is its pressure variation, so rapid alterations in a wave translate to stronger high-frequency components in the wave's spectrum.

The sharp cutoff of airflow that is characteristic of the glottal wave now takes on even more significance. It is an important source of the high-frequency components of the glottal source spectrum. The sharper the cutoff becomes, the stronger those high-frequency compo-

nents should be. It is known that the cutoff becomes sharper as vocal intensity increases. It is also possible to sharpen the cutoff by adjusting the mechanical properties of the vocal folds. Also, of considerable importance to professional voice users, *stronger high harmonics give the voice a perceptually "brighter" sound.* Here, then, is one aspect of voice quality that derives directly from laryngeal adjustment.

Glottal Wave Irregularity

Examination of the amplitude spectrum of a real glottal wave (Fig 11–12) shows it to be different in two significant ways from the ideals we have examined so far. The harmonic lines are not nearly so sharp as we have pictured them thus far, and there is continuous energy that fills in part of the space between them. These differences are the result of two phenomena that we have avoided so far, but that are very much part of any real vocal signal: airflow turbulence and vibrational irregularity.

Turbulence

Airflow through the glottis is not perfectly smooth or (in the language of physics) "laminar." In other words, the air molecules do not all really move in straight lines, like the marchers in a parade. Whenever a flow is forced through a sufficiently narrow opening (like the glottis), there is always a certain amount of random movement or *turbulence*. Also, many individuals do not achieve complete phonatory closure. The arytenoid cartilages may fail to meet at the midline, or

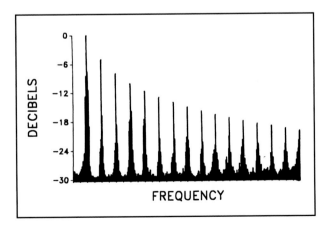

Fig 11–12. Amplitude spectrum of a real glottal wave. Note the thickening of the harmonic lines and the "fill" between them. These result from irregularity of the glottal vibration and airflow turbulence.

they may be angled in such a way that the posterior part of the glottis remains slightly open. In either case, there is often an open pathway by which air can travel around the glottis. This leakage is almost certain to be quite turbulent.

If some of the air molecules are moving in random directions, then there must be randomly oriented pressures acting on them. Since sound is nothing but pressure variation, these erratic pressures contribute randomness to the final acoustic product. That randomness, of course, is noise, and it adds its continuous spectrum characteristics to the line spectrum of the glottal pulsing, partially filling in the spaces between the harmonics.

What is the perceptual effect? Within reasonable limits, added noise in the spectrum produces a sensation of fuzzy softness to the sound, perhaps a velvety quality. A bit more turbulence might be heard as breathiness, or perhaps huskiness, and a lot of turbulence contributes to the perception of hoarseness.

Vibrational Irregularity

Glottal waves are imperfect not only because there are flow turbulences, but also because there is frequency and amplitude *perturbation*: Neither the frequency nor the amplitude of any two successive waves is ever likely to be precisely the same[7] (see Fig 11–13). The average differences are quite small: on the order of 40 μsec for period, and about 0.4 dB for amplitude. Still, if the F_0 and amplitude are varying, then the harmonics (which, let us recall, have frequencies that are integral multiples of F_0) must be varying. This results in thickening of the harmonic lines in the spectrum—an indication that the perturbation has introduced an uncertainty about what the exact frequency value of any given harmonic is.

Normal perturbation does not seem to be measurably lessened by attempts to control the voice or by vocal training. Its irreducibility stems from the fact that it reflects inherent instabilities and irregularities

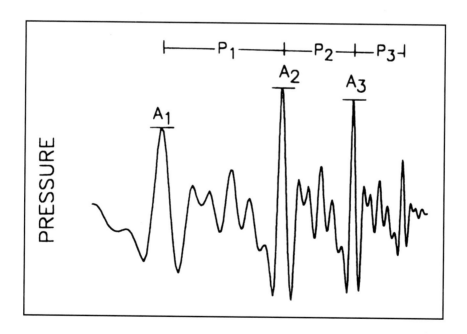

Fig 11–13. Perturbation as shown in the acoustic wave of a vowel. The difference between P(eriod)$_1$, and P$_2$, and between P$_2$ and P$_3$ is called the *frequency perturbation* or *jitter*. The amplitude difference (A$_1$, A$_2$, A$_3$) is the *amplitude perturbation*, or *shimmer*. (For illustrative purposes, the differences shown here have been made greater than would be expected in a normal voice.)

---

[7]In the argot of everyday professional communication, frequency perturbation is referred to as *jitter*, amplitude perturbation as *shimmer*.

in the contractions of the muscles that control the vocal structures. It is not surprising, therefore, that it is one of the factors that give the voice a natural, humanlike quality (a fact appreciated by the creator of the "vox humana" stop on a pipe organ).

Coda

So, at least in outline, we have gone from two flaps of tissue blowing in the pulmonary wind to a palette of acoustic potentials ready to be refined into a baby's cry, a sports fan's cheer, a laborer's grunt, or a Verdi aria.

The voice may be a wondrous thing, but the process of voice production is neither mysterious nor inexplicable. In this chapter, we have been able to explore only the barest outline of the process by which voice is produced, just enough to get the reader started. (There is much that is not understood about laryngeal function, but there is very much that is.) It is obvious, however, that nothing more than perfectly ordinary laws of physics and common principles of physiology are involved.

The mystery, of course, enters with the art.

Bibliography

Of necessity, but unfortunately, this chapter could only touch on the highest of the high points of what is understood about laryngeal function. There is a great deal that the serious student of voice will want to know. This bibliography is intended to help in satisfying that desire.

The listing has been divided by topic to facilitate finding a source for whatever specific information is required. We hope readers will also be encouraged to browse, seeking items that strike a chord resonant with their interests.

Despite its length, this bibliography represents only a very small portion of what is available.

General Introductory Texts

Baken RJ. *Clinical measurement of speech and voice*. Boston: Little, Brown; 1987:518.

Bunch M. *Dynamics of the singing voice*. New York: Springer; 1982:156.

Daniloff R, Schuckers G, Feth L. *The physiology of speech and hearing*. Englewood Cliffs, NJ: Prentice-Hall; 1980:454.

Hirano M. *Clinical examination of voice*. New York: Springer; 1981:100.

Isshiki N. *Phonosurgery: theory and practice*. New York: Springer; 1989:233.

Titze IR: *The principles of voice production*, Englewood Cliffs, NJ: Prentice-Hall. In press.

Zemlin WR. *Speech and hearing science: anatomy and physiology*. Englewood Cliffs, NJ: Prentice-Hall; 1988:603.

Anatomy and Tissue Properties

Bach AC, Lederer RL, Dinolt R. Senile changes in the laryngeal musculature. *Arch Otolaryngol*. 1941;34:47–56.

Baken RJ, Isshiki N. Arytenoid displacement by simulated intrinsic muscle contraction. *Folia Phoniatrica*. 1977;29:206–216.

Biondi S, Biondi-Zappala M. Surface of laryngeal mucosa seen through the scanning electron microscope. *Folia Phoniatrica*. 1974;26:241–248.

Gracco C, Kahane JC. Age-related changes in the vestibular folds of the human larynx: a histomorphometric study. *J Voice*. 1989;3:204–212.

Hast MH. Mechanical properties of the vocal fold muscle. *Practica Oto-Rhino-Laryngologica*. 1967;29:53–56.

Hirano M. Morphological structure of the vocal cord as a vibrator and its variations. *Folia Phoniatrica*. 1974;26:89–94.

Hirano M. Phonosurgery: basic and clinical investigations. *Otologia* (Fukuoka). 1975;21:239–440.

Hirano M. Structure of the vocal fold in normal and disease states. Anatomical and physical studies. In: Ludlow CL, Hart MO, eds. *Proceedings of the Conference on the Assessment of Vocal Pathology*. (ASHA Reports No. 11.) Rockville, Md: The American Speech-Language-Hearing Association;1981:11–30.

Hirano M, Kurita S, Sakaguchi S. Vocal fold tissue of a 104-year-old lady. *Ann Bull Res Inst Logopedics Phoniatrics*. 1988;22:1–5.

Hirano M, Matsuo K, Kakita Y, et al. Vibratory behavior versus the structure of the vocal fold. In: Titze IR, Scherer RC, eds. *Vocal Fold Physiology: Biomechanics, Acoustics and Phonatory Control*. Denver, Colo: The Denver Center for the Performing Arts; 1983:26–39.

Kahane JC. Connective tissue changes in the larynx and their effects on voice. *J Voice*. 1987;1:27–30.

Kahane JC. Histologic structure and properties of the human vocal folds. *Ear, Nose Throat J* 1988;67:322–330.

Koike Y, Ohta F, Monju T. Hormonal and non-hormonal actions of endocrines on the larynx. *Excerpta Medica International Congress Series* 1969; 206:339–343.

Mueller PB, Sweeney RJ, Baribeau LJ. Senescence of the voice: morphology of excised male larynges. *Folia Phoniatrica*. 1985; 37:134–138.

Rossi G, Cortesina G. Morphological study of the laryngeal muscles in man: insertions and courses of the muscle fibres, motor end-plates and proprioceptors. *Acta Otolaryngol*. 1965;59:575–592.

Sataloff, R.T: The human voice, *Scientific American*. 1992; 267(6):108.

Sellars IE, Keen EN. The anatomy and movements of the cricoarytenoid joint. *Laryngoscope*. 1978;88:667–674.

F_0 and Intensity

Atkinson JE. Inter- and intraspeaker variability in fundamental voice frequency. *J Acoustic Soc Am*. 1976;60:440–445.

Bowler NW. A fundamental frequency analysis of harsh vocal quality. *Speech Monog*. 1964;31:128–134.

Coleman RF, Mabis JH, Hinson JK. Fundamental frequency-sound pressure level profiles of adult male and female voices. *J Speech Hearing Res*. 1977;20:197–204.

Colton RH, Hollien H. Phonational range in the modal and falsetto registers. *J Speech Hearing Res*. 1972;15:713–718.

Davis SB. Acoustic characteristics of normal and pathological voices, In: Lass NJ, ed. *Speech and Language: Advances in Basic Research and Practice*. vol. 1 . New York: Academic Press; 1979;271–335.

Dickopf G, Flach M, Koch R, Kroemer B. Varianzanalytische Untersuchungen zur Stimmfeldmessung. *Folia Phoniatrica*. 1988,40: 43–48.

Fairbanks G, Wiley JH, Lassman FM. An acoustical study of vocal pitch in seven- and eight-year-old boys. *Child Dev*. 1949; 0:63–69.

Fitch JL, Holbrook A. Modal vocal fundamental frequency of young adults. *Arch Otolaryngol*. 1970;92:379–382.

Gramming P, Akerlund L. Phonetograms for normal and pathological voices. In: Gramming P, ed. *The Phonetogram: an Experimental and Clinical Study*. Malmö, Sweden: University of Lund; 1988:117–132.

Gramming P, Sundberg J, Ternström S, et al. Relationship between changes in voice pitch and loudness. In: Gramming P, ed. *The Phonetogram: an Experimental and Clinical Study*. Malmö, Sweden: University of Lund; 1988:87–107.

Hacki T. Die Beurteilung der quantitativen Sprechstimmleistungen: Das Sprechstimmfeld im Singstimmfeld. *Folia Phoniatrica*. 1988;40:190–196.

Hiki S. Correlation between increments of voice pitch and glottal sound intensity. *J Acoust Soc Jpn*. 1967;23:20–22.

Hollien H, Jackson B. Normative data on the speaking fundamental frequency characteristics of young adult males. *J Phonetics* 1973;1: 117–120.

Hollien H, Massey K. A male-female coalescence model of vocal change. In: Lawrence VL, ed. *Transcripts of the Fourteenth Symposium: Care of the Professional Voice*, part I. New York: Voice Foundation; 1985:57–60a.

Hollien H, Paul P. A second evaluation of the speaking fundamental frequency characteristics of post-adolescent girls. *Lang Speech*. 1969;12:119–124.

Hollien H, Shipp T. Speaking fundamental frequency and chronologic age in males. *J Speech Hearing Res*. 1972;15: 155–159.

Linville SE. Maximum phonational frequency range capabilities of women's voices with advancing age. *Folia Phoniatrica*. 1987;39:297–301.

McGlone RE, Hollien H. Vocal pitch characteristics of aged women. *J Speech Hearing Res*. 1963;6:164–170.

Michel FJ, Hollien H, Moore P. Speaking fundamental frequency characteristics of 15, 16, and 17 year old girls. *Lang Speech*. 1966;9:46–51.

Mysak ED. Pitch and duration characteristics of older males. *J Speech Hearing Res*. 1959;2:46–54.

Pederson MF, Kitzing P, Krabbe S, Heramb S. The change of voice during puberty in 11 to 16 year old choir singers measured with electroglottographic fundamental frequency analysis and compared to other phenomena of puberty. *Acta Otolaryngol*. 1982;suppl 386:189–192.

Ramig LA, Ringel RL. Effects of physiological aging on selected acoustic characteristics of voice. *J Speech Hearing Res*. 1983;26:22–30.

Ramig LA, Scherer RC, Titze IR. Acoustic correlates of aging. *Recording Res Center Res Rep*. 1985;April:257–277.

Rauhut A, Stürzebecher E, Wagner H, Seidner W. Messung des Stimmfeldes. *Folia Phoniatrica*. 1979;31:119–124.

Robb MP, Saxman IH, Grant AA. Vocal fundamental frequency characteristics during the first two years of life. *J Acoust Soc Am*. 1989; 85:1708–1717.

Saxman JH, Burk KW. Speaking fundamental frequency characteristics of middle-aged females. *Folia Phoniatrica*. 1967;19:167–172.

Stone RE Jr. Ferch PAK. Intra-subject variability in F_0-SPLmin voice profiles. *J Speech Hearing Disord*. 1982;47: 123–134.

Stone RE Jr, Bell CJ, Clack TD. Minimum intensity of voice at selected levels within pitch range. *Folia Phoniatrica*. 1978; 30:113–118.

Perturbation

Beckett RL. Pitch perturbation as a function of subjective vocal constriction. *Folia Phoniatrica*. 1969;21:416–425.

Brown WS Jr, Morris RJ, Michel JF. Vocal jitter in young adult and aged female voices. *J Voice*. 1989;3:113–119.

Cavallo SA, Baken RJ, Shaiman S. Frequency perturbation characteristics of pulse register phonation. *J Commun Disord*. 1984;17:231–243.

Deal RE, Emanuel FW. Some waveform and spectral features of vowel roughness. *J Speech Hearing Res*. 1978;21: 250–264.

Higgins MB, Saxman JH. Variations in vocal frequency perturbation across the menstrual cycle. *J Voice*. 1989;3:233-243.

Horii Y. Fundamental frequency perturbation observed in sustained phonation. *J Speech Hearing Res*. 1979;22:5–19.

Horii Y. Jitter and shimmer in sustained vocal fry phonation. *Folia Phoniatrica*. 1985;37:81–86.

Horii Y. Vocal shimmer in sustained phonation. *J Speech Hearing Res*. 1980;23:202–209.

Iwata S, von Leden H. Pitch perturbations in normal and pathologic voices. *Folia Phoniatrica*. 1970;22:413–424.

Lieberman P. Perturbations in vocal pitch. *J Acoust Soc Am*. 1961;33:597–603.

Lieberman P. Some acoustic measures of the fundamental periodicity of normal and pathologic larynges. *J Acoust Soc Am*. 1963 35: 344–353.

Moore P, von Leden H. Dynamic variaiions of the vibratory pattern in the normal larynx. *Folia Phoniatrica*. 1958;10: 205–238.

Murry T, Large J. Frequency perturbation in singers. In: Lawrence V, ed. *Transcripts of the Seventh Symposium: Care of the Professional Voice*. New York: Voice Foundation; 1978:36–39

Orlikoff RF. Vocal jitter at different fundamental frequencies: a cardiovascular-neuromuscular explanation. *J Voice*. 1989;3:104–112.

Orlikoff RF, Baken RJ . Fundamental frequency modulation of the human voice by the heartbeat: preliminary results and possible mechanisms. *J Acoust Soc Am*. 1989;85: 888–893.

Ramig LA, Shipp T. Comparative measures of vocal tremor and vocal vibrato. *J Voice*. 1987;1:162–167.

Sorensen D, Horii Y. Frequency and amplitude perturbation in the voices of female speakers. *J Commun Disord*. 1983; 16:57–61.

Wilcox KA, Horii Y. Age and changes in vocal jitter. *J Gerontol*. 1980;35:194–198.

Control Mechanisms

Atkinson JE. Correlation analysis of the physiological factors controlling fundamental voice frequency. *J Acoust Soc Am*. 1978;63:211–222.

Baken RJ, Orlikoff RF. Changes in vocal fundamental frequency at the segmental level: control during voiced fricatives. *J Speech Hearing Res*. 1988;31:207–211.

Baken RJ, Orlikoff RF. The effect of articulation on fundamental frequency in singers and speakers. *J Voice*. 1987;1: 68–76.

Baken RJ, Orlikoff RF. Laryngeal and chest-wall responses to step-function changes in supraglottal impedance. *Folia Phoniatrica*. 1986;38:283.

Colton RH. Physiological mechanisms of vocal frequency control: the role of tension. *J Voice*. 1988;2:208–220.

Erickson D, Baer T, Harris KS. The role of the strap muscles in pitch lowering. In: Bless DM, Abbs JH, eds. *Vocal Fold Physiology: Contemporary Research and Clinical Issues*. San Diego, Calif: College-Hill Press, 1983:279–285.

Faaborg-Andersen K. Electromyographic investigation of intrinsic laryngeal muscles in humans. *Acta Physiol Scand*. 1957; 41(suppl. 140):1–150.

Faaborg-Andersen K, Sonninen A. The function of the extrinsic laryngeal muscles at different pitch. *Acta Otolaryngol*. 1960;51:89–93.

Gay T, Hirose H, Strome M, Sawashima M. Electromyography of the intrinsic laryngeal muscles during phonation. *Ann Otol Rhinol Laryngol*. 1972;81:401–410.

Harvey N, Howell P. Isotonic vocalis contraction as a means of producing rapid decreases in F_0. *J Speech Hearing Res*. 1980;23:576–592.

Hast MH. Physiological mechanisms of phonation: tension of the vocal fold muscle. *Acta Otolaryngol*. 1966;62: 309–318.

Hirano M. Behavior of laryngeal muscles of the late William Vennard. *J Voice*. 1988;2:291–300.

Hirano M . The function of the intrinsic laryngeal muscles in singing. In: Stevens KN, Hirano M, eds. *Vocal Fold Physiology*. Tokyo: University of Tokyo Press; 1981:155–167.

Hirano M, Ohala J, Vennard W. The function of laryngeal muscles in regulating fundamental frequency and intensity of phonation. *J Speech Hearing Res*. 1969;12:616–628.

Hirano M, Vennard W, Ohala J. Regulation of register, pitch and intensity of voice. *Folia Phoniatrica*. 1970;22:1–20.

Hixon TJ, Klatt DH, Mead J. Influence of forced transglottal pressure changes on vocal fundamental frequency. *J Acoust Soc Am*. 1971;49 105.

Hollien H. Some laryngeal correlates of vocal pitch. *J Speech Hearing Res*. 1960;3:52–58.

Hollien H. Vocal fold thickness and fundamental frequency of phonation. *J Speech Hearing Res*. 1962;5:237–243.

Hollien H. Vocal pitch variation related to changes in vocal fold length. *J Speech Hearing Res*. 1960;3:150–156.

Hollien H, Colton RH. Four laminagraphic studies of vocal fold thickness. *Folia Phoniatrica*. 1969;21:179–198.

Hollien H, Curtis JF. Elevation and tilting of vocal folds as a function of vocal pitch. *Folia Phoniatrica*. 1962;14:23–36.

Hollien H, Moore GP. Measurements of the vocal folds during changes in pitch. *J Speech Hearing Res*. 1960;3:157–165.

Holmberg EB, Hillman RE, Perkell JS. Glottal airflow and transglottal air pressure measurements for male and female speakers in soft, normal, and loud voice. *J Acoust Soc Am*. 1988;84:511–529.

Horii Y. Acoustic analysis of vocal vibrato: a theoretical interpretation of data. *J Voice*. 1989;3:36–43.

Horii Y, Hata K. A note on phase relationships between frequency and amplitude modulations in vocal vibrato. *Folia Phoniatrica*. 1988;40:303–311.

Isshiki N. Regulatory mechanism of voice intensity variation. *J Speech Hearing Res*. 1964;7:17–29.

Isshiki N. Remarks on mechanism for vocal intensity variation. *J Speech Hearing Res*. 1969;12:665–672.

Isshiki N. Vocal intensity and air flow rate. *Folia Phoniatrica*. 1965;17:92–105.

Keenan JS, Barrett GC. Intralaryngeal relationships during pitch and intensity changes. *J Speech Hearing Res*. 1962;5: 173–177.

Larson CL, Kempster GB. Voice fundamental frequency changes following discharge of laryngeal motor units. In: Titze IR, Scherer RC, eds. *Vocal Fold Physiology: Biomechanics, Acoustics and Phonatory Control*. Denver, Colo: The Denver Center for the Performing Arts; 1983:91–103.

Leonard RJ, Ringel RL, Daniloff RG, Horii Y. Voice frequency change in singers and nonsingers. *J Voice*. 1987;1:234–239.

Lieberman P, Knudson R, Mead J. Determination of the rate of change of fundamental frequency with respect to subglottal air pressure during sustained phonation. *J Acoust Soc Am*. 1969;45:1537–1543.

Löfqvist A, Baer T, McGarr NS, Story RS. The cricothyroid muscle in voicing control. *J Acoust Soc Am*. 1989;85: 1314–1321.

Monsen RB, Engebretson AM, Vemula NR. Indirect assessment of the contribution of subglottal air pressure and vocal-fold tension to changes of fundamental frequency in English. *J Acoust Soc Am*. 1978;64:65–80.

Murry T, Brown WS Jr. Regulation of vocal intensity during vocal fry phonation. *J Acoust Soc Am*. 1971;49:1905–1907.

Niimi S, Horiguchi S, Kobayashi N. The physiological role of the sternothyroid muscle in phonation: an electromyographic observation. *Ann Bull Res Inst Logoped Phoniatr*. 1988;22:163–169.

Nishizawa N, Sawashima M, Yonemoto K. Vocal fold length in vocal pitch change. In: Fujimura O, ed. *Vocal Physiology: Voice Production, Mechanisms and Functions*. New York: Raven Press; 1988:75–52.

Ohala J, Hirano M, Vennard W. An electromyographic study of laryngeal activity in speech and singing. In: *Proceedings of the Sixth International Congress on Acoustics.* Tokyo, 1968:B-5–B-8.

Rubin HJ, LeCover M, Vennard W. Vocal intensity, subglottic pressure and air flow relationships in singers. *Folia Phoniatrica.* 1967;19:393–413.

Shin T, Hirano M, Maeyama T, et al. The function of the extrinsic laryngeal muscles. In: Stevens KN, Hirano M, eds. *Vocal Fold Physiology.* Tokyo,: University of Tokyo Press; 1981:171–180.

Shipp T. Vertical laryngeal position during continuous and discrete vocal frequency change. *J Speech Hearing Res.* 1975;18:707–718.

Shipp T. Vertical laryngeal position in singers with jaw stabilized. In: Lawrence VL, ed. *Transcripts of the Seventh Symposium: Care of the Professional Voice, part I: The Scientific Papers.* New York,: Voice Foundation; 1979:44–47.

Shipp T, McGlone RE. Laryngeal dynamics associated with voice frequency change. *J Speech Hearing Res.* 1971;14: 761–768.

Shipp T, Morrissey P. Physiologic adjustments for frequency change in trained and untrained voices. *J Acoust Soc Am.* 1977;62:476–478.

Sundberg J, Askenfelt A. Larynx height and voice source: a relationship? In: Bless DM, Abbs JH, eds. *Vocal Fold Physiology: Contemporary Research and Clinical Issues.* San Diego, Calif: College-Hill Press; 1983:307–316.

Tanaka S, Tanabe M. Experimental study on regulation of vocal pitch. *J Voice.* 1989;3:93–98.

Titze IR. Control of voice fundamental frequency. *Nat Assoc Teachers of Singing J.* 1988;November/December:6.

Titze IR. On the relation between subglottal pressure and fundamental frequency in phonation. *J Acoust Soc Am.* 1989;85:901–906.

Titze IR, Jiang J, Drucker DG. Preliminaries to the body-cover theory of pitch control. *J Voice.* 1987;1:314–319.

Tizte IR, Luschei ES, Hirano M. Role of the thyroarytenoid muscle in regulation of fundamental frequency. *J Voice.* 1989;3:213–224.

Registers

Allen EL, Hollien H. A laminagraphic study of pulse (vocal fry) register phonation. *Folia Phoniatrica.* 1973,25: 241–250.

Ametrano Jackson MC. The high male range. *Folia Phoniatrica.* 1987;39:18–25.

Colton RH. Spectral characteristics of the modal and falsetto registers. *Folia Phoniatrica.* 1972;24:337–344.

Colton RH. Vocal intensity in the modal and falsetto registers. *Folia Phoniatrica.* 1973;25:62–70

Gougerot L, Grémy F, Marstal N. Glottographie à large bande passante. Application à l'étude de la voix de fausset. *J Physiol.* 1960;52:823–832.

Hirano M, Hibi S, Sawada T. Falsetto, head, chest, and speech mode: an acoustic study with three tenors. *J Voice.* 1989;3:99–103.

Hollien H. On vocal registers. *J Phonet.* 1974;2:125–143.

Hollien H. Three major vocal registers: a proposal. In: Rigault A, Charbonneau R, eds. *Proceedings of the Seventh International Congress of Phonetic Sciences.* The Hague: Mouton, 1972;320–331.

Hollien H, Michel JF. Vocal fry as a phonational register. *J Speech Hearing Res.* 1968;11:600–604.

Hollien H, Brown WS Jr, Hollien K. Vocal fold length associated with modal, falsetto, and varying intensity phonations. *Folia Phoniatrica.* 1971;23:66–78.

Hollien H, Damsté H, Murry T. Vocal fold length during vocal fry phonation. *Folia Phoniatrica.* 1969;21:257–265.

Hollien H, Girard GT, Coleman RF. Vocal fold vibratory patterns of pulse register phonation. *Folia Phoniatrica.* 1977; 29:200–205.

Hollien H, Moore P, Wendahl RW, Michel JF. On the nature of vocal fry. *J Speech Hearing Res.* 1966;9:245–247.

Kitzing P. Photo- and electroglottographic recording of the laryngeal vibratory pattern during different registers. *Folia Phoniatrica.* 1982;34:234–241.

McGlone RE. Air flow during vocal fry phonation. *J Speech Hearing Res.* 1967;10:299–304.

McGlone RE. Air flow in the upper register. *Folia Phoniatrica.* 1970;22:231–238.

McGlone RE, Brown WS Jr. Identification of the "shift" between vocal registers. *J Acoust Soc Am.* 1969;46:1033–1036.

McGlone RE, Shipp T. Some physiologic correlates of vocal-fry phonation. *J Speech Hearing Res.* 1971;14:769–775.

Murry T. Subglottal pressure and airflow measures during vocal fry phonation. *J Speech Hearing Res.* 1971;14: 544–551.

Murry T, Brown WS Jr. Subglottal air pressure during two types of vocal activity: vocal fry and modal phonation. *Folia Phoniatrica.* 1971;23:440–449.

Rohrs M, Pascher W, Ocker C. Untersuchungen über das Schwingungsverhalten der Stimmlippen in verschiedenen Registerbereichen mit unterschiedlichen stroboskopischen Techniken. *Folia Phoniatrica.* 1985;37: 113–118.

Roubeau C, Chevrie-Muller C, Arabia-Guidet C. Electroglottographic study of the changes of voice registers. *Folia Phoniatrica.* 1987;39:280–289.

Schutte HK, Seidner WW. Registerabhangige Differentzierung von Elektrogrammen. *Sprache-Stimme-Gehör.* 1988;12:59–62.

Titze IR. A framework for the study of vocal registers. *J Voice.* 1988;2:183–194.

Welch GF, Sergeant DC, MacCurtain F. Zeroradiographic-electrolaryngographic analysis of male vocal registers. *J Voice.* 1989;3:224–256.

Aerodynamics, Vocal Fold Movement, and Models

Baer T. Observation of vocal fold vibration: measurement of excised larynges. In: Stevens KN, Hirano M, eds. *Vocal Fold Physiology.* Tokyo: University of Tokyo Press; 1981: 119–132.

Baer T, Titze IR, Yoshioka H. Multiple simultaneous measures of vocal fold activity. In: Bless DM, Abbs JH, eds. *Vocal Fold Physiology: Contemporary Research and Clinical Issues.* San Diego, CA: College-Hill; 1983:227–237.

Biever DM, Bless DM. Vibratory characteristics of the vocal folds in young adult and geriatric women. *J Voice.* 1989; 3:120–131.

Brackett IP. The vibration of vocal folds at selected frequencies. *Annal Otol Rhinol Laryngol.* 1948;57:556–558.

Broad DJ. The new theories of vocal fold vibration. In: Lass NJ, ed. *Speech and language: Advances in Basic Research and Practice.* New York,: Academic Press, 1979;2:203–257.

Cavagna GA, Camporesi EM. Glottal aerodynamics and phonation. In: Wyke B, ed. *Ventilatory and Phonatory Control Systems.* New York: Oxford University Press; 1974: 76–87.

Childers DG, Alsaka YA, Hicks DM, Moore GP. Vocal fold vibrations: an EGG model. In: Baer T, Sasaki C, Harris KS, eds. *Laryngeal Function in Phonation and Respiration.* Boston, Mass: Little, Brown; 1987:181–202.

Flanagan JL. Some properties of the glottal sound source. *J Speech Hearing Res.* 1958;1:99–116.

Gauffin J, Liljencrants J. Modelling the airflow in the glottis. *Ann Bull Res Inst Logoped Phoniatr.* 1988;22:39–50.

Hillman RE, Oesterle E, Feth LL. Characteristics of the glottal turbulent noise source. *J Acoust Soc Am.* 1983;74: 691–694.

Holmes, JN. The acoustic consequences of vocal-cord action. *Phonetica.* 1977;34:316–317.

Ishizaka K. Equivalent lumped-mass models of vocal fold vibration. In: Stevens, KN, Hirano M, eds. *Vocal Fold Physiology.* Tokyo: University of Tokyo Press; 1981:231–241.

Isogai Y Horiguchi S, Honda K, et al. A dynamic simulation model of vocal fold vibration. In: Fujimura O, ed. *Vocal Physiology: Voice Production, Mechanisms and Functions.* New York,: Raven Press; 1988:191–206.

Kitzing P, Sonesson B. A photoglottographical study of the female vocal folds during phonation. *Folia Phoniatrica.* 1974;26:138–149.

Kitzing P, Carlborg B, Löfqvist A. Aerodynamic and glottographic studies of the laryngeal vibratory cycle. *Folia Phoniatrica.* 1982;34:216–224.

Koike Y. Sub- and supraglottal pressure variation during phonation. In: Stevens KN, Hirano M, eds. *Vocal Fold Physiology.* Tokyo,: University of Tokyo Press; 1981: 181–189.

Matsushita H. The vibratory mode of the vocal folds in the excised larynx. *Folia Phoniatrica.* 1975;27:7–18.

Monsen, RB, Engebretson AM. Study of variations in the male and female glottal wave. *J Acoust Soc Am.* 1977;62: 981–993.

Rothenberg M. Some relations between glottal air flow and vocal fold contact area. In: Ludlow CL, Hart MO, eds. *Proceedings of the Conference on the Assessment of Vocal Fold Pathology (ASHA Reports no. 11).* Rockville, Md: American Speech-Language-Hearing Association; 1981:88–96.

Rothenberg M, Miller D, Molitor R. Aerodynamic investigation of sources of vibrato. *Folia Phoniatrica.* 1988;40: 244–260.

Saito S, Fukuda H, Kitahara S, Kokowa N. Stroboscopic observation of vocal fold vibration with fiberoptics. *Folia Phoniatrica.* 1978;30:241–244.

Schutte HK. Aerodynamics of phonation. *Acta Oto-rhino-laryngol Belg.* 1986; 40: 344–357.

Schutte HK, Miller DG. Transglottal pressures in professional singing. *Acta Oto-rhino laryngol Belg.* 1986;40: 395–404.

Sonesson B. On the anatomy and vibratory patterns of the human vocal folds. *Acta Otolaryngol.* 1960: suppl. 156: 44–67.

Stevens KN. Modes of vocal fold vibration based on a two-section model. In: Fujimura O, ed. *Vocal Physiology: Voice Production, Mechanisms and Functions.* New York,: Raven Press; 1988:357–371.

Stevens KN. Physics of laryngeal behavior and larynx modes. *Phonetica.* 1977;34:264–379.

Stevens KN. Vibration modes in relation to model parameters. In: Stevens KN, Hirano M, eds. *Vocal Fold Pphysiology.* Tokyo,: University of Tokyo Press; 1981:291–301.

Titze IR. Biomechanics and distributed-mass models of vocal fold vibration. In: Stevens KN, Hirano M, eds. *Vocal Fold Physiology.* Tokyo,: University of Tokyo Press; 1981: 245–264.

Titze IR. The human vocal cords: a mathematical model. *Phonetica.* 1973;28:129–170.

Titze IR. On the mechanics of vocal fold vibration. *J Acoust Soc Am.* 1976;60:1366–1380.

Titze IR. Parameterization of the glottal area, glottal flow, and vocal fold contact area. *J Acoust Soc Am.* 1984;75: 570–580.

Titze IR. The physics of flow-induced oscillation of the vocal folds. I. Small-amplitude oscillations. *Record Res Center Res Rep.* 1985;April:1–49.

Titze IR, Talkin DT. A theoretical study of the effects of various laryngeal configurations on the acoustics of phonation. *J Acoust Soc Am.* 1979;66:60–74.

Neurology

Abo-el-Enein MA, Wyke B. Laryngeal myotatic reflexes. *Nature.* 1966;209:682–686.

Abo-el-Enein MA, Wyke B. Myotatic reflex systems in the intrinsic muscles of the larynx. *J Anat (Lond).* 1966;100: 926–927.

Adzaku FK, Wyke B. Innervation of the subglottic mucosa of the larynx and its significance. *Folia Phoniatrica.* 1979;31: 271–283.

Baer T. Reflex activation of laryngeal muscles by sudden induced subglottal pressure changes. *J Acoust Soc Am.* 1979;65:1271–1275.

Baken RJ. Neuromuscular spindles in the intrinsic muscles of a human larynx. *Folia Phoniatrica.* 1971;23:204–210.

Bowden REM. Innervation of intrinsic laryngeal muscles. In: Wyke B, ed. *Ventilatory and Phonatory Control Systems.* New York,: Oxford University Press; 1974:370–381.

Kurozumi S, Tashiro T, Harada Y. Laryngeal responses to electrical stimulation of the medullary respiratory centers in the dog. *Laryngoscope.* 1971;81:1960–1967.

Larson CR. Brain mechanisms involved in the control of vocalization. *J Voice.* 1988;2:301–311.

Larson CR. The midbrain periaqueductal gray: a brainstem structure involved in vocalization. *J Speech Hearing Res.* 1985;28:241–249.

Larson CR, Kempster GB, Kistler MK. Changes in voice fundamental frequency following discharge of single motor units in cricothyroid and thyroarytenoid muscles. *J Speech Hearing Res.* 1987;30:552–558.

Larson CR, Wilson KE, Luschei ES. Preliminary observations on cortical and brainstem mechanisms of laryngeal control. In: Bless DM, Abbs JH, eds. *Vocal Fold Physiology: Contemporary Research and Clinical Issues.* San Diego, Calif: College-Hill Press; 1983:82–95.

Mallard AR, Ringel RL, Horii Y. Sensory contributions to control of fundamental frequency of phonation. *Folia Phoniatrica*. 1978;30:199–213.

Mårtensson A. Proprioceptive impulse patterns during contraction of intrinsic laryngeal muscles. *Acta Physiol Scand*. 1964;62:176–194.

Ortega JD, DeRosier E, Park S, Larson CR. Brainstem mechanisms of laryngeal control as revealed by microstimulation studies. In: Fujimura O, ed. *Vocal Physiology: Voice Production, Mechanisms and Functions*. New York: Raven Press; 1988:19–28.

Miscellaneous

Abitbol J, de Brux J, Millot G et al. Does a hormonal vocal cord cycle exist in women? Study of vocal premenstrual syndrome in voice performers by videostroboscopy-glottography and cytology on 38 women. *J Voice*. 1989; 3:157–162.

Dmitriev LB, Chernov BP, Maslov VT. Functioning of the voice mechanism in double-voice Touvinian singing. *Folia Phoniatrica*. 1983;35:193–197.

Gossett CW Jr. Electromyographic investigation of the relationship of the effects of selected parameters on concurrent study of voice and oboe. *J Voice*. 1989;3:52–64.

Hamlet SL, Palmer JM. Investigation of laryngeal trills using the transmission of ultrasound through the larynx. *Folia Phoniatrica*. 1974;26:362–377.

Hicks DM, Childers DG, Moore GP, Alsaka J. EGG and the singers' voice. In: Lawrence VL, ed. *Transcripts of the Fourteenth Symposium: Care of the Professional Voice*. New York: The Voice Foundation; 1986:50–56.

King Al, Ashby J, Nelson C. Laryngeal function in wind instruments: the brass. *J Voice*. 1989;3:65–67.

Murry T, Caligiuri MP. Phonatory and nonphonatory motor control in singers. *J Voice*. 1989;3:257–263.

Proctor DF. The physiologic basis of voice training. In: Bouhuys A, ed. *Sound Production in Man* (*Annals of the New York Academy of Sciences*; vol. 155). New York: New York Academy of Sciences; 1968:208–228.

Rosenberg AE. Effect of glottal pulse shape on the quality of natural vowels. *J Acoust Soc Am*. 1971;49:583–588.

Rubin J, Sataloff RT, Korovin G and Gould WJ: *The Diagnosis and Treatment of Voice Disorders*. New York: Igaku-Shoin Medical Publishers, Inc; 1995.

Schutte HK. Efficiency of professional singing voices in terms of energy ratio. *Folia Phoniatrica*. 1984;36:267–272.

Silverman E-M, Zimmer CH. Effect of the menstrual cycle on voice quality. *Arch Otolaryngol*. 1978;104:7–10.

Sundberg J. The source spectrum in professional singing. *Folia Phoniatrica*. 1973;25:71–90.

Sundberg J. *The Science of the Singing Voice*. Dekalb, Ill: Northern Illinois University Press; 1987.

Van Michel C. La courbe glottographique chez les sujets non entrainés au chant. *Comptes Rendus de la Société de Biologie*. 1968;1:583–585.

12

Laryngeal Function During Phonation

Ronald C. Scherer

The larynx performs many functions to aid communication and allow life. As an open flow valve, it permits breathing, blowing, and sucking, as well as yawning, voiceless consonant production, and musical instrument playing. As a transient closed valve, it produces coughing and throat clearing. As a prolonged closed valve, it participates in swallowing and effortful behaviors such as lifting and defecation. As a voiceless repetitive articulator, it valves airflow to produce staccato whistling. As a voiced repetitive articulator, it produces laughter, the singing ornament trillo, and repetitive glottalization of vowels such as the admonition with rising pitch and intensity "a-a-a-ah!" As an incompletely closed voiceless valve, it produces whisper. As a partially or completely closed voicing valve, the larynx produces vowels and prolonged voiced consonants, and as a speech coarticulator, it participates in the production of consonant-vowel strings. For example, the word "seat" begins with an open glottis for the /s/, the glottis acting as an open flow valve allowing airflow under lung pressure to travel through the glottis and through the anterior oral constriction. This is followed by vocal fold approximation for the /i/ vowel, the larynx acting as a partially or completely closed voicing valve. Finally, the glottis opens as an open flow valve to permit the impoundment of air pressure behind the anterior oral /t/-occlusion with the subsequent release of air, creating the characteristic aspiration.

The purpose of this chapter is to describe the larynx as a partially or completely closed voicing valve, that is, as the organ that produces phonation. Neuromuscular, biomechanic, and aeroacoustic characteristics determine phonation duration, pitch, loudness, quality, register, and vocal fold motion, through control of or changes in vocal fold length, mass and tension, vocal fold contour, arytenoid and vocal fold adduc-

tion, subglottal pressure, and vocal tract size and shape. This chapter emphasizes the reasonable hypothesis that effective interventions to help people with voice concerns (whether these involve prevention, rehabilitation, surgery, pharmacology, or training) can be improved by an understanding of basic vocal function.[1,2]

Overview of Basic Characteristics of Phonation

The basic perceptual characteristics of phonation are the presence and change of duration, pitch, register, loudness, and quality. Each of these has one or two primary biomechanical control variables. These will be discussed briefly in this section, followed by discussions of selected topics in greater detail.

Duration of phonation refers to the length of time the vocal folds oscillate during the creation of sound. In the normal larynx, adduction is one of two main control variables for duration; the vocal folds must be sufficiently close to permit oscillation. Subglottal air pressure is also necessary to provide sufficient force to move the vocal folds at the beginning of each vibratory cycle. After phonation commences, to then cease phonation, the arytenoid cartilages can be moved apart (abducted), or moved further together (more highly adducted), both ceasing phonation if the degree of abduction or adduction is great enough. Additional ways to cause phonation to cease are to lower subglottal air pressure, or impound air pressure in the vocal tract above the glottis, until the pressure drop across the glottis is too low to sustain vocal fold vibration.

The perception of pitch, corresponding to the physical measure of fundamental frequency, and vocal register (the very low pitches of vocal fry, the conversational pitches of chest or modal register, and the very high pitches of falsetto), are highly dependent on vocal fold length[3,4] and the associated tension of the vocal fold mucosal cover. The string model for frequency,[5-8]

$$(\text{Equation 1}),\ F_0 = (1/2L)(T/\rho)^{0.5}$$

where T is the tension of the vocal fold mucosal cover, ρ is the density of the tissue, and L is the length of the vibrating vocal folds, is an explanatory model suggesting that tension of the vocal fold cover governs the fundamental frequency (tension T increases faster than vocal fold length L when the vocal folds are lengthened, and ρ is essentially constant regardless of phonatory condition.[8,9]

The loudness of sounds is related to their acoustic intensity, and phonation during speech is primarily dependent upon subglottal pressure. An increase in subglottal pressure changes the characteristics of the airflow that exits the glottis (the glottal volume velocity) during vocal fold vibration, creating an increase in acoustic intensity (see below).

At the glottal level, vocal quality variation, governed primarily by the closeness of the vocal folds, ie, by adduction (separate from tissue or neurologic abnormalities), is related primarily to the perception of normal, breathy, and pressed qualities. Breathiness occurs when the vocal folds are slightly abducted such that they do not close completely during each cycle, allowing some of the glottal volume flow to be unmodulated and turbulent.[10] A breathy voice also can be created by full vocal fold closure (anterior to the vocal processes) but with the posterior glottis open, allowing turbulent air to flow between the arytenoid cartilages. If there is hyperadduction of the vocal folds, but with a significant opening of the posterior glottis, a pressed-breathy (or pressed-leakage) quality can result.[11,12] Pressed or constricted voice quality without breathiness results from full glottal adduction, and little air flows through the posterior glottis.[13]

Intervention strategies to improve voice production require an appreciation of the basic mechanics of phonation. The remainder of this chapter offers a more thorough discussion of basic control characteristics of voice production.

Duration of Phonation

Figure 12–1 illustrates the adductory range of phonation and the corresponding distances between the vocal processes of the arytenoid cartilages, the ventricular folds, and the superomedial eminences of the arytenoid cartilage apexes. Phonation takes place over only a small range of adduction (the *phonatory adductory range*) permitted by movement of the arytenoid cartilages (approximately 14% of the adductory range as shown in the single-subject example of Figure 12–1). From an adductory standpoint, therefore, duration of phonation depends on the potential for the vocal folds to be placed within the phonatory adductory range, and the length of time the vocal folds are actually placed within that range. To discontinue phonation, the arytenoid cartilages can be configured to produce sufficient overcompression of the vocal folds or, alternatively, sufficient abduction.

Phonation requires a certain minimal amount of subglottal air pressure to set the vocal folds into vibration (the *phonatory threshold pressure*[14]) and then to maintain phonation. If the vocal folds are placed in the phonatory adductory range, the subglottal pressure must coordinate with the tissue characteristics of the vocal folds (stiffness, mass, and damping) to cause them to move to begin the first cycle.[14] Lucero[15] suggests, using a theoretical approach, that the pressure threshold should reduce as the vocal folds are brought closer to each other, and as the glottal angle between the vocal folds comes closer to zero or slightly divergent, consistent with Titze[14] and Chan, Titze, and Titze.[16] The threshold pressure typically varies with fundamental frequency, ranging from about 3 cm H_2O (0.3 kPa) for lower pitches to about 6 cm H_2O (0.6 kPa) for higher pitches[17] because of greater tension of the vocal fold cover with vocal fold lengthening. The amount of subglottal pressure at phonation offset is less than the onset pressure, not to exceed about half the onset pressure.[18-22] Because the phonatory threshold pressure is an important measure for glottal efficiency and clinical diagnostics, it is important that it be measured with care.[23]

There also may be an upper limit of subglottal pressure beyond which phonation is prevented or becomes unstable.[14] This upper limit may correspond to the upper limits of the *phonetogram*, a graph of the intensity range versus the fundamental frequency range of phonation for a particular person[24-28] (the recommendation of the term *voice range profile* for the phonetogram was accepted by the Voice Committee of the International Association of Logopedics and Phoniatrics[29]). Subglottal pressures have been measured as high as 30 to 50 cm H_2O in loud phonation[30] (singing loudly at high pitches may produce even greater subglottal pressures[13]), but typically are below 10 cm H_2O for conversational speech.[30,31]

Intervention in voice surgery, therapy, and training often attempts to regain normal thresholds or to low-

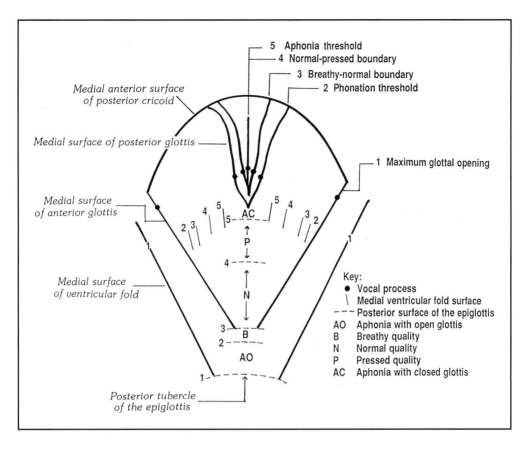

Fig 12–1. Adductory range of the larynx. This figure is a composite from photographs of glottal adductory positions obtained from a single adult male subject using rigid videolaryngoscopy. Positions of the medial surface of the anterior (membranous) glottis, posterior glottis, ventricular folds, and the posterior tubercle of the epiglottis are shown. Stages of glottal positioning include maximum glottal opening (position 1) to full adduction when phonation is not possible (position 5). The other positions (2, 3, and 4) are the position for adductory phonatory threshold and boundary locations between breathy, normal, and pressed voice qualities in this subject, perceptually judged and checked against electroglottograph (EGG) recordings. The adductory phonation range is only about 14% of the entire adductory range (see text).

er existing thresholds, the latter possibly creating less effortful phonation (relative to the employed forces of the respiratory system). Establishment of lower phonation thresholds may correspond to more physiologically efficient phonation and less voice fatigue.

The discussion directly above refers to the dependence that phonation has on subglottal pressure. More appropriately, phonation is dependent upon the *translaryngeal pressure*, defined as the subglottal air pressure minus the supraglottal air pressure for phonation on exhalation. Note that the translaryngeal pressure is the difference between the subglottal and supraglottal pressures acting on the inferior and superior surfaces of the vocal folds, respectively, as well as the pressure difference that drives the air through the glottis. If the translaryngeal air pressure were zero, the pressure would be equal on all surfaces of the vocal folds, air would not pass, and phonation would not occur. This can be approached, for example, with overly prolonged voiced consonants such as /b/, /d/, and /g/ during the complete occlusion of the vocal tract. Prolonging the voicing of these consonants creates buildup of supralaryngeal air pressure until that pressure nearly equals the subglottal pressure, causing cessation of phonation as the translaryngeal pressure drops below the minimum sustaining pressure difference.

Thus, the creation and duration of phonation depend upon how close the vocal folds are to each other and the amount of translaryngeal air pressure (disregarding tissue abnormality). To cease phonation, the vocal folds can be over-adducted or over-abducted, or the translaryngeal pressure can be lowered by decreasing the subglottal pressure or by increasing supraglottal pressure through supraglottal occlusion. All four methods most likely are used in normal speech production, and the ability of a patient to demonstrate all four methods is relevant diagnostically. These mechanisms for phonation cessation potentially can be compromised by arytenoidal, respiratory, or articulatory dysfunction, or by abnormal adductory configuration caused by vocal fold tissue change.

Fundamental Frequency of Phonation

Perceived pitch corresponds (nonlinearly) to the physical measure of fundamental frequency F_0,[32] which in turn corresponds to the number of cycles per second of the glottal motion during phonation. For normal phonation, the motion of the vocal folds is similar from cycle to cycle, giving rise to nearly equal periods of time between glottal closures.

Each phonatory cycle releases time-varying glottal flow (also called the glottal volume velocity) that generates sound. For normal phonation, acoustic excitation is created throughout the varying flow cycle, with a primary location giving the greatest excitation. Figure 12–2 shows two glottal volume velocity cycles of human phonation (top trace). The cycle period is T, which is 10 ms (and thus $F_0 = 1/T = 100$ Hz). The glottal volume velocity (usually given in liters per second, L/s, or cubic centimeters per second, cm³/s) begins to exit the glottis gradually, rises to a peak, and then "shuts off" relatively abruptly. Air exits the glottis from time A to time B during the lateral then medial motion of the membranous vocal folds. The glottis is closed, or nearly so, from B to C. The amount of airflow during the interval B to C (seen as the offset from the horizontal baseline in Figure 12–2) corresponds to air "leakage" when the arytenoid cartilages are separated to some degree.

The lower trace of Figure 12–2 is the time derivative of the volume velocity signal of the upper trace. At any moment in time, the value on the lower trace equals the slope of the volume velocity signal at that moment. The fastest change of the volume velocity in the figure is at time D, and corresponds to the point M on the derivative waveform. The point M corresponds to the moment of time at which the greatest acoustic excitation is created.[33,34]

Perceptual judgments of an unclear voice (rather than confusion of pitch per se) occur when the more prominent moments of acoustic excitation during each cycle are not consistent from one cycle to the next

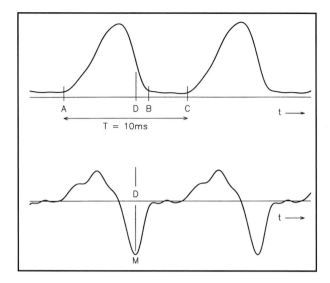

Fig 12–2. Glottal volume velocity waveforms and their derivatives. The top trace is a glottal volume velocity signal, and the bottom trace is the derivative of the top trace, showing the instantaneous slopes of the top trace. Cycle period is T (from time A to time C). "Open" glottis time is from A to B, and "closed" glottis time is from B to C. The moment of the maximum flow shutoff rate, or the maximum negative derivative of the glottal volume velocity signal, occurs at time D and corresponds to point M.

(for a review of cyclic instabilities, see references 32, 35, 36). The time between primary acoustic excitations from one cycle to the next varies a small amount during normal phonation, helping to create a natural voice quality. However, the variation of periods can increase if there are tissue abnormalities such as swelling, nodules, polyps, unilateral stiffness, and so forth, causing kinematic (vocal fold motion) and glottal flow inconsistencies from cycle to cycle. Consecutively varying periods of primary acoustic excitations also can be created by turbulent airflow through the glottis (as in breathy voice), creating added noise to the acoustic signal. Aperiodicities can be measured by jitter, one definition being the average cycle-to-cycle difference in period or equivalent frequency, with large values of jitter corresponding to a sense of vocal roughness.[32] Figure 12–3 illustrates quasi-periodic cycles of the acoustic output of a prolonged vowel with a calculation of the segment's jitter value.

Jitter may be caused by or related to neuromuscular innervation abnormalities[37-40] as well as the structural and turbulence causes given above. Because tension of the vocal folds is highly dependent on the passive lengthening of the vocal fold cover, as suggested by Equation 1, relatively fast abnormal innervation changes to the cricothyroid muscles to lengthen the

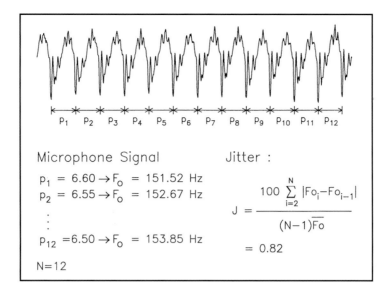

Fig 12–3. Aperiodicity of a microphone signal for a prolonged vowel. The periods of the microphone signal are indicated using the instants of the minimum values, and the calculation of the corresponding jitter is given. This is an example of a measure of voicing perturbation.

vocal folds and to the thyroarytenoid muscles to shorten the vocal folds may cause length and, therefore, tension changes, creating cycle-to-cycle fundamental frequency changes.

Pitch and vocal quality are also affected by changes that occur over longer time lengths than a phonatory cycle. Diplophonia (the existence of two pitches simultaneously[41]) and subharmonics (integer subdivisions of the fundamental frequency) come from multicycle length modulations of the volume velocity signal. These give rise to primary acoustic excitations at varying time intervals as well as about twice (or more) the primary phonatory period.[42-49] Figure 12–4 shows an example of the presence of cycle clustering in the glottal volume velocity signal of a spasmodic dysphonia patient. The cause of this dysfunction appears to be related to hyperadduction or asymmetry of laryngeal muscle function.

In vocal fry and "creaky" voice, pitch may be extremely low and the voice may have varied roughness qualities, depending on the complexity of the low frequency periodicities combined with higher frequency periodicities.[50-54] Figure 12–5 illustrates three different examples of vocal fry[53] (in reference 53, 11 different types of vocal fry and creaky voice are illustrated). For each case, the microphone signal and the electroglottograph signal are displayed. These samples were created intentionally by a single normal adult male subject. The electroglottographic (EGG) signal may

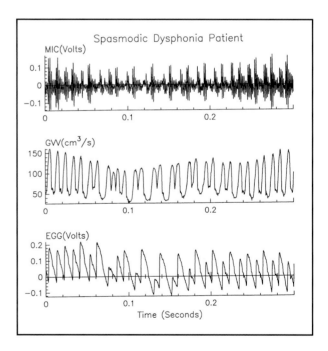

Fig 12–4. Voicing period alterations in a spasmodic dysphonia patient. Microphone, glottal volume velocity, and EGG signals are given, top to bottom. Notice the change from essentially single cycles to cycle clustering of two (and one case of three) cycles. The clustering of two cycles can be seen in all three signals: apparent motion variation of vocal fold contact, double flow pulsing, and double acoustic excitation seen in the microphone signal. (Data courtesy of Dr. Kimberly Fisher)

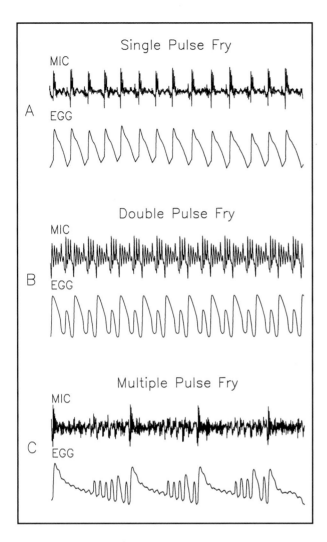

Fig 12–5. Three vocal fry examples. **A.** Single glottal pulses at 30 Hz; **B.** Double glottal pulses at 62 Hz for the period combining the two pulses. **C.** A multiple pulse case with a low frequency of 7.5 Hz and a higher frequency of 93 Hz. In each grouping, the upper trace is the microphone signal and the lower trace is the electroglottograph signal. The examples were produced by a single adult male subject. See reference 53.

folds during each relatively long cycle, with corresponding acoustic excitations.

Pitch can be altered by fluid engorgement (edema). The usual explanation for pitch drop in edema cases is that greater mass creates lower natural frequencies. For example, computer modeling of phonation using biomechanical characteristics of tissue mass, stiffness, and damping relate fundamental frequency to the inverse of the vocal fold mass.[56] Figure 12–6 shows the results of increasing vocal fold mass (only) in a two-mass model of vocal fold function adapted from Ishizaka and Flanagan[57] by Smith.[58] Figure 12–6 shows a decrease in frequency by approximately 5.6 semitones for a doubling of the mass of the vocal folds. For example, for a subglottal pressure of 8 cm H_2O, the change in fundamental frequency for a doubling of the mass is approximately 134 Hz to 97 Hz in the figure.

Subglottal pressure plays a significant role in the control of pitch. Figure 12–6 suggests that an increase in subglottal pressure for a constant vocal fold mass will increase the fundamental frequency. The F_0 changes from 120 Hz to 156 Hz for a mass "M" and subglottal pressure from 4 to 16 cm H_2O for the conditions of Figure 12–6. The literature suggests that a change of 1 cm H_2O subglottal pressure results in a fundamental frequency change of 3-6 Hz.[59-62] The air pressure pushing against the undersurface of the vocal folds moves the vocal fold laterally and somewhat upwardly.[19,63-66] The extent of the lateral excursion is dependent upon the amount of the subglottal pressure and the length of the vocal folds.[6,67,68] Thus, for a constant anterior-posterior length of the glottis, a greater subglottal pressure will literally push the vocal folds to a greater lateral extent, creating a greater maximum *stretch* than for a lower subglottal pressure. Greater maximum stretch creates higher effective tension and thus a higher fundamental frequency.[6] Intonational (pitch) changes during conversational speech appear to be caused by a significant combination of the passive vocal fold stretch by both the cricothyroid muscles and the subglottal pressure[69,70] (refer especially to the general discussion at the end of reference 70).

Tension of the vocal fold cover may be changed (and therefore fundamental frequency changed) by external adjustments affecting the length of the vocal folds. Anterior pull of the hyoid bone by suprahyoid muscles may help tilt the thyroid cartilage forward to position its inferior border closer to the superior border of the anterior cricoid cartilage (similar to the function of the cricothyroid muscle), thus increasing vocal fold length and raising the fundamental frequency, as shown by Honda.[71] Alternatively, a suggestion is put forward by Sundberg et al[72] that the cricoid cartilage may be tilted down posteriorly, shortening the vocal

correspond to the contact area between the vocal folds when they touch each other during each cycle.[32,55] Figure 12–5A illustrates vocal fry of low and specific pitch. Each cycle shows a single primary acoustic excitation. This excitation corresponds to the fast upward movement of the EGG signal which corresponds to glottal closure and, therefore, to the glottal volume velocity "shutoff." Figure 12–5B illustrates the typical bimodal electroglottograph signal for vocal fry, with corresponding double acoustic excitations during each (low pitch) cycle. Figure 12–5C illustrates an extreme case of multiple cyclic motions of the vocal

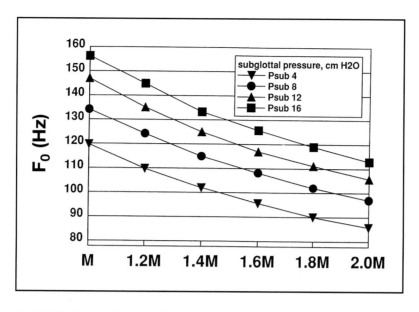

Fig 12–6. Vocal fold mass effect on fundamental frequency. As the amount of mass of the vocal fold in vibration increases, the fundamental frequency decreases. The abscissa ranges from a value of M = 0.16 g to twice that. The figure also indicates that fundamental frequency is dependent upon subglottal pressure. (Figure courtesy of Dr. Marshall Smith, who used an adaptation of the Ishizaka and Flanagan simulation.[57,58])

fold length, by an inferior tracheal pull. This would come about by lowering the diaphragm with higher lung volume levels (or by coactivation of the diaphragm during phonation), inducing a pitch drop unless compensated for by increased cricothyroid muscle activity.

The above discussion emphasizes the contribution to pitch control through tension change of the vocal fold cover through passive stretch or by increasing subglottal pressure. The fundamental frequency is also dependent upon the activity of the vocalis (thyroarytenoid) muscle.[73,74] The vocalis muscle acts antagonistically to the cricothyroid muscle relative to length change of the cover.[73,75,76] Thus, if only the cover is vibrating, as in soft, high-pitch phonation, increase in vocalis contraction should shorten and reduce the tension of the mucosal cover, and thereby lower the fundamental frequency. However, if the vocalis muscle participates in the motion of the vocal fold to a significant degree, as in loud, low-pitch phonation, increase in vocalis muscle contraction will increase the effective tension of the entire tissue in motion as a primary effect, and thereby raise the fundamental frequency. The effect on F_0 change related to vocalis muscle involvement conceptually depends on the relative amount of vocalis muscle participating in the vibratory mass, the tension within the vocalis mus-

cle portion of the mass in motion, and the relative activity level of the vocalis muscle, as Titze, Jiang, and Drucker[73] analytically describe. In general then, pitch is controlled by many combinations of cricothyroid muscle contraction (to passively stretch the tissue in motion), vocalis muscle contraction (to passively shorten the cover and actively increase the tension of the vibratory vocalis portion), and subglottal pressure increase (to increase the amount of vocal fold mass placed into vibratory motion and passively stretch the tissue in motion). As a general rule, fundamental frequency would be expected to rise if there is greater tension (passive plus active) of the tissue in motion or less mass of the tissue in motion. Intervention strategies dealing with pitch alteration need to take into consideration these physiologic and aerodynamic bases.

As a segue to the next section on loudness and vocal quality, it is noted that various combinations of cricothyroid and vocalis muscle contraction, with adduction, may change vocal quality, especially relative to the medial shaping of the vocal fold. Greater vocalis muscle contraction tends to round (and medialize) the medial contour of the vocal fold,[74,77,78] potentially decreasing the vibratory threshold pressure[14] and creating a relatively longer closed time of the vocal folds each cycle,[79] which may change the voice spectra to reflect a brighter, louder sound.

Loudness and Quality of Phonation

Loudness and quality of phonation are perceptual correlates to the physical measures of intensity and acoustic spectra, respectively.[13,32,80,81] Both perceptions depend upon the glottal volume velocity waveform characteristics and vocal tract resonance structure. We will emphasize the glottal volume velocity here.

Figure 12–7 illustrates a typical glottal volume velocity waveform in modal register with corresponding schematized glottal motion. The general shape of the glottal volume velocity waveform shows that the flow typically begins more gradually than when it is shut off, and the flow maximum is produced after the time when the maximum of the glottal area occurs. This flow delay characteristic (or *skewing* to the right relative to the glottal area) is related to the inertance of the airway, glottal wall motion, and glottal shape. The inertive effect[82,83] refers to the fact that the air within the vocal tract has mass. When the glottis just opens, the air (being driven by the translaryngeal air pressure) moves through the glottis to meet the column of air of the vocal tract. The air coming through the glottis must literally move other air already within the vocal tract, and this requirement slows the motion of the air as it first comes out of the glottis.[2,84] Corresponding to this event is the increase in air pressure just above the glottis as air moves through the glottis into the air above, thus typically reducing the translaryngeal pressure drop.[2,85-89] If the vocal tract were modeled as a uniform tube, greater glottal airflow skewing would be created from greater inertance by elongating the vocal tract (through larynx lowering or lip protrusion) or by narrowing the cross-sectional vocal tract area.[89,90] Fant[86] showed analytically that skewing increases not only with an increase of the vocal tract inertance (which changes with certain vowels and is higher with a constriction at the false fold level), but also with an increase in the maximum glottal excursion during the phonatory cycle, a faster glottal closing time, a lower subglottal pressure, and a smaller glottal kinetic flow factor k (the latter is derived in detail in references 91 and 92), concepts fruitful for clinical and training considerations. After the moment of maximum flow, the airflow will reduce to zero or to its minimum value as the two vocal folds come together at the end of glottal closing.

Skewing of the glottal volume velocity is related to the motion of the vocal folds according to a numerical model by Alipour and Scherer.[93] The lower margin of the vibrating vocal fold may have a different amplitude of motion than the upper margin, and the two margins may vary in their relative phase during the cycle. Skewing of the glottal volume flow appears to increase as the amplitude of the lower margin increas-

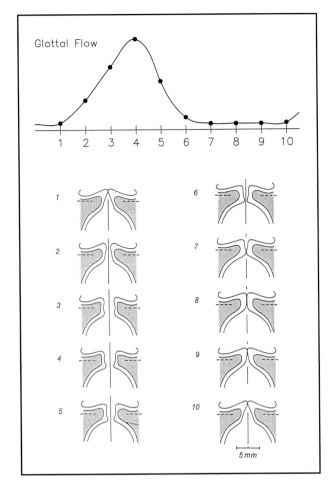

Fig 12–7. Glottal volume velocity waveform and corresponding glottal motion. The specific phases of the glottal cycle shown in the motion schematic are suggested on the glottal volume velocity waveform. (Adapted with permission from Hirano, M. *Clinical Examination of Voice.* Copyright 1981, Springer-Verlag.[30])

es relative to the upper margin, and decreases as the phase lead of the lower margin increases relative to the upper margin. This suggests that there may be an optimal compromise between amplitude and phase differences between the lower and upper glottal margins to maximize the skewing of the glottal volume velocity.

As Figure 12–7 shows, the glottis takes on a number of shapes during the vibratory cycle. A duct that expands in shape (a diffuser shape as suggested in steps 4, 5, and 6 of Fig 12–7) can have less resistance to flow than one of the same but constant (uniform) diameter.[91,92,94,95] The minimum flow resistance may occur when the glottis creates a diffuser shape of small angle (estimated to be between 5° and 10°[96,97]), which would most likely occur just past the time of the maximum glottal area. Therefore, when the glottis takes on the shape of a small-angled diffuser, the flow resistance may be less than at maximum glottal opening, and greater flow may then exit the glottis, to help skew the flow to the right relative to glottal area.

In general, then, if greater skewing of the glottal volume velocity is desired (as would be the case for any clinical or training condition needing greater energy in higher harmonic frequencies, see below), physiologic maneuvers should be considered to bring about the following: increase in the inertance of the vocal tract, increase in the lateral excursion of the vocal folds, decrease in the phase lead of the lower margin relative to the upper margin, and increase in the speed of glottal closure. These maneuvers would depend upon adjustments of the vocal tract shaping and length, level of glottal adduction (see below), level of subglottal pressure, and alteration in differential thyroarytenoid muscle contraction. These coordinations for optimal shaping and sizing of the glottal volume velocity waveform are central themes of needed research.

The qualities of the voice depend upon the glottal volume velocity waveform. Figure 12–8 shows an example of breathy (hypoadducted), normal, and pressed (hyperadducted) phonations in a normal adult male. The figure demonstrates typical variations of the glottal flow, the spectrum of the glottal flow, and the electroglottograph (EGG) waveforms for these qualities (the signals are not exactly time aligned). A Glottal Enterprises wide-band pneumotach system was used to acquire the inverse filtered (glottal) flow, and a Synchrovoice Laryngograph was used to obtain the EGG signal. Breathy voice is characterized by a more sinusoidal flow waveform than for normal phonation, with a significant flow bias. The flow bias is seen as a shift of the waveform away from the zero-flow baseline, indicating that there is always some flow exiting the glottis because of nonclosure throughout the cycle (the bias is also called the *DC flow*). In pressed phonation, the peaks of the flow are significantly smaller than for normal phonation, and the

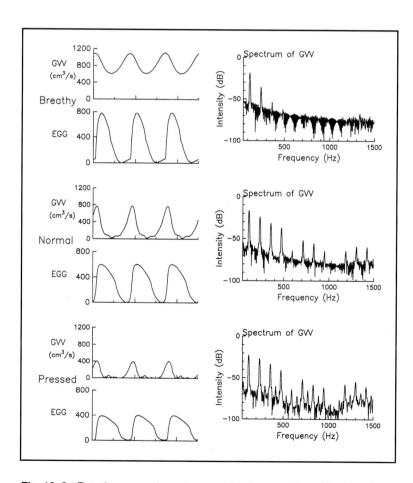

Fig 12–8. Breathy, normal, and pressed voice qualities. Glottal volume velocity and EGG waveforms are shown, as well as the spectrum of the glottal volume velocity waveforms. The subject was a normal adult male.

amount of time within the cycle during which the air exits the glottis is relatively short. Spectrally, the breathy quality example has energy primarily in the first two partials, whereas greater energy is distributed to higher harmonic frequencies in the normal and pressed quality examples. Up to 1000 Hz, the spectral slope is relatively steep at –17.3 dB/octave for breathy voice, less steep at –14.4 dB/octave for normal, and flattest at –10.8 dB/octave for the pressed condition for the examples in Figure 12–8. Notice the relative reduction in the level of the fundamental frequency compared to the first overtone from breathy to normal to pressed. The EGG waveforms suggest that there was a relatively large change of contact area between the surfaces of the two vocal folds during the breathy voicing, as seen by the relatively large amplitude (note that the greater the extent of the EGG waveform, the more vocal fold contact area change there is presumed to be[55]). However, the time during which the glottis was open, shown by the baseline length of the waveform, was relatively long in the breathy phonation compared to the other two qualities. The height of the pressed quality EGG waveform is shortest, suggesting relatively less dynamic contact of the vocal fold surfaces. This was explained by viewing the subject's larynx with stroboscopy; in pressed voice, the compression allowed only a restricted anterior glottal region to vibrate, thus resulting in the relatively short amplitudes because less of the total medial vocal fold surface participated in the vibration.

The overall intensity or sound pressure level (SPL) of the output sound may increase with increase in the maximum rate of change of the glottal volume velocity "shutoff" (the value M shown in Figure 12–2).[12,98-100] The maximum rate of change of the glottal flow is also the maximum negative slope, or the maximum flow declination rate. Greater maximum slope has the spectral effect of raising the energy of the partials primarily within the region of the first formant,[101] usually the most important spectral portion for overall SPL. This is like "turning [up] the volume control"[12(p562)] (see also reference 102). A doubling of the maximum negative slope corresponds empirically to an approximate increase of 5-9 dB in overall SPL.[12] Increased skewing of the glottal flow (discussed above) through increased vocal tract inertance and greater vocal fold motion should raise the overall SPL. For example, in their numerical study, Alipour and Scherer[93] found that increasing the amplitude of the lower glottal margin alone by 50% produced an increase in closing slope of more than 50%. These suggestions of acoustic (inertance) and kinematic (vocal fold motion) aides to enhance the desired characteristics of the glottal volume velocity need to be explored with human subject

studies to eventually improve treatment and training of people with voice concerns.

It is of importance to note some other spectral effects of differences in the glottal volume velocity waveform. The amount of time the waveform shows air exiting the glottis (time A to time B in Figure 12–2) divided by the period of the cycle (time A to time C in Figure 12–2) is called the *open quotient*. The open quotient typically decreases when changing adduction from a more breathy to a more normal quality voice, and with increase in loudness.[14] When the open quotient decreases, there may be a minor reduction (a few dB) of the intensity of the fundamental frequency and possibly a minor boost (a few dB) of the intensity of the first overtone (an octave above the fundamental frequency).[102,103] Also, the greater the amplitude of the volume velocity waveform (or the greater the area under the volume velocity waveform), the greater is the amplitude of the fundamental frequency.[12,101,104] A doubling of the amplitude of the waveform corresponds to an increase of approximately 3 to 7 dB in the spectral level of the fundamental frequency. When the flow has nearly completely shut off, that is, when the flow has nearly reached the baseline just before glottal closure, there is a "shutoff corner." The sharpness of this corner is related to the energy generated in the overtones of the voice, according to the modeling by Fant and his colleagues.[101,103] A change from a well-rounded corner to a very sharp corner can cause the intensity of the overtones to increase by up to 10 to 20 dB, undoubtedly affecting the quality of the sound[102,103] (changing glottal adduction from a breathy voice quality to a normal quality would sharpen this flow shutoff corner considerably). This concept needs exploration relative to how the vocal folds come together and to the perception of vocal quality, especially taken in the context of clinical intervention and vocal performance instruction.

The intensity and spectra of the glottal airflow are dependent on subglottal air pressure and fundamental frequency. As subglottal air pressure increases for a constant level of glottal adduction, the maximum (peak) airflow through the glottis increases. This follows from the greater maximum glottal width that is created when subglottal air pressure increases (see discussion above) and the greater driving pressure across the larger opening (see, eg, reference 105). As the maximum value of the volume velocity waveform increases, the intensity level of the fundamental frequency increases, as discussed above.[12] Also, if the peak flow increases, the maximum flow derivative should typically increase as the flow must reduce to zero (or near zero) from a greater value if the time during which the flow decreases remains the same.[100] An increase in the maximum flow derivative will increase the overall SPL and augment the spectrum, as indicated above. In addition, the increase in subglottal pressure may cause the vocal folds to come back together faster (or perhaps alter their dynamic phasing) after their larger maximum excursion, creating a sharper flow shutoff corner near the baseline, raising the overall spectrum of the overtones. Therefore, greater subglottal pressure may contribute to increasing the flow peak, increasing the maximum flow derivative, and sharpening the baseline flow shutoff corner. These effects change the flow spectrum shape by increasing the intensity level of the fundamental frequency and increasing the intensity of the overtones, thus raising the overall intensity of the voice. Titze and Sundberg[99] show explicitly how a doubling of subglottal pressure (more precisely, a doubling of the difference between subglottal pressure and threshold pressure) raises source acoustic power by 6 dB. Fant[86] broke down the intensity increase relative to the contributions of increased air velocity, increased maximum glottal area during the cycle, reduced time the glottis is open, faster glottal closing, and an increased flow derivative, totaling approximately 6 dB in intensity gain for a doubling of subglottal pressure. The early literature showed that voice intensity is strongly associated with subglottal pressure,[106-110] and this discussion has attempted to offer what has been suggested as an explanation as to how the subglottal pressure increase affects the sound source volume velocity waveform and the resultant increase of intensity.

Intensity is affected strongly by the fundamental frequency of voice production. Titze and Sundberg[99] show that the glottal power output will increase by 6 dB for an octave rise in fundamental frequency (all else the same), caused by the increase in the maximum flow derivative as the fundamental frequency rises (the same waveform shape with a shorter cycle period has a larger maximum flow derivative). At this point, one might ask why females, who speak at about 9 to 10 semitones above the fundamental frequency of men,[32] typically do not sound louder than men, and indeed do not differ substantially from men in intensity.[111] The just-mentioned effect of the higher frequency for women (about a ratio of 1.7 to 1) is potentially offset by a larger amplitude of glottal volume velocity for males (a ratio of about 2 to 1) so that the SPL for females is only 1 to 2 dB lower than for males.[99,111] In possible support, it is noted that Sapienza and Stathopoulos[112] found that the maximum flow derivative was essentially the same between men and women when they produced the same SPL values. On the other hand, Sulter and Wit[113] found that at normal and loud levels, the maximum flow derivative for untrained men was

approximately double that for untrained women at comparable SPL levels. These conflicting data suggest that this area of study is unresolved.

Because vocal sound is created by the glottal volume velocity, intervention strategies should attempt to improve the glottal airflow waveform, as mentioned above. There may be combinations of voicing variables that produce optimally efficient voice production from acoustic and physiologic orientations. Titze[114] has reported maximal intensity production in excised dog larynges for vocal processes that are placed very near each other, with less intensity (ranging to a few dB) for greater and less adduction. Sundberg[13] (also see Reference 104) has proposed the term *flow mode*, a type of phonation in which the glottal volume velocity amplitude is relatively large with high efficiency of laryngeal function. This is further emphasized, perhaps diagnostically, by examining the value of the flow amplitude divided by the subglottal pressure (the *glottal permittance*[100]). This ratio allows a clear separation between a pressed (constricted) voice versus normal and "flow" phonations (for a limited number of subjects[100]) because of the greater flow amplitudes for the same subglottal pressure in the normal and "flow" types. It is of considerable importance (theoretically and clinically) that professional (classically trained) male singers may produce voiced sounds at higher intensity levels than male nonsingers for the same subglottal pressures, caused primarily by greater glottal flow amplitudes (from adjusted flow impedance).[14,99] In addition, performance training strategies have emphasized vocal tract adjustments to match lower voicing partials with the first formant[115] or to create an enhanced higher formant region[116,117] by clustering formants numbers 3, 4 and 5, strategies that boost the output energy of certain partials of the voice, creating a "bright" or "carrying" voice with desirable performance qualities. These tactics are not dissimilar to strategies employed in voice pathology (eg, references 118 and 119).

Vocal Fold Motion During Phonation

Although it is important to realize that the creation of the sound of voicing is within the airflow exiting the glottis, and not in the motion of the vocal folds per se, the motion of the vocal folds helps to determine the characteristics of the airflow.

Basic kinematic (motion) aspects of normal vocal folds include the effects of increased subglottal pressure, vocal fold elongation, and glottal adduction. Increased subglottal pressure produces increased lateral pressures on the medial surfaces and vertical pressures on the undersurface of the vocal folds, creating greater maximum excursion during the vibratory cycle (as discussed above). Elongation of the vocal folds by increased contraction of the cricothyroid muscles and/or decreased contraction of the thyroarytenoid muscles modifies the cross-sectional shape of the vocal fold (with no change of total vocal fold mass) to form a reduced vocal fold thickness (measured in the vertical direction),[120-123] giving rise to potentially less vocal fold tissue contact during vocal fold closure. For the same subglottal pressure and glottal adduction, vocal fold lengthening would affect the glottal volume velocity waveform by increasing the open quotient and decreasing the maximum flow derivative. Increased adduction will affect the motion of the vocal folds by creating more contact between the vocal folds and a longer glottal closed time within each cycle.[48,124-128] Any abnormality of tissue morphology (swelling, stiffness, or growth along the vocal fold), unilaterally or bilaterally, may alter the vibratory motion to create different glottal volume velocity waveforms from cycle to cycle, or from cycle group to cycle group (refer to the earlier discussion on perturbation). Severe laryngitis associated with extreme edema creates the well-known response of aphonia (inability to phonate or absence of phonation), which may be explained by the mass being too great to permit vibration, and the rounded glottal shaping causing less-effective intraglottal pressures during phonation.[129] Refer to Hirano and Bless[130] for photographs of vibratory patterns for a number of vocal pathologies including nodules, polyps, cysts, and others.

These kinds of structural changes to the vocal folds lead to the question: How is the vibration of the vocal folds maintained? That is, what allows them to remain in oscillation? A response to this question will now be explored.

The mechanical phonatory motion of the vocal folds depends upon the folds being driven by air pressures within the glottis,[91,96,131-136] such air pressure forces working with the biomechanical characteristics of the vocal folds (mass, stiffness, damping) to overcome the damping losses within the tissue.[22,57,66,137-142] The *intraglottal pressures* are extremely important, then, in the maintenance of vocal fold oscillation.[2,8,142] If the intraglottal pressures are positive, they act to push the vocal folds away from each other. If the intraglottal pressures are negative, they pull the vocal folds toward each other. The polarity (positive or negative) of the intraglottal pressure depends upon both the dynamic air pressures directly above and below the glottis and the shape of the glottal airway, as will now be discussed (see references 2 and 90).

The acoustic air pressure just above the glottis may be important for maintaining vocal fold oscillation. As the glottis nears closure during a normal vibratory cycle, the airflow through the glottis decreases relatively quickly. The air that has already passed through the glottis continues to travel up the vocal tract, creating greater distance between itself (the air) and the glottis. This air momentum produces a negative rarefaction pressure directly above the glottis as the particles of air separate more and more from each other. Negative pressure at the glottal exit location would create pressures that are negative within the glottis (at least within the glottal duct near the exit) if the glottis has not closed at the lower glottal edge. The intraglottal negative pressure, located at least near the glottal exit, thus should facilitate the final closing of the glottis by pulling the two folds together (aided by the closing momentum of the tissue itself). The amount of the negative intraglottal pressure would depend upon the value of the maximum negative supraglottal pressure.

As the glottis opens during a vibratory cycle, the airflow through the glottis meets the mass of air directly above it, creating compression of the air and positive air pressure. The positive air pressure directly above the glottis would raise the air pressure within the glottis, at least near the glottal exit. This increased pressure caused by the positive supraglottal pressure would therefore facilitate glottal opening by allowing more push on the vocal folds to help separate them. Thus, during opening, supraglottal positive pressure may aid glottal opening, and during closing, supraglottal negative pressure aids glottal closing.

The glottis takes on two primary shapes during (exhalatory) phonation, *convergent* and *divergent* (see Fig 12–9).[18,143-145] During glottal opening, the convergent glottal shape is produced with a wider opening at glottal entrance and a narrower opening at glottal exit (Fig 12–7). Because of the convergent shape, a pressure drop (from a higher value to a lower value, Fig 12–9) is created from the positive tracheal pressure to the pressure existing at the glottal exit location,[96] which may be close to positive (as discussed above) or near atmospheric. Thus, the glottal convergent shape (itself) creates a positive pressure within the glottis, and this positive pressure pushes on the vocal folds, facilitating glottal opening. This pressure decrease within the converging glottis follows directly from the Bernoulli equation (for steady flow).

During glottal closing, the divergent glottal shape may be most prominent; the configuration has a narrower opening at glottal entrance than at glottal exit (Fig 12–9). Divergent glottal duct shapes are similar to mechanical diffusers in that the expanding area allows pressures within the duct to increase between the upstream inlet and the downstream outlet.[94,96,97] The pressure at glottal entry is, therefore, lower than at exit, and is negative within the glottis if the glottal exit pressure is atmospheric (zero) or negative (per the discussion above on glottal closing). This negative pressure is caused by the divergent shape of the glottis, with the minimal duct diameter formed at entry, creating the lowest pressure there (at entry) essentially in accordance with the Bernoulli equation. The negative intraglottal pressure would pull on the vocal fold surfaces, facilitating glottal closure.

The "Bernoulli effect" refers to the existence of negative pressure in a narrowed location of a duct through which air (fluid) is flowing. This is the result of the trade-off (described by the Bernoulli equation) between air pressure and air particle velocity for different size sections of the duct (lower pressure and higher velocity exist in a narrower section). The Bernoulli effect has been used historically to help "explain" phonation (Tonndorf was an important ear-

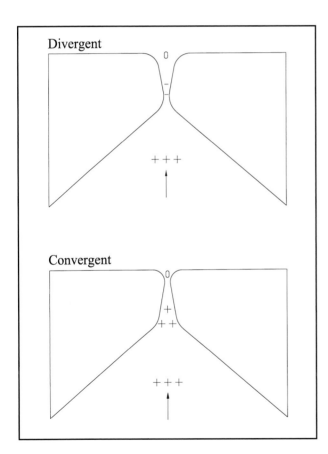

Fig 12–9. Pressures within the glottis relative to glottal shape. In the convergent glottis (lower sketch), the air pressures are positive in the entrance of the glottis and decrease to zero (or to the pressure just above the glottis). In the divergent glottis (upper sketch), the air pressures are negative in the entrance of the glottis and increase to zero (or to the pressure just above the glottis).

ly proponent of this concept for the maintenance of vocal fold oscillation, see reference 146). That is, as the air particles speed up as they enter the glottis from the trachea, the air pressure supposedly would become negative throughout the glottis because it would constitute a smaller opening than the trachea, and then the negative pressure would suck the folds toward each other regardless of the glottal shape. This explanation is incomplete. During glottal opening, when the glottis has a convergent shape and the minimal glottal diameter is at the glottal exit, the Bernoulli energy equation does help to explain the pressure reduction from the glottal entrance to the glottal exit, but the intraglottal pressure is positive, not negative, despite the glottis being smaller than the trachea, because the pressure lowers from the positive tracheal value to the positive or near zero value at glottal exit. During glottal closing when the glottis forms a divergent (diffuser) shape, the pressure reduction from the trachea to glottal entry may follow the Bernoulli equation for the most part, but the application of the Bernoulli equation within the glottis would essentially apply only in the special case of no flow separation from the glottal walls. *Flow separation*, in which the air flows away from the glottal wall rather than staying close to the wall, occurs when there is a sufficient pressure rise in the diverging glottal duct. This creates a condition where the Bernoulli equation no longer applies beyond the flow separation point.[96,132,133,147] The pressure will increase from a negative value at the entrance to the glottis to a rather constant value (equal to the air pressure just downstream of the glottis) a short distance past the air separation location for these divergent glottis conditions.[147] These concepts are based on steady (constant) flow modeling with static glottal shapes of many angles.[97]

The pressure on the medial vocal folds during vibration is more complex than indicated above. During phonation the glottis viewed superiorly is rather elliptical in shape, with greatest amplitude of motion near the middle of the membranous glottis. Pressures appear to vary the most during the cycle within the glottis at the location of the maximum motion, with cyclic pressure variations decreasing anteriorly and posteriorly to this location.[136] These dynamic glottal pressure changes are called *bidirectional pressure gradients*.[136]

Another interesting complexity of glottal pressures is that, even when the glottis forms a symmetric convergent or divergent duct, the pressures on the two vocal folds may not be identical because of flow separation only on one side of the glottis and not the other side, or because the flow bends to one side downstream of the glottis.[97,147] However, there may not be time to develop these glottal wall pressure differences during phonation because the geometry changes so quickly.[148-150] When the glottal duct is slanted to one side, as can be seen in some normal and abnormal phonations in which the two vocal folds vibrate out of phase with each other,[151-153] the pressures on the two sides of the glottis may be substantially different.[147] These pressure differences may promote the out-of-phase motion of the two vocal folds.

The actual interdependence among dynamic (time-varying) glottal shaping, translaryngeal pressures, and intraglottal pressures, and the application of equations of mechanics, require precise empirical measurement of glottal shaping, flows, and pressures during phonation, research yet to be adequately performed. In addition, the relationship among these aspects, the particle velocities that make up the glottal flow, and the resulting acoustic signal[33,154-164] extend this matter to the necessary and interfacing aeroacoustic level of phonation.

Conclusion

This chapter has reviewed basic aspects of laryngeal function during phonation. The concepts underlying the understanding of duration, frequency, intensity, spectra, and vocal fold motion during phonation are the bases with which to make effective intervention decisions for laryngeal and voice change. These underlying concepts are applicable to both clinical and training practices.

Acknowledgments The author is grateful to and would like to thank Chwen Guo and Daoud Shinwari for their help with the figures, Kimberly Fisher for the use of her spasmodic dysphonia data, Marshall Smith for his figure dealing with vocal mass and fundamental frequency change, Tamara Field for help in preparing Figure 12–1, and David Kuehn for an anatomical discussion. This project was prepared with support from NIDCD grants P60 DC00976 RTC and R01 DC03577, and is dedicated to the memory and mentorship of Dr. Wilbur James Gould.

References

1. Scherer RC. Aerodynamic assessment in voice production. In: Cooper JA, ed. *Assessment of Speech and Voice Production: Research and Clinical Applications.* NIDCD Monograph Vol 1-1991. Bethesda, Md: National Institute on Deafness and Other Communication Disorders, NIH; 1991:112–123.

2. Scherer RC. Physiology of phonation: A review of basic mechanics. In: Ford CN, Bless DM, eds. *Phonosurgery: Assessment and Surgical Management of Voice Disorders.* New York, NY: Raven Press; 1991:77–93.

3. Hollien H, Moore GP. Measurement of the vocal folds during changes in pitch. *J Speech Hear Res.* 1960;3:157–165.

4. Nishizawa N, Sawashima M, Yonemoto K. In: Fujimura O, ed. *Vocal Physiology: Voice Production, Mechanisms, and Function.* New York, NY: Raven Press; 1988:75–82.

5. Backus J. *The Acoustical Foundations of Music.* 2nd ed. New York, NY: WW Norton & Co; 1977.

6. Titze IR, Durham PL. Passive mechanisms influencing fundamental frequency control. In: Baer T, Sasaki C, Harris KS, eds. *Laryngeal Function in Phonation and Respiration.* San Diego, Calif: College-Hill Press; 1987:304–319.

7. Colton RH. Physiological mechanisms of vocal frequency control: the role of tension. *J Voice.* 1988;2(3):208–220.

8. Titze IR. *Principles of Voice Production.* Englewood Cliffs, NJ: Prentice Hall; 1994.

9. Perlman AL, Titze IR. Development of an in vitro technique for measuring elastic properties of vocal fold tissue. *J Speech Hear Res.* 1988;31/2:288–289.

10. Colton RH, Casper JK. *Understanding Voice Problems.* Baltimore, Md: Williams & Wilkins; 1990.

11. Hammarberg B, Fritzell B, Gauffin J, Sundberg J. *Acoustic glottogram, subglottic pressure, and voice quality during insufficient vocal fold closure phonation: Proceedings of the International Conference on Voice,* Kurume, Japan. 1986:28–35.

12. Gauffin J, Sundberg J. Spectral correlates of glottal voice source waveform characteristics. *J Speech Hear Res.* 1989;32:556–565.

13. Sundberg J. *The Science of the Singing Voice.* Dekalb, Il: Northern Illinois University Press; 1987.

14. Titze IR. Phonation threshold pressure: a missing link in glottal aerodynamics. *J Acoust Soc Am.* 1992;91(5): 2926–2935.

15. Lucero JC. Optimal glottal configuration for ease of phonation. *J Voice.* 1998;12:151–158.

16. Chan RW, Titze IR, Titze MR. Further studies of phonation threshold pressure in a physical model of the vocal fold mucosa. *J Acoust Soc Am.* 1997;101:3722–3727.

17. Verdolini-Marston K, Titze I, Druker D. Changes in phonation threshold pressure with induced conditions of hydration. *J Voice.* 1990;4(2):142–151.

18. Baer T. *Investigation of Phonation Using Excised Larynges* [dissertation]. Cambridge, Mass: Massachusetts Institute of Technology; 1975.

19. Baer T. Observation of vocal fold vibration: Measurement of excised larynges. In: Stevens KN, Hirano M, eds. *Vocal Fold Physiology.* Tokyo, Japan: University of Tokyo Press; 1981:119–133.

20. Draper MH, Ladefoged P, Whitteridge D. Expiratory pressures and air flow during speech. *British Med* J. 1960;18:1837–1843.

21. Berry DA, Herzel H, Titze IR, Story BH. Bifurcation in excised larynx experiments. *J Voice.* 1996;10:129–138.

22. Lucero JC. A theoretical study of the hysteresis phenomenon at vocal fold oscillation onset-offset. *J Acoust Soc Am.* 1999;105:423–431.

23. Fisher KV, Swank PR. Estimating phonation threshold pressure. *J Speech Hear Res.* 1997;40:1122–1129.

24. Coleman RF, Mabis JH, Hinson JK. Fundamental frequency-sound pressure level profiles of adult male and female voices. *J Speech Hear Res.* 1977;20:197–204.

25. Klingholz F, Martin F. Die quantitative Auswertung der Stimmfeldmessung. Sprache-Stimme-Gehor. 1983;7:106–110.

26. Titze IR. Acoustic interpretation of the voice range profile (phonetogram). *J Speech Hear Res.* 1992;35:21–34.

27. Coleman RF. Sources of variation in phonetograms. *J Voice.* 1993;7(1):1–14.

28. Gramming P. The Phonetogram: An Experimental and Clinical Study. Malmo, Sweden: Department of Otolaryngology, University of Lund; 1988.

29. Bless DM, Baken RJ, Hacki T, et al. International Association of Logopedics and Phoniatrics (IALP) Voice Committee discussion of assessment topics. *J Voice.* 1992;6(2):194–210.

30. Hirano M. *Clinical Examination of Voice.* New York, NY: Springer-Verlag; 1981.

31. Hirose H, Niimi S. The relationship between glottal opening and the transglottal pressure differences during consonant production. In: Baer T, Sasaki C, Harris KS, eds. *Laryngeal Function in Phonation and Respiration.* San Diego, Calif: College-Hill Press; 1987:381–390.

32. Baken RJ. *Clinical Measurement of Speech and Voice.* Boston, Mass: College-Hill Press, Little, Brown & Co; 1987.

33. Kakita Y. Simultaneous observation of the vibratory pattern, sound pressure, and airflow signals using a physical model of the vocal folds. In: Fujimura O, ed. *Vocal Physiology: Voice Production, Mechanisms, and Function.* New York, NY: Raven Press Ltd.; 1988:207–218.

34. Fant G. Some problems in voice source analysis. *Speech Commun.* 1993;13:7–22.

35. Kiritani S, Hirose H, Imagawa H. High-speed digital image analysis of vocal cord vibration in diplophonia. *Speech Commun.* 1993;13:23–32.

36. Pinto NB, Titze IR. Unification of perturbation measures in speech signals. *J Acoust Soc Am.* 1990;87(3):1278–1289.

37. Larson C, Kempster G, Kistler M. Changes in voice fundamental frequency following discharge of single motor units in cricothyroid and thyroarytenoid muscles. *J Speech Hear Res.* 1987;30:552–558.

38. Kempster GB, Larson CR, Kistler MK. Effects of electrical stimulation of cricothyroid and thyroarytenoid muscles on voice fundamental frequency. *J Voice.* 1988;2(3):221–229.

39. Titze IR. A model for neurologic sources of aperiodicity in vocal fold vibration. *J Speech Hear Res.* 1991;34(3):460–472.

40. Baer T. Vocal jitter: A neuromuscular explanation. In: Lawrence V, Weinberg B, eds. *Transcripts of the Eighth Symposium on Care of the Professional Voice.* New York, NY: The Voice Foundation; 1979:19–22.

41. Cavalli L, Hirson A. Diplophonia reappraised. *J Voice.* 1999;13:542–556.

42. Isshiki N, Ishizaka K. Computer simulation of pathological vocal cord vibration. *J Acoust Soc Am.* 1976;60:1193–1198.

43. Moon FC. *Chaotic Vibrations.* New York, NY: John Wiley & Sons; 1987.

44. Gerratt BR, Precoda K, Hanson D, Berke GS. Source characteristics of diplophonia. *J Acoust Soc Am.* 1988;83:S66.

45. Wong D, Ito MR, Cox NB, Titze IR. Observation of perturbations in a lumped-element model of the vocal folds with application to some pathological cases. *J Acoust Soc Am.* 1991;89:383–394.

46. Berke GS, Gerratt BR. Laryngeal biomechanics: an overview of mucosal wave mechanics. *J Voice.* 1993;7(2):123–128.

47. Titze IR, Baken RJ, Herzel H. Evidence of chaos in vocal fold vibration. In: Titze IR, ed. *Vocal Fold Physiology: Frontiers in Basic Science.* San Diego, Calif: Singular Publishing Group; 1993:143–188.

48. Scherer R, Gould WJ, Titze I, Meyers A, Sataloff R. Preliminary evaluation of selected acoustic and glottographic measures for clinical phonatory function analysis. *J Voice.* 1988;2:230–244.

49. Omori K, Kojima H, Kakani R, Slavit DH, Blaugrund SM. Acoustic characteristics of rough voice: subharmonics. *J Voice.* 1997;1:40–47.

50. Hollien H, Moore P, Wendahl RW, Michel JF. On the nature of vocal fry. *J Speech Hear Res.* 1966;9:245–247.

51. Keidar A. Vocal Register Change: An Investigation of Perceptual and Acoustic Isomorphism [dissertation]. Iowa City: The University of Iowa; 1986.

52. Titze IR. A framework for the study of vocal registers. *J Voice.* 1988;2(3):183–194.

53. Scherer RC. Physiology of creaky voice and vocal fry. *J Acoust Soc Am.* 1989;86(S1):S25(A).

54. Blomgren M, Chen Y, Ng ML, Gilbert HR. Acoustic, aerodynamic, physiologic, and perceptual properties of modal and vocal fry registers. *J Acoust Soc Am.* 1998;103:2649–2658.

55. Scherer RC, Druker DG, Titze IR. Electroglottography and direct measurement of vocal fold contact area. In: Fujimura O, ed. *Vocal Physiology: Voice Production, Mechanisms, and Function.* New York, NY: Raven Press, Ltd; 1988:279–291.

56. Ishizaka K, Matsudaira M. Analysis of the vibration of the vocal cords. *J Acoust Soc Jap.* 1968;24:311–312.

57. Ishizaka K, Flanagan JL. Synthesis of voiced sounds from a two-mass model of the vocal cords. *Bell Sys Tech J.* 1972;51(6):1233–1268.

58. Smith ME, Berke GS, Gerratt BR, Kreiman J. Laryngeal paralysis: theoretical considerations and effects on laryngeal vibration. *J Speech Hear Res.* 1992;35:545–554.

59. Rothenberg M, Mahshie J. Induced transglottal pressure variations during voicing. *Speech Commun.* 1986;14(3-4):365–371.

60. Baer T. Reflex activation of laryngeal muscles by sudden induced subglottal pressure changes. *J Acoust Soc Am.* 1979;65:1271–1275.

61. Cheng YM, Guerin B. Control parameters in male and female glottal sources. In: Baer T, Sasaki C, Harris KS, eds. *Laryngeal Function in Phonation and Respiration.* San Diego, Calif: College-Hill Press; 1987:219–238.

62. Baken RJ, Orlikoff RF. Phonatory response to step-function changes in supraglottal pressure. In: Baer T, Sasaki C, Harris KS, eds. *Laryngeal Function in Phonation and Respiration*. San Diego, Calif: College-Hill Press; 1987: 273–290.

63. Saito S, Fukuda H, Isogai Y, Ono H. X-ray stroboscopy. In: Stevens KN, Hirano M, eds. *Vocal Fold Physiology*. Tokyo, Japan: University of Tokyo Press; 1981:95–106.

64. Saito S, Fukuda H, Kitahara S, et al. Pellet tracking in the vocal fold while phonating—experimental study using canine larynges with muscle activity. In: Titze IR, Scherer RC, eds. *Vocal Fold Physiology: Biomechanics, Acoustics and Phonatory Control*. Denver, Colo: The Denver Center for the Performing Arts; 1985:169–182.

65. Fukuda H, Saito S, Kitahara S, et al. Vocal fold vibration in excised larynges viewed with an x-ray stroboscope and an ultra-high-speed camera. In: Bless DM, Abbs JH, eds. *Vocal Fold Physiology, Contemporary Research and Clinical Issues*. San Diego, Calif: College-Hill Press; 1983:238–252.

66. Alipour-Haghighi F, Titze IR. Simulation of particle trajectories of vocal fold tissue during phonation. In: Titze IR, Scherer RC, eds. *Vocal Fold Physiology: Biomechanics, Acoustics and Phonatory Control*. Denver, Colo: The Denver Center for the Performing Arts; 1985:183–190.

67. Muta H, Fukuda H. Pressure-flow relationship in the experimental phonation of excised canine larynges. In: Fujimura O, ed. *Vocal Physiology: Voice Production, Mechanisms, and Function*. New York, NY: Raven Press, Ltd; 1988:239–247.

68. Titze IR, Luschei ES, Hirano M. Role of the thyroarytenoid muscle in regulation of fundamental frequency. *J Voice*. 1989;3(3):213–224.

69. Gelfer CE, Harris KS, Collier R, Baer T. Is declination actively controlled? In: Titze IR, Scherer RC, eds. *Vocal Fold Physiology: Biomechanics, Acoustics and Phonatory Control*. Denver, Colo: The Denver Center for the Performing Arts; 1985:113–126.

70. Gelfer CE, Harris KS, Baer T. Controlled variables in sentence intonation. In: Baer T, Sasaki C, Harris KS, eds. *Laryngeal Function in Phonation and Respiration*. San Diego, Calif: College-Hill Press; 1987:422–435.

71. Honda K. Relationship between pitch control and vowel articulation. In: Bless DM, Abbs JH, eds. *Vocal Fold Physiology, Contemporary Research and Clinical Issues*. San Diego, Calif: College-Hill Press; 1983:286–297.

72. Sundberg J, Leanderson R, von Euler C. Activity relationship between diaphragm and cricothyroid muscles. *J Voice*. 1989;3(3):225–232.

73. Titze IR, Jiang J, Drucker DG. Preliminaries to the body-cover theory of pitch control. *J Voice*. 1988;1(4):314–319.

74. Choi HS, Berke GS, Ye M, Kreiman J. Function of the thyroarytenoid muscle in a canine laryngeal model. *Ann Otol Rhinol Laryngol*. 1993;102:769–776.

75. Arnold GE. Physiology and pathology of the cricothyroid muscle. *Laryngoscope*. 1961;71:687–753.

76. Fujimura O. Body-cover theory of the vocal fold and its phonetic implications. In: Stevens KN, Hirano M, eds. *Vocal Fold Physiology*. Tokyo, Japan: University of Tokyo Press; 1981:271–288.

77. Hirano M. Phonosurgery: Basic and clinical investigations. *Otologia (Fukuoka)*. 1975;21:239–442.

78. Hirano M. The laryngeal muscles in singing. In: Hirano M, Kirchner JA, Bless DM, eds. *Neurolaryngology, Recent Advances*. Boston, Mass: A College-Hill Publication, Little, Brown & Co; 1987:209–230.

79. Titze IR. A four-parameter model of the glottis and vocal fold contact area. *Speech Commun*. 1989;8:191–201.

80. Plomp R. *Aspects of Tone Sensation*. New York, NY: Academic Press; 1976.

81. Strong WJ, Plitnik GR. *Music Speech Audio*. Provo, UT: Soundprint; 1992.

82. Rothenberg M. Acoustic interaction between the glottal source and the vocal tract. In: Stevens KN, Hirano M, eds. *Vocal Fold Physiology*. Tokyo, Japan: University of Tokyo Press; 1981:305–328.

83. Rothenberg M. An interactive model for the voice source. In: Bless DM, Abbs JH, eds. *Vocal Fold Physiology, Contemporary Research and Clinical Issues*. San Diego, Calif: College-Hill Press; 1983:155–165.

84. Titze IR. The physics of small-amplitude oscillation of the vocal folds. *J Acoust Soc Am*. 1988;83:1536–1552.

85. Kitzing P, Lofqvist A. Subglottal and oral pressures during phonation—preliminary investigation using a miniature transducer system. *Med Biolog Eng*. 1975;13(5):644–648.

86. Fant G. Preliminaries to analysis of the human voice source. *STL-QPRS*. 1983;(4)1982:1–27.

87. Miller DG, Schutte HK. Characteristic patterns of sub- and supra-glottal pressure variations within the glottal cycle. In: Lawrence VL, ed. *Transcripts of the XIIIth Symposium: Care of the Professional Voice*. New York, NY: The Voice Foundation; 1984:70–75.

88. Cranen B, Boves L. A set-up for testing the validity of the two mass model of the vocal folds. In: Titze IR, Scherer RC, eds. *Vocal Fold Physiology: Biomechanics, Acoustics and Phonatory Control*. Denver, Colo: The Denver Center for the Performing Arts; 1985:500–513.

89. Olson HF. *Solutions of Engineering Problems by Dynamical Analogies*. 2nd ed. New York, NY: D Van Nostrand Co; 1966.

90. Titze IR. Mean intraglottal pressure in vocal fold oscillation. *J Phonetics*. 1986;14:359–364.

91. Scherer RC, Guo CG. *Laryngeal modeling: translaryngeal pressure for a model with many glottal shapes*. ICSLP Proceedings, 1990 International Conference on Spoken Language Processing. Vol 1. The Acoustical Society of Japan, Japan; 1990:3.1.1–3.1.4.

92. Scherer RC, Guo CG. Generalized translaryngeal pressure coefficient for a wide range of laryngeal configurations. In: Gauffin J, Hammarberg B, eds. *Vocal Fold Physiology: Acoustic, Perceptual, and Physiological Aspects of Voice Mechanisms*. San Diego, Calif: Singular Publishing Group; 1991:83–90.

93. Alipour F, Scherer RC. Pulsatile flow within an oscillating glottal model. *J Iran Mech Eng*. 1998;3:73–81.

94. Kline SJ. On the nature of stall. *ASME J Basic Eng*. 1959;81:305–320.

95. Miller DS. *Internal Flow, a Guide to Losses in Pipe and Duct Systems.* Cranfield, UK: British Hydromechanics Research Association; 1971.

96. Guo CG, Scherer RC. Finite element simulation of glottal flow and pressure. *J Acoust Soc Am.* 1993;94(2)(pt 1): 688–700.

97. Scherer RC, Shinwari D. Glottal pressure profiles for a diameter of 0.04 cm. *J Acoust Soc Am.* 2000;107(5)(pt 2): 2905.

98. Scherer R, Sundberg J, Titze I. Laryngeal adduction related to characteristics of the flow glottogram. *J Acoust Soc Am.* 1989;85(S1):S129(A).

99. Titze IR, Sundberg J. Vocal intensity in speakers and singers. *J Acoust Soc Am.* 1992;91:2936–2946.

100. Sundberg J, Titze I, Scherer R. Phonatory control in male singing: a study of the effects of subglottal pressure, fundamental frequency, and mode of phonation on the voice source. *J Voice.* 1993;7(1):15–29.

101. Fant G, Liljencrants J, Lin Q. A four-parameter model of glottal flow. *STL-QPSR.* 1985;(4):1–13.

102. Gobl C, Karlsson I. Male and female voice source dynamics. In: Gauffin J, Hammarberg B, eds. *Vocal Fold Physiology: Acoustic, Perceptual, and Physiological Aspects of Voice* Mechanisms. San Diego, Calif: Singular Publishing Group; 1991:121–128.

103. Fant G, and Lin Q. Comments on glottal flow modeling and analysis. In: Gauffin J, Hammarberg B, eds. *Vocal Fold Physiology: Acoustic, Perceptual, and Physiological Aspects of Voice* Mechanisms. San Diego, Calif: Singular Publishing Group; 1991:47–56.

104. Sundberg J, Gauffin J. Waveform and spectrum of the glottal voice source. In: Lindblom B, Ohman S, eds. *Frontiers of Speech Communication Research.* New York, NY: Academic Press; 1979:301–322.

105. Scherer RC, Titze IR, Curtis JF. Pressure-flow relationships in two models of the larynx having rectangular glottal shapes. *J Acoust Soc Am.* 1983;73:668–676.

106. Ladefoged P, McKinney NP. Loudness, sound pressure, and subglottal pressure in speech. *J Acoust Soc Am.* 1963;35:454–460.

107. Isshiki N. Regulatory mechanism of voice intensity variations. *J Speech Hear Res.* 1964;7:17–29.

108. Isshiki N. Remarks on mechanism for vocal intensity variation. *J Speech Hear Res.* 1969;12:665–672.

109. Rubin HJ, LeCover M, Vennard W. Vocal intensity, subglottic pressure, and airflow relationships in singers. *Folia Phoniatr.* 1967;19:393–413.

110. Bouhuys A, Mead J, Proctor D, Stevens K. Pressure-flow events during singing. *Ann NY Acad Sci.* 1968;155: 165–176.

111. Holmberg EB, Hillman RE, Perkell J. Glottal airflow and transglottal air pressure measurements for male and female speakers in soft, normal, and loud voice. *J Acoust Soc Am.* 1988;84:511–529.

112. Sapienza CM, Stathopoulos ET. Comparison of maximum flow declination rate: children versus adults. *J Voice.* 1994;8:240–247.

113. Sulter AM, Wit H. Glottal volume velocity waveform characteristics in subjects with and without vocal train-ing, related to gender, sound intensity, fundamental frequency, and age. *J Acoust Soc Am.* 1996;100:3360–3373.

114. Titze IR. Regulation of vocal power and efficiency by subglottal pressure and glottal width. In: Fujimura O, ed. *Vocal Physiology: Voice Production, Mechanisms, and Function.* New York, NY: Raven Press, Ltd; 1988:227–238.

115. Raphael BN, Scherer RC. Voice modifications of stage actors: acoustic analyses. *J Voice.* 1987;1:83–87.

116. Bartholomew WT. A physical definition of "good voice quality" in the male voice. *J Acoust Soc Am.* 1934;6: 25–33.

117. Sundberg J. Articulatory interpretation of the "singing formant." *J Acoust Soc Am.* 1974;55:838–844.

118. Perkins WH. *Voice Disorders.* New York, NY: Thieme-Stratton Inc; 1983.

119. Verdolini K, Druker DG, Palmer PM, Samawi H. Laryngeal adduction in resonant voice. *J Voice.* 1998;12: 315–327.

120. Hollien HF, Curtis JF. A laminagraphic study of vocal pitch. *J Speech Hear Res.* 1960;3:361–371.

121. Hollien HF. Vocal fold thickness and fundamental frequency of phonation. *J Speech Hear Res.* 1962;5(3):237–243.

122. Hollien HF, Colton RH. Four laminagraphic studies of vocal fold thickness. *Folia Phoniatr.* 1969;21:179–198.

123. Hollien HF, Coleman RF. Laryngeal correlates of frequency change: A STROL study. *J Speech Hear Res.* 1970;13(2):271–278.

124. Scherer RC, Vail VJ, Rockwell B. Examination of the laryngeal adduction measure EGGW. In: Bell-Berti F, Raphael LJ, eds: *Producing Speech: Contemporary Issues: A Festshrift for Katherine Safford Harris.* Woodbury, NY: American Institute of Physics; 1995:269–290.

125. Hess MM, Verdolini K, Bierhals W, Mansmann U, Gross M. Endolaryngeal contact pressure. *J Voice.* 1998;12:50–67.

126. Verdolini K, Chan R, Titze IR, Hess M, Bierhals W. Correspondence of electroglottographic closed quotient to vocal fold impact stress in excised canine larynges. *J Voice.* 1998;12:415–423.

127. Verdolini K, Hess MH, Titze IR, Bierhals W, Gross M. Investigation of vocal fold impact stress in human subjects. *J Voice.* 1999;13:184–202.

128. Yamana T, Kitajima K. Laryngeal closure pressure during phonation in humans. *J Voice.* 2000;14:1–7.

129. Scherer RC, DeWitt K, Kucinschi BR. Effect of exit vocal radii on intraglottal pressure distributions in the convergent glottis. *J Acoust Soc Am.* 2001;110:1253–1256.

130. Hirano M, Bless DM. *Videostroboscopic Examination of the Larynx.* San Diego, Calif: Singular Publishing Group; 1993.

131. Berg Jw van den, Zantema JT, Doornenbal P Jr. On the air resistance and the Bernoulli effect of the human larynx. *J Acoust Soc Am.* 1957;29:626–631.

132. Scherer RC. Pressure-flow relationships in a laryngeal airway model having a diverging glottal duct. *J Acoust Soc Am.* 1983;73(S1):S46(A).

133. Scherer RC, Titze IR. Pressure-flow relationships in a model of the laryngeal airway with a diverging glottis. In: Bless DM, Abbs JH, eds. *Vocal Fold Physiology, Contemporary Research and Clinical Issues.* San Diego, Calif: College-Hill Press; 1983:179–193.

134. Gauffin J, Binh N, Ananthapadmanabha TV, Fant G. Glottal geometry and volume velocity waveform. In: Bless DM, Abbs JH, eds. *Vocal Fold Physiology: Contemporary Research and Clinical Issues.* San Diego, Calif: College-Hill Press; 1983:194–201.

135. Ishizaka K. Air resistance and intraglottal pressure in a model of the larynx. In: Titze IR, Scherer RC. eds. *Vocal Fold Physiology: Biomechanics, Acoustics and Phonatory Control.* Denver, Colo: The Denver Center for the Performing Arts; 1985:414–424.

136. Alipour R, Scherer RC. Dynamic glottal pressures in an excised hemilarynx model. *J Voice.* 2000;14:443–454.

137. Ishizaka K, Matsudaira M. *Fluid mechanical considerations of vocal cord vibration.* SCRL Monograph No. 8, April 1972.

138. Titze IR. The human vocal cords: a mathematical model. Part I. *Phonetica.* 1973;28:129–170.

139. Titze IR. The human vocal cords: a mathematical model. Part II. *Phonetica.* 1974;29:1–21.

140. Titze IR. On the mechanics of vocal fold vibration. *J Acoust Soc Am.* 1976;60(6):136–138.

141. Titze IR. Biomechanics and distributed-mass models of vocal fold vibration. In: Stevens KN, Hirano M, eds. *Vocal Fold Physiology.* Tokyo, Japan: University of Tokyo Press; 1981:245–270.

142. Alipour F, Titze IR. A finite element simulation of vocal fold vibration. In: *Proceedings of the Fourteenth Annual Northeast Bioengineering Conference.* Durham, NC; IEEE publications #88-CH2666-6; 1988:86–189.

143. Schonharl E. *Die Stroboskopie in der praktischen Laryngologie.* Stuttgart, Germany: Thieme; 1960.

144. Stevens KN, Klatt DH. Current models of sound sources for speech. In: Wyke B, ed. *Ventilatory and Phonatory Control Systems, an International Symposium.* New York, NY: Oxford University Press; 1974:279–292.

145. Hirano M. Structure and vibratory behavior of the vocal folds. In: Sawashima M, Cooper FS, eds. *Dynamic Aspects of Speech Production.* Tokyo, Japan: University of Tokyo Press; 1977:13–27.

146. Cooper DS. Voice: a historical perspective (Woldemar Tonndorf and the Bernoulli effect in voice production). *J Voice.* 1989;3(1):1–6.

147. Scherer RC, Shinwari D, DeWitt K, Zhang C, Kucinschi B, Afjeh A. Intraglottal pressure profiles for a symmetric and oblique glottis with a divergence angle of 10 degrees. *J Acoust Soc Am.* 2001;109:1616–1630.

148. Pelorson X, Hirschberg A, van Hassel RR, Wijnands APJ. Theoretical and experimental study of quasi-steady-flow separation within the glottis during phonation. Application to a modified two-mass model. *J Acoust Soc Am.* 1994;96:3416–3431.

149. Pelorson X, Hirschberg A, Wijnands APJ, Bailliet H. Description of the flow through in vitro models of the glottis during phonation. *Acta Acustica.* 1995;3:191–202.

150. Hofmans GCJ. *Vortex Sound in Confined Flows* [dissertation]. Eindhoven: CIP-Data Library Technische Universiteit Eindhoven; 1998.

151. von Leden H, Moore P, Timcke R. Laryngeal vibrations: measurements of the glottic wave. Part III: the pathologic larynx. *Arch Otolaryngol.* 1960;71:16–35.

152. Koike Y, Imaizumi S. Objective evaluation of laryngostroboscopic findings. In: Fujimura O, ed. *Vocal Physiology: Voice Production, Mechanisms and Functions.* New York, NY: Raven Press, Ltd; 1988:433–442.

153. Svec JG, Schutte HK. Videokymography: high-speed line scanning of vocal fold vibration. *J Voice.* 1996;10: 201–205.

154. Kaiser J. Some observations on vocal tract operation from a fluid flow point of view. In: Titze IR, Scherer RC, eds. *Vocal Fold Physiology: Biomechanics, Acoustics and Phonatory Control.* Denver, Colo: The Denver Center for the Performing Arts; 1985:358–386.

155. Teager H, Teager S. Active fluid dynamic voice production models, or there is a unicorn in the garden. In: Titze IR, Scherer RC, eds. *Vocal Fold Physiology: Biomechanics, Acoustics and Phonatory Control.* Denver, Colo: The Denver Center for the Performing Arts; 1985: 387–401.

156. McGowan RS. An aeroacoustic approach to phonation. *J Acoust Soc Am.* 1988;88:696–704.

157. McGowan RS. Phonation from a continuum mechanics point of view. In: Gauffin J, Hammarberg B, eds. *Vocal Fold Physiology: Acoustic, Perceptual, and Physiological Aspects of Voice Mechanisms.* San Diego, Calif: Singular Publishing Group; 1991:65–72.

158. Berke GS, Moore DM, Monkewitz PA, Hanson DG, Gerratt BR. A preliminary study of particle velocity during phonation in an in vivo canine model. *J Voice.* 1989;3(4):306–313.

159. Shadle CH, Barney AM, Thomas DW. An investigation into the acoustic and aerodynamics of the larynx. In: Gauffin J, Hammarberg B, eds. *Vocal Fold Physiology: Acoustic, Perceptual, and Physiological Aspects of Voice Mechanisms.* San Diego, Calif: Singular Publishing Group; 1991:73–80.

160. Alipour F, Fan C. Pulsatile flow in a three-dimensional model of larynx. In: Biewener AA, Goel VK, eds. *Proceedings of 1993 ASB Meeting.* 1993:221–222.

161. Davies POAL, McGowan RS, Shadle CH. Practical flow duct acoustics applied to the vocal tract. In: Titze IR, ed. *Vocal Fold Physiology: Frontiers in Basic Science.* San Diego, Calif: Singular Publishing Group; 1993:93–134.

162. Scherer R. Practical flow duct acoustics applied to the vocal tract: Response. In: Titze IR, ed. *Vocal Fold Physiology: Frontiers in Basic Science.* San Diego, Calif: Singular Publishing Group; 1993:134–142.

163. Alipour F, Scherer RC. Pulsatile airflow during phonation: an excised larynx model. *J Acoust Soc Am.* 1995; 97:1241–1248.

164. Zhao W. *A Numerical Investigation of Sound Radiated From Subsonic Jet With Application to Human Phonation* [dissertation]. West Lafayette, Ind: Purdue University; 2000.

13

Vocal Tract Resonance

Johan Sundberg

Generation of Vocal Sound

The human voice organ consists of three parts, as is illustrated schematically in Figure 13–1. One is the breathing apparatus, which acts as a compressor: it compresses the air contained in the lungs. The second is the pair of vocal folds, which act as a sound generator: by vibrating they chop the airstream from the lungs into a sequence of air pulses, which is actually a sound. It sounds like a buzz and contains a complete set of harmonic partials. The third part is the cavity system constituted by the pharynx and mouth cavities, or the "vocal tract": it acts as a resonator, or a filter, which shapes the sound generated by the vocal folds. In producing nasal sounds, we lower the velum, and so supplement the vocal tract resonator by the nasal cavity, called the "nasal tract." Of the three parts, the breathing apparatus, the vocal folds, and the vocal tract, only the latter two contribute directly to forming vocal timbre. In other words, the acoustic characteristics of the voice are determined by two factors, (1) the voice source (ie, the functioning of the vocal folds} and (2) the vocal tract. This chapter will focus on the role of the vocal tract resonator.

The voice source passes through the vocal tract resonator, which thereby shapes it acoustically. The nature of this shaping depends on the vocal tract configuration. The act of changing the shape of the vocal tract is called "articulation." The structures that we use to arrange the shape of the vocal tract in different ways are called "articulators." For example, the tongue is an articulator.

The vocal tract is a *resonator* or, in other words, an object in which resonance occurs. Resonance is a phenomenon created by synchronization of input and reflected energy. To realize the meaning of this, it is helpful to imagine what will happen if one hits one end of a very long tube with both ends closed. A clap-like sound will be generated that runs to the opposite end where it is reflected. After a while, it returns and is reflected again; and the process is repeated. Thus, the clap sound will travel back and forth in the tube. The result is that we will hear a repeated clap. The time intervals between the claps are determined by the distance that the sound has to travel to the opposite end and back; the longer the tube, the longer the intervals between the sounds (ie, the lower the frequency of the claps). Because some sound energy is consumed during the travel, the returning clap sounds gradually will become softer. If one or both ends of the tube are open, reflection still occurs; but the decay will be quicker, because more sound energy is lost at an open end than at a closed end.

This is exactly what happens in tube resonators. The resonator responds with a tone that dies rather quickly. The frequency of the tone is determined by the time it takes for the sound to travel to the opposite end and back. In the case of the vocal tract, the distance is short, so the frequency of a response to a clap is comparatively high, about 500 Hz, if the tube is cylindrical. Thus, if one flicks one's neck above the larynx with a finger with closed glottis and open mouth, one can hear a quickly-decaying tone; it sounds similar to the sound produced when one hits an empty bottle, which, incidentally, is another example of a resonator.

Imagine now that you hit the end of the long tube repeatedly with a time interval that equals the intervals between the returning clap sounds and furthermore that you hit it exactly when a clap sound returns. Then, the new and the returned clap sound will cooperate so that a loud clap sound is produced. This is exactly what resonance is: the sound fed into the resonator is helped by the sound that is traveling back and forth in the resonator. The result is that you obtain

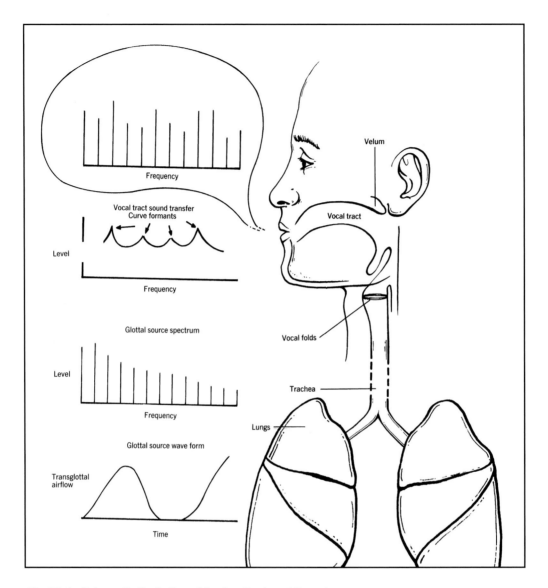

Fig 13–1. Schematic illustration of the functioning of the voice organ.

loud sound with little effort. This will, however, happen only at a particular frequency, the resonance frequency, which depends on the length of the tube; the longer the tube, the lower the resonance frequency.

However, resonance occurs not only at one particular frequency. It is perfectly possible to hit the tube end at higher frequencies and still keep synchrony between the hits and the returning clap sounds. In this case, there are several claps traveling in the tube, but they do not disturb each other. Thus, a resonator possesses several resonance frequencies.

Things do not get much more complicated if the sound fed into a tube resonator is a sine wave rather than an impulse sound. If the frequency of an input sine wave is moved toward a resonance frequency, the

amplitude of the tone in the resonator will increase gradually, culminating at the resonance frequency, because input and reflected sound are then in perfect synchrony. Likewise, if the frequency of an input sine wave is moved away from a resonance frequency, the amplitude will decrease gradually. Figure 13–2 illustrates this in terms of an experiment in which a sine wave of increasing frequency is fed into the closed end of a tube resonator. The sound picked up at the opposite open end increases in amplitude as the sine wave frequency approaches a resonance frequency and then decreases.

In the case of the vocal tract resonator, however, the resonances are called "formants" and the resonance frequencies are referred to as "formant frequencies."

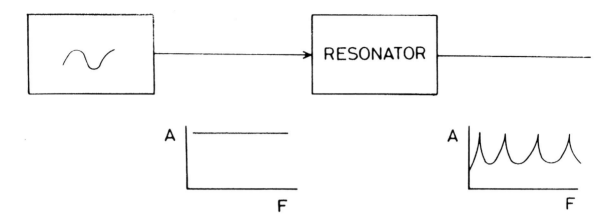

Fig 13–2. Schematic illustration of the phenomenon of "resonance." If a sine wave of constant amplitude (A) sweeps from low to high frequency (F), the frequency-dependent sound transferability of the resonator imposes great variations in the amplitude. The amplitude culminates at the resonance frequencies.

Formants are of paramount importance to the voice. In the vocal tract, there are four or five formants of interest. The frequencies of the two lowest formants determine most of the vowel quality, whereas the third, fourth and fifth formants are of greater significance to personal voice timbre.

We are very skilled in tuning our formant frequencies. We do this by changing the shape of the vocal tract (ie, by moving our articulators). In this way, the vocal tract may assume a great variety of shapes. The mandible is one articulator that may be raised or lowered. The tongue is another one that may constrict the vocal tract at almost any location from the hard palate to the deep pharynx. The lip opening is a third articulator, which may be widened or narrowed. The larynx can be raised or lowered. The latter two variations also affect vocal tract length. Finally, the side walls of the pharynx can be moved.

The vocal tract length affects all formant frequencies. Adult males have a tube length of about 17 to 20 centimeters (cm). Assuming a cylindrical vocal tract shape of length $l = 17.5$ cm, the formant frequencies occur near the odd multiples of 500 Hz: 500, 1500, 2500 Hz, and so on. Because of sex differences in vocal tract length, a similar articulatory configuration gives formant frequencies that are about 40% higher in children than in adult males. Because adult females have shorter vocal tracts than adult males, their formant frequencies are on the average 15% higher than those of adult males.

Tuning formant frequencies is achieved by adjusting the vocal tract shape, as mentioned. A reduction of the lip opening and a lengthening of the vocal tract by a lowering of the larynx or by protruding the lips lowers all formant frequencies. Similarly, constricting the

vocal tract in the glottal region leads to an increase of the formant frequencies.

Some articulators are particularly efficient in tuning certain formant frequencies. The mandible, which expands the vocal tract in the lip region and constricts it in the laryngeal region, raises the frequency of the first formant. In vowels produced by male adults, the first formant varies between approximately 200 and 800 Hz. The second formant is particularly sensitive to the tongue shape. The second formant frequency in male adults varies within a range of about 500 to 2500 Hz. The significance of the jaw opening and the tongue shape to the first and second formant frequencies is illustrated in Figure 13–3, which shows results from an articulatory model of the vocal tract. The figure shows that widening the jaw opening causes increase of the first formant frequency, while changing the tongue shape from [i] to [u] to [a] mainly affects the second formant.

The third formant is sensitive especially to the position of the tip of the tongue or, when the tongue is retracted, to the size of the cavity between the lower incisors and the tongue. In vowels produced by male adults, the third formant varies between approximately 1600 and 3500 Hz.

The relationships between the vocal tract shape and the fourth and fifth formants are more complicated and difficult to control by particular articulatory means. However, they seem to be very dependent on vocal tract length and also on the configuration in the deep pharynx. In vowels produced by adult males, the fourth formant frequency is generally in the vicinity of 2500 to 4000 Hz and the fifth approximately 3000 to 4500 Hz.

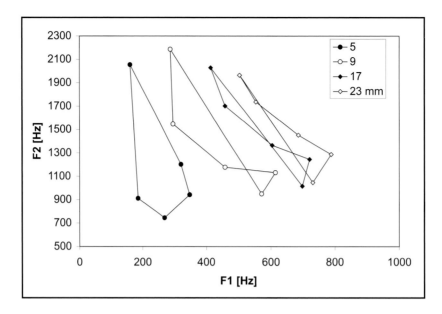

Fig 13–3. Effect on the two lowest formant frequencies of changing the tongue shape from the configuration for the vowel [i] to the configuration for the vowel [u] to the configuration for the vowel [a] and back to the configuration for the vowel [i] at the jaw openings indicated.

It is evident that the formant frequencies must have a great effect on the spectrum, as the vocal tract resonator filters the voice source (see Fig 13–1). At intermediate degrees of vocal loudness, the spectrum envelope of the voice source slopes off at a rate of approximately 12 decibels (dB) per octave, if measured in airflow units. The spectrum of a radiated vowel, however, is characterized by peaks and valleys; because the partials lying closest to a formant frequency get stronger than adjacent partials in the spectrum. In this way, the vocal tract resonances "form" the vowel spectrum; hence the term formants. Recalling that formants are vocal tract resonances, we realize that it is by means of vocal tract resonance that we form vowels.

Various vowels correspond to different articulatory configurations attained by varying the positions of the articulators, [1] as illustrated in Figure 13–4. In the vowel /i:/ (as in heed), the tongue bulges so that it constricts the buccal part of the vocal tract. As a consequence of this, the first formant is low while the second formant is high. In the vowel /u:/ (as in the word who'd), the first and second formant frequencies are both low; and in the vowel /a:/ (as in the Italian word *caro*), the first formant is high and the second takes an intermediate position.

Figure 13–5 shows typical formant frequencies for various spoken vowels as produced by male and female children and adults.[2] Figure 13–5A shows that females have higher formant frequencies than males and that children have higher formant frequencies than adults. The graphs also show what vowel will result if the frequencies of the two lowest formants are combined in specific ways. For example, if the first and second formants are near 600 and 1000 Hz, respectively, the vowel will be an /a:/. Note that, in Figure 13–5B, the vowels are distributed within a triangular contour, the three corners of which are the vowels /i:/, /a:/, and /u:/. The vowel /oe:/ (as in heard) is located in the center of the triangle. The "islands" imply that the vowel marked will result, provided the frequencies of the first and second formants remain within that island. The exact position of the two lowest formant frequencies for a given vowel depends on the individual morphology of the speaker's vocal tract, among other things, and also on habits of pronunciation.

Formant Frequencies in Singing

Singer's Formant

With regard to the loudest possible tones, remarkably, there is no clear difference between a trained singer and a nonsinger when measured under identical conditions. This can be seen in Figure 13–6, which shows

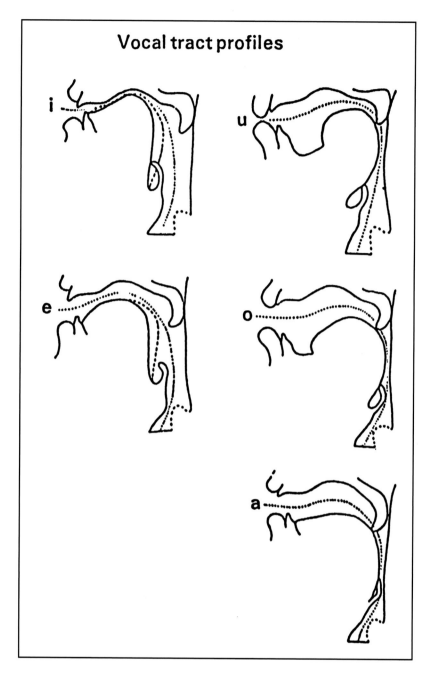

Fig 13–4. Tracings of x-ray profiles of the vocal tract showing articulatory configurations for some vowels. (After G. Fant[1].)

average maximum and minimum sound levels as functions of frequency for professional male singers and nonsingers.[3] Thus, a singer's fortissimo does not necessarily reach a higher sound level than a nonsinger's loudest possible voice production. Why, then, can we hear a singer so clearly even when he is accompanied by a loud orchestra?

The answer can be found in the spectral characteristics, which differ considerably between male singers and nonsingers. Also, vowels spoken and sung by

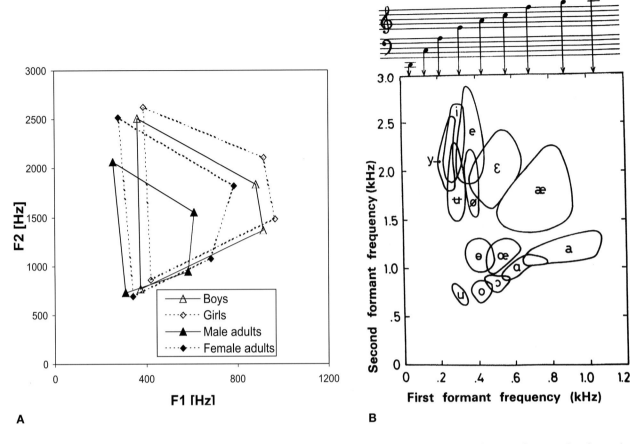

A

B

Fig 13–5. A. Typical formant frequencies for various spoken vowels as produced by male and female adults and 10-year-old children (children's data from White[2]). **B.** Typical mean values for the two lowest formant frequencies for various spoken vowels as produced by male and female adults. The first formant frequency is given in musical notation at the top.

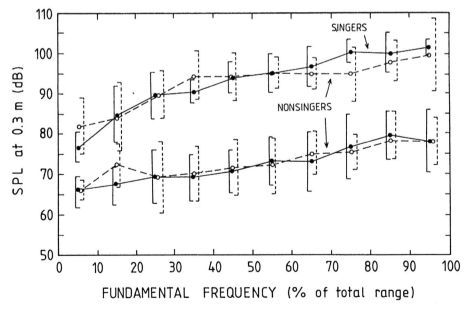

Fig 13–6. Average maximum and minimum sound pressure level at 0.3 meter distance in anechoic room as produced by 10 professional singers and 10 nonsingers. The bars represent ± one standard deviation. (From Gramming et al[3] with permission.)

male singers typically differ with regard to the spectrum characteristics. Figure 13–7 illustrates the most apparent difference, called the "singer's formant." This is a prominent spectrum envelope peak appearing in the vicinity of 3 kHz in all vowel spectra sung by male singers. It is associated with the typical features of a vowel sung in the classical style of singing.

The center frequency of the singer's formant varies depending on the voice category. In bass singers, it is often found around 2.4 kHz, in baritones around 2.6, and in tenors around 2.8; but there are great individual variations. These frequency differences contribute significantly to the timbral differences between these voice categories.[4] Female singers, on the other hand, have a much lower spectrum level in this frequency region than male singers; and usually there are two peaks.[5] It appears that, in the case of sopranos, these peaks are produced by nothing but a perfectly normal third and fourth formant.

Regardless of voice category, the level of the singer's formant also varies with loudness of phonation,[6,7] as illustrated in Figure 13–8. In the case shown in the figure, a sound pressure level (SPL) increase of 10 dB is accompanied by an increase of 17 dB in the singer's formant.[8] This effect derives from the voice source, the sound generated by the pulsating glottal flow.

The presence of the singer's formant in the spectrum of a vowel sound is an advantage in that it helps the singer's voice to be heard through a loud orchestral accompaniment. In the spectrum of the sound from a symphony orchestra, the partials near 500 Hz tend to be loudest; above this frequency region, the

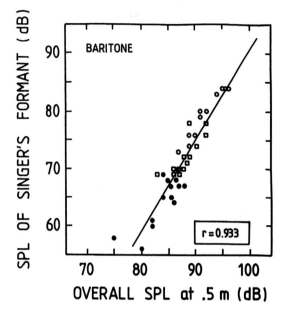

Fig 13–8. Level of the singer's formant as function of loudness of phonation. (From Cleveland & Sundberg[7] with permission.)

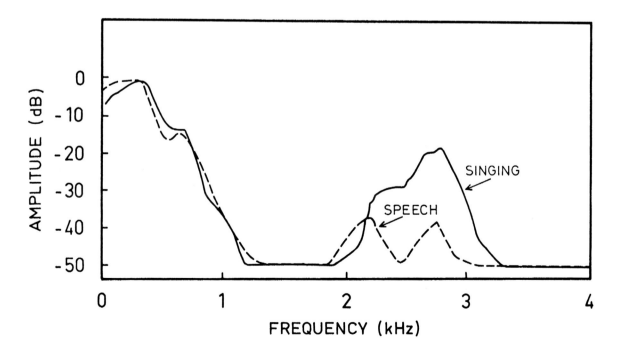

Fig 13–7. Illustration of the "singer's formant," a prominent peak in the spectrum envelope appearing in the vicinity of 3 kHz in all vowel spectra sung by male singers and also by altos.

levels of the spectrum components decrease with rising frequency. This is illustrated by the long-term-average spectrum of orchestral music shown in Figure 13–9 where the slope above 500 Hz is about 9 dB per octave.[9] The perceptual point with a singer's formant is, then, to enhance the spectrum partials in a frequency range where the sound of the accompaniment offers less severe acoustic competition. This effect cannot be achieved by a normal speaking voice, because its long-term-average spectrum slope above 500 Hz is similar to that of a symphony orchestra.

How do singers generate this spectrum peak in voiced sounds? The answer is, "by resonance!" If it is assumed that the third, fourth, and fifth formants are close in frequency, thus forming a formant cluster, the "singer's formant" peak can be explained as an articulatory phenomenon that can be produced with a normal voice source. In Figure 13–10, formant frequency measurements compatible with this assumption for vowels sung by professional singers are compared with those typical for normal speech. As can be seen, the fifth formant in the sung vowels is lower than the fourth formant in the spoken vowels. Thus, five for-

mants appear in the same frequency range as four formants in spoken vowels. In the vicinity of the singer's formant, the density of formants is high in the sung vowels.

The acoustic consequence of clustering formants is that the spectrum partials in the frequency range of the cluster are enhanced in the radiated spectrum as is illustrated in Figure 13–11. In other words, the singer's formant is compatible with the normal concept of voice production, provided a clustering of the higher formants is possible.

The plausibility of the assumption that formants 3, 4, and 5 can be clustered was examined in an experiment in which a singer's vocal tract shape for a sung [a] was measured by magnetic resonance imaging.[10] Measurement of the formant frequencies of this vocal tract revealed that formants 3, 4, and 5 were clustered in a 1000-Hz wide frequency band. Moreover, experiments with acoustic models of the vocal tract showed that such a clustering of formants could be attained if the pharynx is wide as compared with the entrance to the larynx tube. In this case, the larynx tube acts as a separate resonator with a resonance in the vicinity of

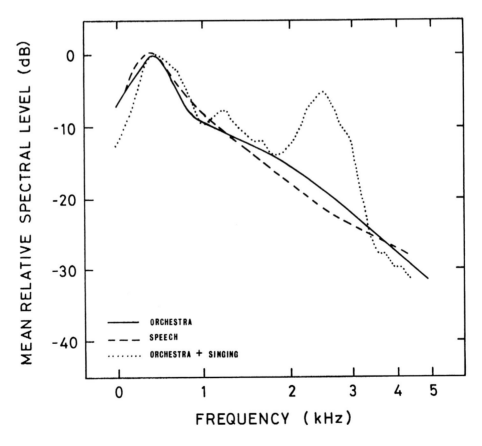

Fig 13–9. Long-term-average spectrum of orchestral music with and without a solo singer's voice. (From Sundberg[9] with permission.)

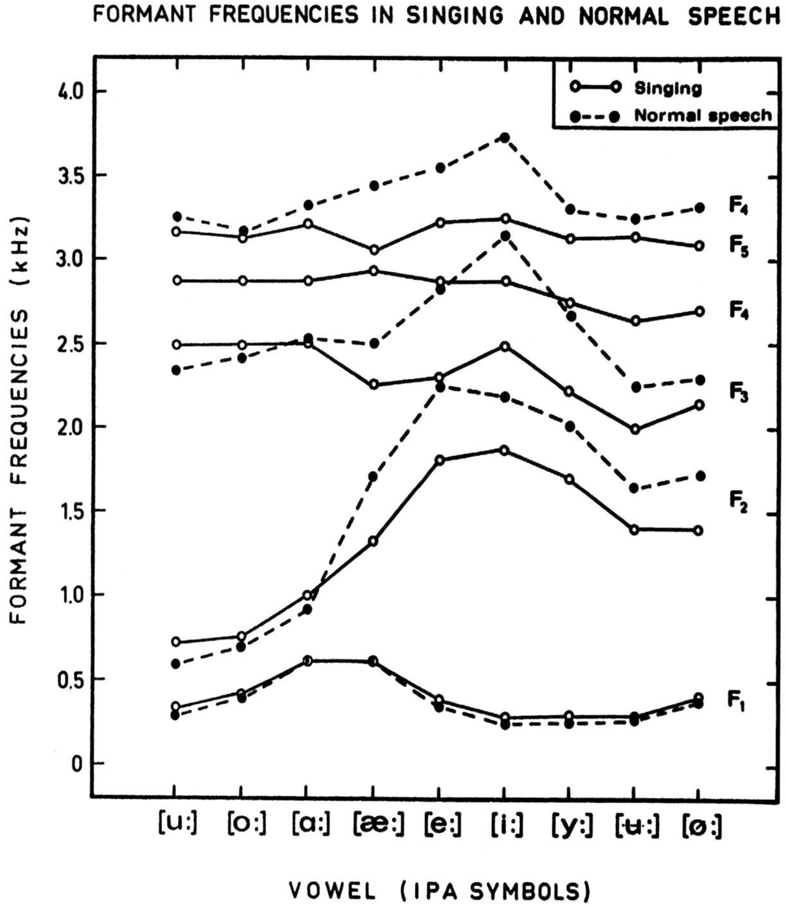

FORMANT FREQUENCIES IN SINGING AND NORMAL SPEECH

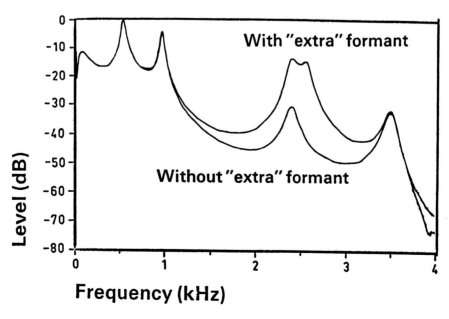

Fig 13–10. Average formant frequencies for vowels spoken normally and sung by professional singers.

Fig 13–11. The effect of clustering formants 3, 4, and 5 on the idealized spectrum envelope.

2.5 kHz.[11] It seems that in many singers this effect is obtained by a lowering of the larynx.

There also may be other, as yet unknown, ways of generating a singer's formant. A Chinese researcher, S. Wang, found that in classical Beijing opera singing and in the type of singing typically used for medieval music, a singer's formant was produced without a lowering of the larynx.[12] He hypothesized that the peak was produced by an acoustic interaction between the voice source and the vocal tract resonator. However, the criteria applied by Wang for the presence of a singer's formant seem controversial, and attempts to replicate his findings on classical Beijing opera singers have failed.

The particular arrangements of the vocal tract that generate vowels with a singer's formant have certain consequences for the vowel quality as well. This is illustrated in Figure 13–10. We can see that the second and third formant of /i/ are low, in fact, almost as low as in the German vowel /y/. This is in accordance with the common observation that vowels are "colored" in singing. This coloring can be seen as a price the singer pays in order to buy his singer's formant.

The singer's formant is found in the classical operatic style of singing but not among artists singing in nonclassical, or so-called popular styles, such as country or rock. It is interesting that in performances of music in these styles, the singer is provided with an amplification system that ensures that the voice of the soloist can be heard over the accompaniment. Under these conditions, the singer does not need a singer's formant.

Summarizing, we see that resonance is of decisive relevance to singing, because it creates major characteristics of the male Western operatic singing voice

especially. It should be observed that all of this resonance takes place within the vocal tract. It has not been possible to demonstrate any acoustic significance at all from the vibration sensations in the chest, skull, and face that singers reportedly feel during singing.

Super Pitch Singing

So far, we have reviewed typical formant (or resonance) frequency differences between speech and singing in male singers and altos. However, the formant frequency differences between spoken and sung vowels are much greater in singing at high pitches. While a bass singer is not required to go higher than 330 Hz fundamental frequency, the maximum for a high soprano may be as high as 1500 Hz (pitch F6).

Let us now recall Figure 13–5B, which showed the formant frequencies for various vowels. The scale for the first formant frequency was given in the usual frequency unit Hz, but also, at the top of the graph, in musical pitch symbols. From this we can see that the fundamental frequency in singing is often higher than the first formant frequency. For example, the first formant of /i:/ and /u:/ is about 250 Hz, which is close to the frequency corresponding to the pitch of C4, and the highest value for the first formant in a vowel occurs at 900 Hz for the vowel /a:/, which is close to the pitch of C6, approximately.

It is difficult to determine formant frequencies accurately when the fundamental frequency is high. The spectrum partials of voiced sounds are equidistantly spaced along the frequency axis, as shown in Figure 13–12, because they form a harmonic series. This

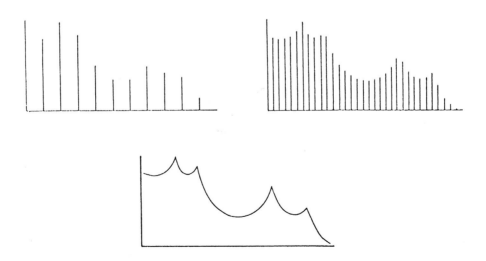

Fig 13–12. Illustration of the differing difficulty of determining formant frequencies in spectra with a high (*top left*) and a low (*top right*) fundamental frequency. Both spectra were generated using the same formant frequencies represented by the idealized spectrum envelope below.

implies that the partials are densely spaced along the frequency axis only when fundamental frequency is low. In that case, the formants easily can be identified as spectrum envelope peaks. If the pitch is high, the frequency distance between adjacent partials is large; and then formant peaks are often impossible to discern, particularly if there is no partial near the formant frequency. It is certainly for this reason that voice researchers have analyzed male voices much more frequently than female voices. Still, attempts have been made to determine the formant frequencies in female singers using various experimental techniques.

One method was to use external excitation of the vocal tract by means of a vibrator while the singer silently articulated a vowel. Another method was to take an x-ray picture of the vocal tract in profile while the singer sang different vowels at different pitches. A third method was to excite the singer's vocal tract during singing with a well-defined sound and measure the vocal tract response to this sound.[13] For obvious reasons, the number of subjects in most of these studies has been low, only one or two. Still the results were encouraging in that they agreed surprisingly well. This supports the assumption that they are probably typical.

Some formant frequency values for a soprano singer are shown in Figure 13–13. These results can be idealized in terms of lines, also shown in the figure, relating the first, second, third, and fourth formant frequencies to the fundamental frequency. Also shown are the subject's formant frequencies in speech. The main principle seems to be as follows. As long as fundamental frequency is lower than the normal value of the vowel's first formant frequency, this formant frequency is used. At higher pitches, the first formant is raised to a value somewhat higher than the fundamental frequency. In this way, the singer avoids having the fundamental frequency exceed the first formant frequency. With rising fundamental frequency, the second formant of front vowels is lowered, while that of back vowels is raised to a frequency just above the second spectrum partial; the third formant is lowered, and the fourth is raised.

What articulatory means do the singers use to achieve these great pitch-dependent rearrangements of the formant frequencies? A frequently used tool is jaw opening. Formal measurements on singers' jaw opening have shown that, under controlled experimental conditions, the jaw opening is systematically widened with rising fundamental frequency.[14] This rule is illustrated in Figure 13–14A, which shows the jaw opening of professional singers as a function of the frequency separation between the fundamental and the frequency value of the first formant that the subject used at low pitches. The graph shows that most

singers began to widen their jaw opening when the fundamental was about 4 semitones below the normal first formant.

Figure 13–14B shows the corresponding data for the vowel [e]. For this vowel, most subjects started to widen the jaw opening when the fundamental was about 4 semitones above the normal first formant. It is likely that below this pitch singers increase the first formant by other articulatory means than the jaw opening. A plausible candidate in front vowels is the degree of vocal tract constriction; a reduced constriction increases the first formant. There are also other articulators that can be recruited for the same purpose. One is the lip opening. By retracting the mouth corners, the vocal tract is shortened; and hence the frequencies of the formants will increase. The vocal tract can also be shortened by raising the larynx, and some professional female singers take advantage of this tool when singing at high pitches. Figure 13–15 gives an example. It is interesting that most singing teachers regard such a pitch-dependent variation of larynx height as a sign of a deficient singing technique. Perhaps these teachers do not mean larynx elevation in general, but rather a larynx elevation that is associated with an audible shift in the mode of phonation and vowel quality. In normal speech, a raised larynx is generally associated with a pressed type of phonation, like in screaming. Figure 13–16 shows that the tongue shape also may be modified in a pitch-dependent manner. In this subject, the vowels /a:/ /i:/, and /u:/ were produced with differentiated tongue shapes at the fundamental frequencies of 230 Hz and 465 Hz (pitches B3 and B4, approximately) but with a similar tongue shape at 960 Hz (pitch B5). Still, with these wide jaw openings and at that high pitch, a small difference in tongue shape is not likely to affect the formant frequencies to an audible extent.

This principle of tuning formant frequencies depending on the fundamental frequency has been found in all singers who encounter the situation that the normal value of the first formant is lower than their highest pitches. In fact, all singers except basses encounter this situation at least for some vowels sung at high pitches. As the first formant frequency varies between vowels, the case depends on the vowel. In the highest range of a baritone, the vowels /i/, /y:/, /u:/ would need pitch-dependent first formant frequencies. In the top part of an alto's range, all vowels except /a:/ and /ae:/ need modification of the first formant frequency. However, near the upper limit of their pitch range, in the so-called flageolet register, sopranos have been found to have their first formant frequency lower than the fundamental.[15]

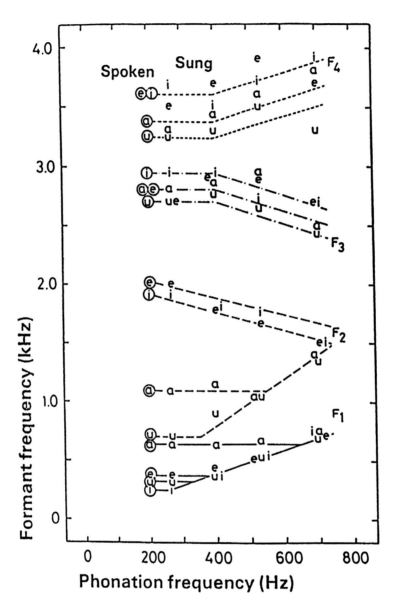

Fig 13–13. The vowel symbols show formant frequency estimates of the first, second, third, and fourth formant frequencies for various vowels as sung by a professional soprano singer. The circled vowel symbols represent the corresponding data measured when the vowels were pronounced by the same subject in a speech mode. The lines represent an idealization of how the formant frequencies changed with fundamental frequency.

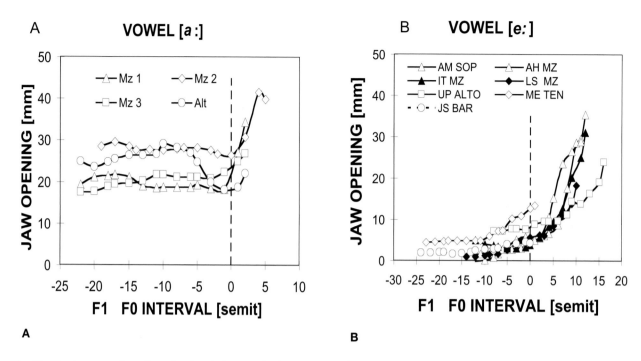

Fig 13–14. Jaw opening of professional singers singing an ascending scale on the vowel [a] and [e] (**A** and **B**, respectively). The horizontal axis shows the frequency separation, in semitones, between the fundamental and their first formant used for the respective vowels at speaking pitches. (From Sundberg and Skoog[15] with permission.)

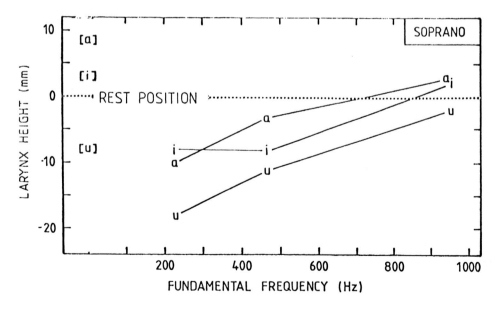

Fig 13–15. Vertical laryngeal position as determined from x-ray profiles of the vocal tract of a professional soprano singing the indicated vowels at various fundamental frequencies.

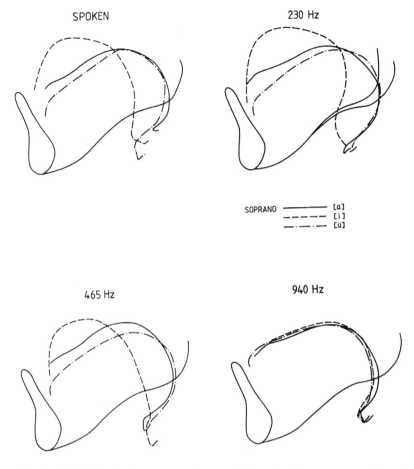

SPOKEN

230 Hz

SOPRANO ——————— [ɑ]
- - - - - - - [i]
- · — · — · — [u]

465 Hz

940 Hz

Fig 13–16. Midsagittal tongue contours as determined from x-ray profiles of the vocal tract of a professional soprano singing the indicated vowels at various fundamental frequencies shown. (From Sundberg[11] with permission.)

The benefit of these arrangements of the formant frequencies is great. They imply that the sound level of the vowels increases enormously in some cases. Figure 13–17 shows the gain in sound level attained by means of the pitch-dependent choice of formant frequencies that was shown in Figure 13–13. In some cases, the gain is no less than 30 dB. This is a truly huge increase in sound level, which the singer gains by sheer resonance.

Choral Singing

An often-discussed question is to what extent choral singing requires the same vocal technique as solo singing. Choir directors tend to maintain that there are no important differences, whereas many singing teachers see highly important differences.

Because the singer's formant apparently serves the purpose of helping the individual singer's voice to be heard through a loud orchestral accompaniment, it can be hypothesized that the singer's formant is not indicated in choral singing. This hypothesis was supported by experiments in which male singers, experienced in both choir and solo performance, were asked to sing in a choral and in a soloistic framework.[16] In the solo singing condition, they heard over earphones the piano accompaniment of a solo song that they were to sing. In the choir singing condition, they heard the sound of a choir that they were asked to join. As shown in Figure 13–18A, the subjects had a singer's formant that was more prominent in solo than in choir singing; and the lowest spectrum partials, below the first formant, were weaker in solo singing. The higher level of the singer's formant in solo singing was associated with a denser clustering of the third, fourth, and fifth formant frequencies. These subjects, unlike average choral singers, were also excellent solo singers. It can be assumed that the differences between solo and choir singing are generally greater than was revealed by this experiment.

A corresponding experiment was also performed with soprano subjects.[17] Disregarding the fact that it

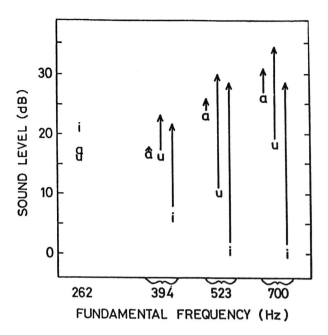

Fig 13–17. Gain in sound level at different fundamental frequencies resulting from the pitch-dependent tuning of formant frequencies that were represented by the lines in Figure 13–13.

seems inadequate to speak of a singer's formant in soprano singing,[18] the result was similar. As can be seen in Figure 13–18B, the mean spectrum level between 2 and 3 kHz was clearly higher when the singers sang in a solo mode. This suggests that even female solo singers profit from high levels of the higher spectrum partials. This assumption was further supported by the fact that two opera sopranos of world fame were found to sing with a clearly higher level of the partials in the 2- to 4-kHz range than the singers who worked both as choral and solo singers (Fig 13–18C). These measurements seem to indicate that solo and choral singing differ with respect to vocal technique.

Overtone Singing

In some music cultures, a very special type of singing is practiced, in which the voice pitch remains constant, as in a drone, while the musical interest is carried by melodic patterns formed by salient high overtones. The vocal technique underlying this phenomenon has been studied.[19] Figure 13–19 shows an example of a vowel spectrum produced in this type of singing where the salient pitches were produced by the sixth and seventh partial (ie, pitches lying two octaves plus a fifth or a seventh above the fundamental). In view of the spectrum,

the salience of these partials is not surprising. These partials are quite outstanding in the spectrum.

The underlying vocal technique seems based on formant tuning. The singers tune the second and third formants so that both are quite close to the partial to be enhanced. The other formants are tuned carefully to avoid enhancing any of the other partials. As a result, one single partial becomes much stronger than the others, so that its pitch stands out of the timbral percept. The articulatory tools used seem to be the shape of the tongue body, the position of the tongue tip, and the lip opening. The tongue tip is often raised while the tongue body is pulled anteriorly or posteriorly. In addition, the voice source characteristics seem to be adjusted so that the fundamental is suppressed, presumably by shifting the type of phonation toward pressed phonation.

A more modest form of overtone singing is rather simple to practice and learn. The point is to keep the fundamental constant at a rather high frequency, say 300 Hz, and then to vary articulation by changing the tongue shape and lip opening rhythmically in several steps between the /u:/ and the /i:/ positions. If the rhythmical pattern is repeated, the ear will soon catch individual overtones. Then, it is rather easy to moderate articulation to enhance the effect.

Head Resonance

In the preceding sections, we discussed several examples of the enormous significance of resonance in singing. So far, the only type of resonance dealt with has been the formants, the resonances of the vocal tract. Face or skull resonances have not been reviewed. There is no doubt, however, that the voice sets up forceful vibrations in the structures limiting the voice organ, such as the chest wall, the throat, the face, and the skull. However, except at the lowest pitches of a bass singer, these vibrations are much too feeble to compete with the sound radiation from the open mouth. In other words, such vibrations do not contribute acoustically to the formation of vowel sounds. This is not to say that they cannot be used as a proprioceptive feedback helping singers to control their voice production.

Conclusions

The vocal tract resonances, or formants, are of paramount significance to voice and vowel quality. The two lowest formants determine vowel quality; whereas the higher formants determine much of the personal voice characteristics, including voice classification. In classically trained male singers, the third, fourth,

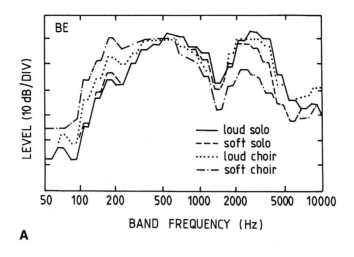

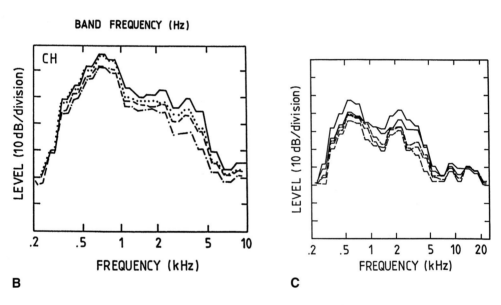

Fig 13–18. Long-term-average spectra of male (**A**) and female (**B**) singers singing as soloists and as members of a choir. In **A** and **B**, solid, dashed, dotted, and chain-dashed lines pertain to loud and soft solo and loud and soft choral singing, respectively. In **C**, the solid curves represent the spectra of two opera sopranos of international fame and the dashed curves pertain to sopranos who sang professionally both as soloists and as choir singers. (From Rossing et al[16,17] with permission.)

and fifth formants constitute the singer's formant, which helps the singer's voice to be heard through a loud accompaniment. During singing at high pitches, where the fundamental is higher than the normal value of the first formant, the frequency of this formant is increased to a frequency somewhat higher than the fundamental. This increases the loudness of the voice considerably. It is also possible to make small articulatory adjustments with formants to have them "show" individual partials to the listener.

However, the great relevance of vocal tract reso-nance to singing should not conceal the fact that there are other factors of great importance, too. Thus, the voice source (ie, the chopped airstream through the vibrating vocal folds) is as decisive to voice quality, as are the formants. Of course, the resulting great variability complicates the work of both singers and singing teachers; there are many parameters that the singer needs to bring under proper control. Nevertheless, the reward is generous. The abundant timbral variability that may result certainly offers the singer access to one of the most flexible musical instruments.

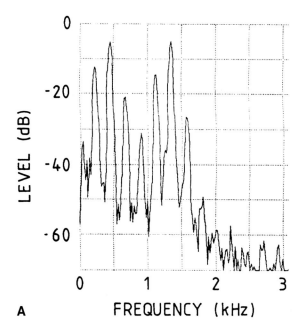
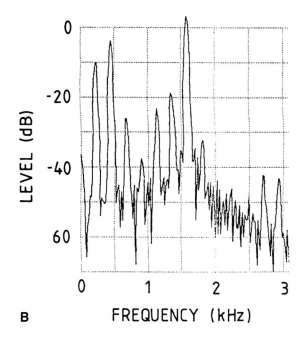

Fig 13–19. Vowel spectrum produced in two cases of overtone singing performed by one of the members in The Harmonic Choir. In **A**, the sixth harmonic partial was perceived as an extra tone in the spectrum, two octaves plus a fifth above the fundamental. In **B**, the seventh harmonic partial was perceived as an extra tone, two octaves plus a seventh above the fundamental.

References

1. Fant G. *Acoustic Theory of Speech Production.* The Hague, The Netherlands,: Mouton; 1960.

2. White P. Acoustic and Aerodynamic Measurements of Children's Voice [dissertation]. London, UK: University of Surrey; 1997.

3. Gramming P, Sundberg J, Ternström S, et al. Relationships between changes in voice pitch and loudness. *J Voice.* 1988;2:118–126.

4. Berndtsson G, Sundberg J. Perceptual significance of the center frequency of the singer's formant. *Scand J Logoped Phoniatr.* 1995;20:35–41.

5. Seidner W, Schutte H, Wendler J, Rauhut A. Dependence of the high singing formant on pitch and vowel in different voice types. In: Askenfelt A, Felicetti S, Jansson E, Sundberg J, eds. *Proceedings of the Stockholm Music Acoustics Conference (SMAC 83).* Stockholm: Royal Swedish Academy of Music; 1985;46(1):261–268

6. Bloothooft G, Plomp R. The sound level of the singer's formant in professional singing. *J Acoust Soc Am.* 1986; 79:2028–2033.

7. Cleveland T, Sundberg J. Acoustic analysis of three male voices of different quality. In: Askenfelt A, Felicetti S, Jansson E, Sundberg J, eds. *Proceedings of the Stockholm Music Acoustics Conference (SMAC 83).* Stockholm: Royal Swedish Academy of Music; 1985;46(1):143–156.

8. Sjölander P, Sundberg J. Spectrum effects of subglottal pressure variation on professional baritone singers. *J Acoust Soc Am.* 2004;115:1270–1273.

9. Sundberg J. *The Science of the Singing Voice.* DeKalb, Ill: Northern Illinois University Press; 1987.

10. Sundberg J. The singer's formant revisited. *Voice.* 1995;4: 106–119.

11. Sundberg J. Articulatory interpretation of the "singing formant." *J Acoust Soc Am.* 1974;55:838–844.

12. Wang S. Singing voice: Bright timbre, singer's formant and larynx positions. In: Askenfelt A, Felicetti S, Jansson E, Sundberg J, eds. *Proceedings of the Stockholm International Music Acoustics Conference (SMAC 83).* Stockholm: Royal Swedish Academy of Music; 1985;46(1):313–322.

13. Joliveau E, Smith J, Wolfe J. Tuning of vocal tract resonance by sopranos. *Nature.* 2004;427:116

14. Miller DG, Schutte H. Physical definition of the "flageolet register." *J Voice.* 1993;7:206–212.

15. Sundberg J, Skoog, J. Dependence of jaw opening on pitch and vowel in singers. *J Voice.* 1997;11:301–306

16. Rossing, TD, Sundberg J, Ternström S. Acoustic comparison of voice use in solo and choir singing. *J Acoust Soc Am.* 1986;79:1975–1981.

17. Rossing, TD, Sundberg J, Ternström S. Acoustic comparison of soprano solo and choir singing. *J Acoust Soc Am.* 1987;82:830–836.

18. Barnes, JJ, Davis P, Oates J, Chapman J. The relationship between professional operatic soprano voice and high range spectral energy. *J Acoust Soc Am.* 2004;116:530–538.

19. Bloothooft G, Bringman E, van Cappellen M, et al. Acoustics of overtone singing. *J Acoust Soc Am.* 1992;92: 1827–1836.

14

Chaos in Voice Research

Rajeev Bhatia, Mary J. Hawkshaw,
and Robert Thayer Sataloff

Nonlinear dynamics theory provides a means of describing the complex interactions of mathematical, physical, and biological systems that exhibit nonlinear characteristics. The distinct and complementary mathematical concepts of fractals and chaos are central to nonlinear dynamics theory. Gleick[1] has provided a particularly good introduction to fractals and chaos theory with other nontechnical introductions also available.[2-7]

Application of Fractals in Biomedical Research

Inspired by the successful early application of nonlinear dynamics theory to the electrophysiology of the heart and frustrated by the failure of conventional statistical or stochastic approaches to compute the inherent morphological or temporal nonlinearities present in biological systems, biomedical researchers have turned to fractals (particularly the use of the fractal dimension) as a method of quantifying these inherent nonlinearities.

A wide variety of methods are employed to calculate the fractal dimension.[8] Researchers seeking to quantify morphological (geometric) nonlinearities in biological systems have typically computed the fractal dimension using the box-counting algorithm for digitized data.[9] Temporal nonlinearities have been successfully quantified in biological systems by computing the fractal dimension using the D2 algorithm developed by Grassberger and Proccacia for discrete time data samples.[10] Examples of the use of fractals in quantifying the morphological and temporal nonlinear complexity in biological systems are growing in number and importance.

Today, modern chaos theory has wide application to various biological phenomena. Fractal analysis is being used as a measurement of complexity. It is being applied by scientists, researchers, and physicians as we continue to study changes in humans, from fetal life through senescence. Review of the literature yields many biological applications of chaos theory.[11-47] Fractal analysis appears useful in understanding and quantifying structure, function, and texture of various body systems that have previously been difficult or impossible to study adequately. It seems particularly important at the cellular level where scientists are looking at structure, ion exchange, protein sequences and their dynamics, DNA genetics, fluidity and transport, and diffusion kinetics. Scientifics and physicians continue to pursue explanations for currently unexplainable events, for example, sudden death due to ventricular fibrillation. Current investigations of chaotic dynamics and fractal architectures in the human body are shedding light on such occurrences, challenging long-held principles of medicine and revealing possible methods of predicting disease.

Voice Analysis

Research into the application of nonlinear dynamics theory to the analysis of voice has been motivated primarily by the failure of objective measures based on perturbation analysis in capturing salient features of the acoustic or electroglottographic (EGG) signal associated with pathologic voice. As an example, consider the abrupt spectral characteristics of the acoustic and EGG signal associated with neurological dysphonias. Hertrich et al[48] report that prevailing perturbation measures (jitter, shimmer, and harmonic-to-noise ratio) fail to provide a reliable quantitative account of these abrupt spectral changes. They reported that abrupt shifts in spectral characteristics impede accurate determination of pitch, which is paramount to the accurate calculation of the above-stated perturbation measures. Furthermore, they found that in the calculation of these perturbation measures an assumption is made that observed acoustic instabilities can be modeled as random alterations of an underlying periodic signal. The research conducted by Baken, Herzel, Titze et al suggests that this assumption is false.[49-52]

Titze[53] established the following categorization of "quasi-periodic" acoustic voice signals:

Type 1 signals: nearly periodic signals that display no qualitative changes in the analysis segment; if modulating frequencies or subharmonics are present, their energies are an order of magnitude below the energy of the fundamental frequency

Type 2 signals: signals with qualitative changes (bifurcations) in the analysis segment, or signals with subharmonic frequencies or modulating frequencies whose energies approach the energy of the fundamental frequency, there is therefore no obvious single fundamental frequency throughout the segment.

Type 3 signals: signals with no apparent periodic structure. These signals may be further classified mathematically as being chaotic or random.

The acoustic voice signal generated by "normal" phonation is categorized as a Type 1 signal. The acoustic voice signal generated by pathologic phonation may be categorized as being either Type 1, 2, or 3. Titze notes that objective voice measures based on perturbation analysis may be applied to Type 1 signals but are not applicable to the characterization of Type 2 and 3 acoustic voice signals.

Given the limited application of perturbation analysis to the overall categorization of the "quasi-periodic" acoustic voice signal, Bhatia proposes the following guidelines in the formulation of alternative objective measures:

- New objective measures must not explicitly rely on the accurate estimation of the fundamental frequency and must be robust enough to be applicable to Titze's Type 1, 2 and 3 signals.
- New objective measures must address the non-stationary nature of the acoustic voice signal.
- New objective measures must address only the pathophysiological mechanisms of voice disorders. Acoustic characteristics that may be considered

irrelevant to the perceptual categorization of the acoustic signal may be important with respect to pathophysiological classification and therefore should not be discarded from consideration. If the goal of voice analysis is to predict the perception of voice quality, then features extracted from an accurate auditory model must be further considered (masking and frequency sensitivities, etc.).[54]

The following section provides a basic introduction to nonlinear dynamics theory and describes its applicability to the characterization of voice quality as an alternative to perturbation analysis. Finally, as a demonstration of the viability of nonlinear systems analysis methods, an overview of the Bhatia neural classifier is presented. The Bhatia neural classifier discriminates normal voice quality from pathologic voice quality using feature extraction methods based on nonlinear dynamics theory and the spectrogram time-frequency representation of the acoustic voice signal.

Nonlinear Dynamics Theory and State Space Analysis

Let x(t) be a univariate time series representation of a measured signal for a system under analysis. The fundamental assumption of nonlinear time series analysis is that the measured signal x(t) contains multivariate information about the generating process. Using Takens'[55] time-delay embedding theorem, it is possible to reconstruct a representation of the generating system dynamics in the form of state (phase) space trajectories. These state space trajectories (orbits) are multidimensional maps of the multivariate information contained in the measured signal.

In general, the geometric structures of the state space trajectories differ for various types of measured signals (periodic, quasi-periodic, chaotic, and random). Figure 14–1 shows a state space reconstruction of a periodic signal. For a pure sinusoidal time series, the orbits generated in the state space reconstruction are well organized with no variability with respect to orbital divergence. When noise in added to the sinusoidal signal as in Figure 14–2, the orbits generated in the state space reconstruction become less organized with variability due to noise clearly present. Figure 14–3 shows the state space reconstruction of a chaotic time series. The cohesive orbital structure generated in the state space reconstruction of a chaotic time series helps to distinguish it from the state space reconstruction of a pure random time series signal, as shown in Figure 14–4, which completely lacks orbital structure. Interestingly, a cross selection of the state space reconstruction of a chaotic time series will often appear in

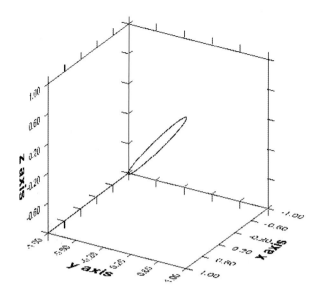

Fig 14–1. State space reconstruction of a sinusoidal time series.

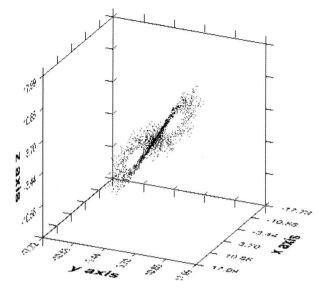

Fig 14–3. State space reconstruction of a chaotic time series.

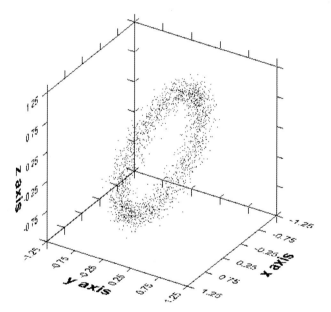

Fig 14–2. State space reconstruction of a noisy sinusoidal time series.

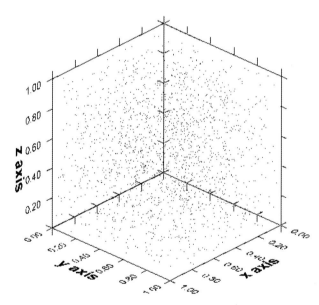

Fig 14–4. State space reconstruction of a random time series.

the form of a strange attractor having a fractal structure with a fractal dimension.[56]

Applying nonlinear dynamics theory to the analysis of the acoustic voice signal yields some interesting results. The state space reconstruction of a normal and pathologic voice sample of a sustained /ɑ/ sampled at 50 kHz are shown in Figures 14–5 and 14–6. The state space trajectories of a normal phonation of /ɑ/ are

well organized with some variability (orbital divergence) present. In contrast the state space trajectories of a pathological phonation of /ɑ/ are not well organized, with greater variability (orbital divergence) clearly present.

The Lyapunov exponents are the measure of the average exponential rates of divergence or convergence of nearby trajectories in state space. The number

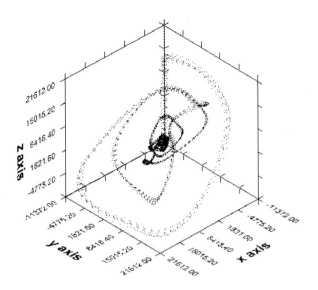

Fig 14–5. State space reconstruction of a normal voiced /ɑ/ time series.

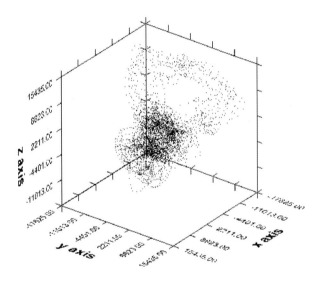

Fig 14–6. State space reconstruction of a pathologically voiced /ɑ/ times series.

of Lyapunov exponents (the Lyapunov Spectrum) equals the embedding dimension of the state space reconstruction. Negative Lyapunov exponents are characteristic of dissipative or nonconservative systems (ie, damped harmonic oscillators). Any system containing at least one positive Lyapunov exponent is defined to be chaotic.

The fractal dimension measure and the Lyapunov exponents are examples of objective measures that can be applied to the analysis of Titze's Type 1, 2, and 3 acoustic voice signals, because they do not explicitly

rely on the estimation of the fundamental frequency. However, these measures are not invariant to the nonstationary nature of the acoustic signal; and great care should be taken in their application.

The Bhatia Neural Classifier

The Bhatia neural classifier is a nonparametric, artificial neural-network-based classification system designed to discriminate normal voice samples from pathological voice samples. Figure 14–7 shows the general architecture of the Bhatia neural classifier. A digitized time series representing a sustained /ɑ/ phonation generated by a test subject sampled at 50 KHz serves as input to the Bhatia neural classifier. The nonlinear dynamics present in the input time series are quantified using features extracted in the time domain, the state space domain, and the time-frequency domain using a spectrogram. The features generated from each of these domains of analysis are used to form a composite feature vector that serves as input to a nonparametric artificial neural network pattern classifier. The artificial neural-network pattern classifier uses the composite feature vector to generate a model of normal and pathological voice during the training phase. Subsequently, the generated model is validated in the testing phase by having the artificial neural-network classify a test voice sample.

Using features based on nonlinear dynamics theory, the Bhatia neural classifier achieved a 95% correct classification result. A neural classifier designed to use features based on perturbation analysis achieved an 89% correct classification result. The results obtained from the Bhatia classifier suggest that features based on nonlinear dynamics theory can provide a viable alternative to perturbation analysis in the characterization of voice quality.

Survey of Nonlinear Dynamics in Vocal Production

The application of chaos to voice analysis has already proven to be exciting and promising. Voice research has been plagued by numerous apparently random, unpredictable aspects of phonation. These have defied measurements and study. Chaos theory has helped address these problems. As Titze, Baken, and Herzel point out, it is important to remember that the existence of a noninteger fractal dimension by itself is not an indicator that the nonlinearity exhibited by a biological system can be characterized as being chaotic.[57] They remind us that the following criteria must be satisfied before the behavior of a nonlinear system can be classified as being chaotic:

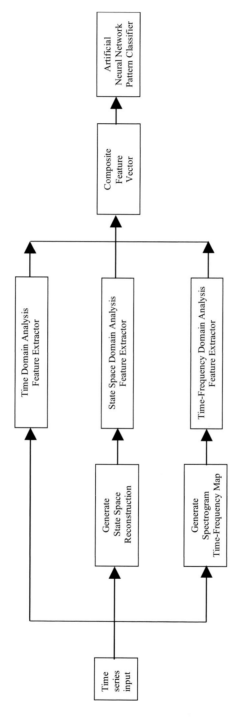

Fig 14–7. Bhatia Neural Classification System architecture.

1. The behavior of the system is the product of a deterministic nonlinear system. There must be some nonlinear rule(s) that govern the behavior of the system.
2. Despite the determinism of the generating system, the output of the system must nonetheless be unpredictable.
3. The behavior of the system must be sensitive to initial conditions.

From an implementation perspective, for a system to be considered chaotic, it must have not only a non-integer fractal dimension but, more importantly, its behavior must be describable by the presence of strange attractors as generated by phase plane plots, or return maps, or it must show evidence of bifurcations of bifurcations.

Baken et al further report that several researchers working independently have yielded evidence of the chaotic nature of voice production.[57] Bifurcation behavior has been observed in mathematical models of phonatory function, normal infant cry, and the abnormal phonation of adults with demonstrable laryngeal disorders. Awrejcewicz has shown that an important class of laryngeal models is chaotic, producing bifurcations.[50] Wong and colleagues have demonstrated that a hybrid of Ishizaka-Flanagan and Titze models is also chaotic and produces outputs that mimic important characteristics of the voices of pathological larynges.[51] In addition, evidence of bifurcations of subharmonic breaks and turbulence observed in infant's cries has been reported by Mende et al.[52] A few early works are worthy of particular attention.

In "Evidence of Chaos in Vocal Fold Vibration,"[57] Titze, Baken, and Herzel describe the need in voice science for a method of summarizing all the dynamic properties of the vocal folds. Predictable physical phenomena are easily described by classic modeling methods. Unpredictable or unstable phenomena have proven highly refractory to such descriptions. Years of research have shown that vocal fold motion exhibits orderliness and underlying unity. The authors review the essential properties of chaotic systems, starting with a review of Poincaré's seminal papers in topology, which date back to 1891 and the early work of Mandelbrot in the late 1960s. The authors reviewed the development of the science of nonlinear dynamics and fractal geometry. Their research efforts have certified the applicability of nonlinear dynamics to understanding vocal function.

In "Analysis of Vocal Disorders of Methods from Nonlinear Dynamics"[58] Herzel and colleagues present simple techniques that will aid all voice researchers in the identification of nonlinear dynamics and voice signals. Within the context of chaos theory, these authors attempt to clarify and standardize some of the terms that have been used in the literature to describe abnormal voice. It appears as if much of the terminology used to describe vocal roughness can be unified using nonlinear dynamics. They also suggest directions for future research. This practical article provides a first step in the transaction between more complex chaos theory and the clinical setting. It is essential for the leaders in the field of chaos theory to provide such practical simplification. Only in this way will these new concepts be applied. Moreover, only such application and analysis of the resultant clinical data will clarify the true importance and utility of chaos theory in voice care.

This research has obvious applications for our understanding of control of phonation. Considering the speed at which phonatory events occur, the maximal speed of any given system has obvious implications for its ability to control specific phonatory functions. In addition, it is clinically important to note the nature of neural communication systems such as this. They are obviously involved in respiration and phonation. Because of their speed, the activities that they control must be slow relative to phonatory events such as high frequency vibratory margin vibration, but they are probably important. One may hypothesize that anything that further slows conduction might have a disproportionate effect on a system that is also relatively slow in comparison with other body systems. This may help explain some of the disproportionately great voice effects seen on patients who seem to have relatively minor pulmonary, thoracic, or abdominal disease or injury, particularly those which alter rib cage and related functions.

Herzel, in "Bifurcations and Chaos in Voice Signals,"[59] examines speech production through speech synthesis and recognition. He reviews bifurcation and chaotic behavior that are apparent in voice signals. He also reviews the basic physiologic mechanism of speech production, including the bifurcations seen in the newborn infant's cry and during voicing. He believes that there is convincing evidence of voice bifurcations and low dimensional attractors in the voice signal and that fractal analysis will aid in the diagnosis of voice disorders and vocal fold pathology.

Steinecke reaffirms that normal voice contains periodic signals, and pathologic voice sounds contain many signal irregularities.[60] Acoustical analysis has shown voice to be a highly nonlinear, dynamic system. All existing models of vocal fold vibration exhibit chaos and bifurcations at different parameter values.

Steinecke discusses a left-to-right asymmetry in a two-mass model, and has shown through bifurcation analysis that the system is relatively stable against small deviations from normal parameters. However, sufficiently large right-left tension imbalances induce bifurcations to subharmonic regimes, toroidal oscillations, and chaos. Bifurcations are located in parameter planes such as vocal fold stiffness and subglottal pressure.

In our opinion, these observations are consistent with clinical observations that the phonatory system can compensate for small, or even substantial, variations from normal. Since variations and the initial condition of this magnitude might be expected to cause greater effect in a predominantly chaotic system, this model helps clarify the combined effect of chaotic and periodic phenomena within the phonatory system. Intuitively, it also may help explain why minor changes in vocal fold condition are tolerated much more poorly by patients who have vocal fold injury. One might infer that, when such an injury impairs the periodic function of normal vocal fold vibration by inducting structural asymmetries, then the chaotic activity becomes more dominant, and any change in initial condition or phase plane thereafter results in greater effect on phonatory output.

In *Vocal Fold Pathology: Frontiers in Basic Science,* Titze summarizes his research findings, which indicate that an understanding of pathological voices can be augmented through the application of nonlinear dynamics.[61] Many observed phenomena such as resonances, Torsades, or chaos can be observed and understood at the borderline of the 1:1 synchronization zone of oscillating models. The exact identification of the essential modes and their relevant nonlinearities are not yet clear. He speculates that a great deal of what is known about voice will be gleaned from diagrams of the voice signal's bifurcations and resultant sophisticated models.

Herzel, Berry, Titze, and Steinecke, in "Nonlinear Dynamics of the Voice: Signal Analysis and Biomechanical Modeling,"[62] point out that vocal irregularities are related to the intrinsic nonlinearities in vocal fold vibrations. Narrow band spectrograms were used to analyze bifurcations and chaos in voice signals. They found that human voice source exhibits several essential nonlinearities that include:

1. Nonlinear stress-strain characteristics of vocal fold tissue,
2. A highly nonlinear relation between pressure and glottal area,
3. Collision of the vocal folds, and
4. Vortices and jet instabilities.

In simulations utilizing the two-mass model, these researchers have shown that the various bifurcations

appear to be due to the synchronization of the right and left vocal fold for overcritical asymmetry. The resulting instabilities are similar to those seen in patients with vocal fold paralysis.

From our clinical perspective, assuming that the nonlinearities are important in vocal function and in the distinct and desirable acoustic output of the vocal mechanism in some situations, this research provides particularly interesting insights for the clinician. It shows that not only are chaotic activities present and potentially measurable, but they are also intimately related to vocal fold synchronization and symmetry. It also is essential for the physician to understand exactly which degree of symmetry is necessary to maintain such effects, and which aspects of vocal fold motion are critical. Such considerations are key in designing vocal fold therapy, especially surgery; and measurement of nonlinear functions restored following treatment may prove a valuable measure of the success of each technique.

Fletcher notes that the property of nonlinearity, seen in nearly all biological systems, suggests the possibility of complex behavior and, thus, the need for special control strategies for satisfactory function or performance.[63] In the vocal system, nonlinearity is observed in the multidimensional vocal fold vibrations and in the aerodynamics of flow through the vocal fold opening. It is encountered in the interaction between these two quantities, as well. Considering the physical features of the vocal system that lead to complex behavior, Fletcher suggests some strategies of control that need to be employed to produce desired sound.

In "Coupling of Neural and Mechanical Oscillators in Control of Pitch, Vibrato and Tremor"[64] Titze suggests that conceptualizing voice production as active and passive systems is no longer viable. He suggests that each normal mode of a single vocal fold should be thought of as a distinct oscillator, just as each vocal tract formant represents an oscillator. Neurologic oscillators override the mechanical and acoustic oscillators. He believes there is growing evidence that vocal vibrato, for example, may be a cultivated vocal tremor. In our opinion, clarifying these issues may be extremely helpful clinically. First, Titze's model adds to our understanding of function of the vocal folds themselves. Second, his concepts make it easier to approach interactions between the vocal fold and other parts of the body. For example, there is good reason to believe that various pathologic conditions are due to central loop dysfunction. Laryngeal dystonia is probably one such disorder. Current treatment is fairly gross, such as paralyzing muscles with botulinum toxin or surgery. For many conditions, there is no effective treatment. Understanding neurological and mechanical oscillators and their interactions should allow more precise diagnoses, and more scientific, specific, and effective intervention.

In "Possible Mechanisms of Vocal Instabilities,"[65] Herzel adds to his important contributions in this area. Voice instabilities/abnormalities include hoarseness, which Herzel says still remains the overall description for deviation from a normal voice; breathiness, which is turbulent noise quantified by the degree of high frequency noise and/or the weakness in harmonics of the pitch; and roughness, which is a result of irregular vibrations of the vocal folds. Herzel has found that roughness especially can be analyzed using the framework of bifurcation theory and chaos. He believes that convincing evidence exists that a rough voice is intimately related to nonlinear dynamics such as period doubling. The goal of his research has been an attempt to achieve quantitative agreement between observations and computer simulation, developing methods for the quantification of irregularities commonly seen in vocal fold pathology such as hoarseness, paralysis, and masses. He employs two-parameter bifurcation diagrams, mode concept, excised larynx studies, and high speed digital imaging. This work focused on subharmonics and oscillations. The presence of subharmonics indicates that there is something going on other than random, turbulent noise. Herzel points out that voice disorders associated with some neurologic conditions such as Huntington's chorea, tremor, pathological jitter and shimmer, and sometimes with normal vibrato, may show subharmonics. Various vibratory asymmetries result in subharmonics that are easily identifiable on spectrograms.

Herzel's work is particularly important and interesting. It provides the clinician with the opportunity to understand the importance of asymmetries, the nature of their interference with phonatory function, and perhaps to quantify the degree of symmetry required for clinically satisfactory phonatory function. When asymmetries are present at the vocal fold level, bifurcations and subharmonics are seen in areas of instability. There is also a relationship between the degree of asymmetry and subglottal pressure. Recognizing these phenomena provide the clinician with not only a new set of behaviors that are helpful for diagnostic purposes, but also a new set of measures to allow pretreatment and posttreatment comparisons for assessment of therapeutic efficacy.

Baken believes that the strongest available proof of the chaotic nature of voice production lies in the obvious bifurcations that are seen as described in his, "Epilogue: Into a Chaotic Future."[66] He reiterates that bifurcation has been observed in three different con-

texts: (1) in the normal infant cry, (2) in the mathematical models of phonatory function; and, (3) in the abnormal phonation patterns of adults with pathological voices. Mathematical models can predict very peculiar vocal behaviors, and these behaviors are observable in the infant's immature voice as well as in the abnormal adult voice. These behaviors cannot be explained by any of the widely accepted theories of vocal fold physiology. Maintaining that the phonatory system is highly nonlinear, chaos theory should predict strange vocal attributes. Nonlinear dynamics offers tools for evaluating, as well as quantifying, specific characteristics of the dynamic phonatory system that have remained mysterious, so far.

The artificial voice source differs from the human voice source in that human speech involves small wave forms and spectral fluctuations. It has been shown that recurrent neural networks with arbitrary feedback are highly nonlinear dynamic systems. In "APOLONN Brings Us to The Real World: Learning Nonlinear Dynamics and Fluctuations in Nature,"[67] Sato et al hypothesize that if recurrent networks could learn the voice source waveforms, and if they could reproduce them under some control, a recurrent net-driven synthesizer could yield synthetic speech. They tested their idea in computer simulation utilizing APOLONN, the recurrent network they chose. APOLONN was trained to generate voice-source waveforms and to produce fluctuations of frequency and amplitude among 32 pitches. They provided a fascinating report with excellent computer graphics. Earlier synthesizers such as MUSA have been invaluable educational aids that have enhanced our understanding of voice. This later generation synthesizer promises to do the same. In so doing, it allows clinicians to understand more discretely exactly which phenomenon produces any specific auditory effect. Hence, the physician understands more clearly which functions are most important to restore. This work also raises interesting speculation about applications in human artificial laryngeal replacement in future years. With this degree of sophistication, it should be possible for the synthesizer to acquire not only the nuances of speech, but also the nuances of timbre of an individual's speech. When the technology has been developed and microminiaturized, it might prove to be an important part of the next generation of artificial larynges. Additional concepts and research on this subject are reviewed in chapter 15.

Conclusions

It is clear that chaos theory and fractal analysis have been employed successfully in characterizing nonlinear behavior of biological systems. Technical and factual advances in this field by molecular biologists, cardiologists, ophthalmologists, and others are likely to be valuable to voice researchers, who should be able to apply information learned from other disciplines. Initial applications of chaos theory in voice research have confirmed the presence of important nonlinearities in voice function and have shown great promise for further understanding of voice through the application of nonlinear dynamics. The new insights obtained through such research and technological advances in clinical instrumentation that are likely to follow have exciting potential for advancing rational medical care of the human voice. Continued basic research and early application in clinical research and treatment settings should be encouraged.

References

1. Gleick J. *Chaos: Making a New Science*. New York, NY: Viking Penguin Inc; 1987.
2. Goldberger A, Rigney D, West B. Chaos and fractals in human physiology. *Sci Am.* 1990;43-49.
3. Gulick D. *Encounters with Chaos*. New York, NY: McGraw-Hill, Inc; 1992.
4. Denton T, Diamond G, Helfant R, Khan S, Karagueuzian H. Fascinating rhythm: a primer on chaos theory and its application to cardiology. *Am Hear J.* 1990;120(6)(Pt 1):1419-1439.
5. Mandelbrot BB. *Fractals: Form, Chance and Dimension*. New York, NY: Freeman Press; 1977.
6. Stewart I. *Does God Play Dice? The Mathematics of Chaos*. New York, NY: Basil Blackwell, Ltd; 1989.
7. Bascum PAJ, Cobbold RFC, Roeloff BHM. Influence with spectral broadening on continuous wave Doppler ultrasound spectra: a geometric approach. *Ultrasound Med Biol.* 1986;12:387-395.
8. Schepers H, Beek VJ, Bassingthwaighte J. Four methods to estimate the fractal dimension from self-affine signals. *IEEE Engineer Med Biol.* 1992;57-64.
9. Liebovitch LS, Toth, TA. A fast algorithm to determine fraction dimensions by box counting. *Phys Lett A.* 1989;141:386-390.
10. Grassberger P, Procaccia I. Measuring the strangeness of strange attractors. *Physica 9D.* 1983;183-208.
11. Skinner JE, Molnar M, Vybiral P, Mitra M. The application of Chaos theory to biology and medicine. *Integrative Physiologic Behavioral Sci.* 1992;27(1):39-53.
12. Sadana A, Madagula A. A fractal analysis of external diffusion limited first-order kinetics for the binding of antegin by immobilized antibody. *Biosensors Bioelectronics.* 1994;9:45-55.
13. Bassingthwaighte J, King R, Sambrook JE, Stenewyn BS. Fractal analysis of blood-tissue exchange kinetics. *Adv Exper Med Biol.* 1988;222:15-23.

14. Solovyev VD. Fractal graphical representation and analysis of DNA and protein sequences. *Biosystems.* 1993;30:137-160.
15. Li H, Li Y, Zhao H. Fractal analysis of protein chain confirmation. *Internal J Biol Macro Mol.* 1990;12:6-8.
16. El-Jaick LJ, Wajnberg E. Fractal analysis of photolosis of nitrosal hemaglobin at low temperatures. *Intl J Biol Macro Mol.* 1993;15:119-123.
17. Liebovitch LS, Sullivan JM. Fractal analysis of a voltage-dependent potassium channel from cultured mouth hippocampal neurons. *Biophys J.* 1987;52:979-988.
18. Smith TG, Marks WB, Lange GD, Sherrif WH, Neale EA. A fractal analysis of cell images. *J Neurosci Methods.* 1989;27:173-180.
19. MacAulay C, Palcic B. Fractal texture features based on optical density of surface area used in imaging analysis of cervical cells. *Analytical Quantitative Cytol Histol.* 1990;12(6):394-398.
20. Glenny RW, Robertson HT, Yamashiro S, Bassingthwaighte JB. Applications of fractal analysis to physiology. *J Appl Physiol.* 1991;70:2351-2367.
21. Janse M: Is there Chaos in cardiology? *Brit Heart J.* 1992;67(1):3-4.
22. Rambihar V. Jurrasic heart: from the heart to the edge of chaos. *Can J Cardiol.* 1993;9(9):787-788.
23. Stein K, Kligfield P. Application of fractal geometry to the analysis of ventricular premature contractions. *J Electrocardiol.* 1990;23(suppl):82-84.
24. Berenfeld O, Sadeh D, Abboud S. Modeling of the heart's ventricular conduction system using fractal geometry: spectral analysis of the QRS complex. *Ann Biomed Engineer.* 1993;21:125-134.
25. Yamashiro SM, Flaas DW, Reneman RS, Tangelder GJ, Bassingthwaighte JB. Fractal analysis of vasomotion. *Ann N Y Acad Sci.* 1990;591:410-416.
26. Herzel H, Seidel H, Warzel H. Heart rate, respiration, and baroreflex: entrainment, bifurcations, and chaos. *Wiss Z Humboldt-Universitat zu Berlin, R. Medizin.* 1992;41(4):51-57.
27. Warzel H, Seidel H, Herzel H. Heart rate, respiration, and baroreflex: motivation and expirations. *Wiss Z Humboldt-Universitat zu Berlin, R. Medizine.* 1992;41(4):59-61.
28. Seidel H, Herzel H. Modelling heart rate variability due to respiration and baroreflex. In: Mosekilde E, Mouritsen OG, eds. *Modelling the Dynamics of Biological Systems.* New York, NY: Springer-Verlag; 1995:205-229.
29. Griffith TM, Edwards DH. Fractal analysis of role of smooth muscle CA^{2+} fluxes in genesis of chaotic arterial pressure oscillations. *Amer J Physiol.* 1994;226(Heart Circ Physiol, 35):H1801-H1811.
30. Gough N. Fractal analysis of fetal heart rate variability. *Physiol Meas.* 1993;14:309-315.
31. Verhoeven JTM, Thijssen JM. Potential fractal analysis for lesion detection in echographic images. *Ultrasonic Imaging.* 1993;15:304-323.
32. Bullmore E, Branmer M, Alarcon G, Binnie C. A new technique for fractal analysis applied to human, intracerebrally recorded, ictal electroencephalographic signals. *Neurosci Lett.* 1992;146:227-230.

33. Mandelbrot B. *Fractal Geometry of Nature*. New York, NY: WH Freeman; 1982.

34. Porter R, Ghosh S, Lange GD, Smith TG. A fractal analysis of parametal neurons in mamillion motor cortex. *Neurosci Lett*. 1991;130(1):112-116.

35. Cross SS, Start RC, Silcocks PD, Bull AD, Cotton DWK, Underwood JC. Quantitation of the renal arterial tree by fractal analysis. *J Pathol*. 1993;170:479-484.

36. Morigawa K, Tauchi M, Fukuda Y. Fractal analysis of ganglion cell dendritic branching patterns of the rat and cat retina. *Neurosci Res*. 1989;10(suppl):S131-S140

37. Smith TG, Behar TN. Comparative fractal analysis of cultured glia derived from optic nerve and brain demonstrate different rates of morphological differentiation. *Brain Res*. 1994;634:181-190.

38. Smith TG, Lange GD, Marks WD, Sheriff WH, Behar TN. The fractal analysis of cultured rats' optic nerve glial growth and differentiation. *Neuroscience*. 1991; 41(1):159-166.

39. Wingate R, Fitsbiggon T, Thompson ID. Lucifer yellow, retrograde tracers, and fractal analysis characterize adult ferret retina ganglion cells. *J Comp Neurol*. 1992; 323(4):449-474.

40. Boxt LM, Katz J, Liebovitch LS, Jones R, Esser TD, Reid L. Fractal analysis of pulmonary arteries: the fractal dimension is lower in pulmonary hypertension. *J Thorac Imaging*. 1994;9(1):8-13.

41. Witten ML, McKee JL, Lantz RC, Haze AM, Quan SS, Sobonya RE, Lemen RJ. Fractal and morphometric analysis of lung structures after canine adenovirus-induced bronchiolitis in beagle puppies. *Pediatric Pulmonary*. 1993;16:62-68.

42. Lynch JA, Hawkes DJ, Bucklind-Wright JC. Analysis of texture in macroradiographs of osteoarthritic knees using the fractal signature. *J Phys Med Biol*. 1991; 36(6):709-722.

43. Landini G, Misson G, Murray PI. Fractal analysis of the normal human retinal fluorescine angiogram. *Current Eye Res*. 1993;12(1):23-27.

44. Grant PE, Lumsden CJ. Fractal analysis of renal cortical perfusion. *Invest Radiol*. 1994;29:16-23.

45. Priebe CE, Solka JL, Lorey RA, Rogers GW, Poston WL, Kallergi M, Qian W, Clarke LP, Clark RA. The application of fractal analysis to mammographic tissue classification. *Cancer Lett*. 1994;77:183-189.

46. Oshida Y, Munoz C, Winkler MM, Hashem A, Itoh M. Fractal dimension analysis of aluminum oxide particle for sandblasting dental use. *Biomed Materials Engineering*. 1993;3(3):117-126.

47. Wang YY, Wang WQ. Fractal concept and its analysis method for Doppler ultrasound signals. *Ultrasound Med Biol*. 1993;19(8):661-666.

48. Hertrich I, Lutzenberger W, Spieker S, Ackermann H. Fractal dimension of sustained vowel productions in neurological dysphonias: an acoustic and electroglottographic analysis. *J Acoustic Soc Am*. 1997;102(1):652–654.

49. Baken RJ. Irregularity of vocal periodicity and amplitude: a first approach to the fractal analysis of voice. *J Voice*. 1990;4:185-197.

50. Awrejcewicz J. Bifurcation portrait of the human vocal cord oscillations. *J Sound Vibr*. 1990;136:151-156.

51. Wong D, Ito MR, Cox NB Titze IR. Observation of perturbations in a lumped-element model of the vocal folds with application to some pathological cases. *J Acous Soc Amer*. 1991;89:383-391.

52. Mende W, Herzel H, Wermke K. Bifurcations and chaos in newborn infant cries. *Phys Lett A*. 1990;145:418-424.

53. Titze I. *Summary Statement: Workshop on Acoustic Voice Analysis*. Denver, Colo: National Center for Voice and Speech; 1994.

54. Davis P, Fletcher N. *Vocal Fold Physiology: Controlling Complexity and Chaos*. San Diego, Calif.: Singualr Publishing Group, Inc; 1996:253–261.

55. Takens F. *Detecting Strange Attractors in Turbulence. Lecture Notes in Math*. New York, NY: Springer Publishing Group; 1981.

56. Rowlands G., Sprott J. *Chaos Data Analyzer: The Professional Version*. New York, NY: American Institute of Physics; 1995.

57. Titze IR, Baken RJ, Herzel H. Evidence of chaos in vocal fold vibration. In: Titze IR, ed. *Vocal Fold Physiology: New Frontiers in Basic Science*. San Diego, Calif: Singular Publishing Group, Inc; 1993:143.

58. Herzel H, Berry DA, Titze IR, Saleh M. Analysis of vocal disorders of methods from nonlinear dynamics. *J Speech Hear Res*. 1994;37:1008-1019.

59. Herzel M. Bifurcations and chaos in voice signals. *Appl Mechans Rev*. 1993;46:399-413.

60. Steinecke I. Bifurcations in an asymmetric vocal fold model. *J Acoust Soc Amer*. 1995;97:1-11.

61. Titze IR, ed. *Vocal Fold Physiology: New Frontiers in Basic Science*. San Diego, Calif: Singular Publishing Group, Inc; 1993.

62. Herzel H, Berry D, Titze I, Steinecke I. Nonlinear dynamics of the voice: signal analysis and biomechanical modeling. *Am Inst Physics*. 1995;5(1):30-34.

63. Fletcher N. Nonlinearity, complexity and control. In: Davis P, Fletcher N, eds: *Vocal Fold Physiology: Controlling Complexity and Chaos*. San Diego, Calif: Singular Publishing Group, Inc; 1996.

64. Titze IR. Coupling of neural and mechanical oscillators in control of pitch, vibrato and tremor. In: Davis P, Fletcher N. *Vocal Fold Physiology: Controlling Complexity and Chaos*. San Diego, Calif: Singular Publishing Group, Inc; 1996.

65. Herzel H. Possible mechanisms of vocal instabilities. In: Davis P, Fletcher N. *Vocal Fold Physiology: Controlling Complexity and Chaos*. San Diego, Calif: Singular Publishing Group, Inc; 1996.

66. Baken RJ. Epilogue: Into a chaotic future. In: Rubin JS, Satlaoff RT, Korovin GS, Gould WJ, eds. *Diagnosis and Treatment of Voice Disorders*. New York, NY:Igaku-Shoin; 1995:502-509.

67. Sato M, Joe K, Hirahara T. APOLONN brings us to the real world: learning nonlinear dynamics and fluctuations in nature. *Proc IJCNN*. 1990;1:I581-I586.

15

Dynamical Disorders of Voice: A Chaotic Perspective on Vocal Irregularities

Ronald J. Baken

The modern era of voice research might fairly be said to have begun about 50 years ago, with the elaboration of a crucial understanding: phonation results from and is governed by the biomechanical characteristics of vocal fold tissue interacting with glottal aerodynamic properties. That insight was the heart of the myoelastic-aerodynamic theory of phonation,[1-3] a construct that physiologic observation of vocal fold behavior has amply validated. Numerous mathematical models of vocal fold function that were founded upon it[4-5] have generally had extraordinarily impressive predictive and explanatory power. As a result, the process of normal phonation is quite well understood.

Unfortunately, despite very serious efforts by many of our best researchers over a significant period of time, there are still large gaps in our comprehension of laryngeal phonatory behavior. Nowhere are these lacunae wider than in our understanding of many of the anomalies encountered in abnormal vocal function, and (when one actually looks for them) even in the normal voice.[6] The increase of frequency and amplitude perturbation that is so characteristic of dysphonia, for example, remains only poorly explained, despite several hypotheses of varying attractiveness.[7-13] The "pitch breaks" of the adolescent also lack a coherent explanatory model, as has the "biphonation" of the infant's cry.[14-15]

Even less well explained is the kind of situation illustrated in Figure 15–1A, which shows the fundamental frequency (F_0) of successive periods during a sustained vowel by an 81-year-old female with a diagnosis of spasmodic dysphonia. Her F_0 undergoes

a relatively slow cyclic variation at a rate of about 4 cycles per second, most likely caused by tremor of the laryngeal muscles. There is also, however, a much faster frequency variation that is sometimes observable at the peaks of the slower oscillations. This is harder to explain. However, most striking are the outbreaks of "diplophonia"—more properly, subharmonic oscillation—that occur in the "valleys" of the F_0 pattern and that persist halfway up the next peak. We have had no easy explanation for this kind of behavior. Even less have we been able to offer coherent and parsimonious explanations for the more complex patterns of F_0 change, like that of Figure 15–1B, that are not uncommon in dysphonic voices. While we have developed a fairly clear picture of the mechanisms of the phonationally regular, we have not done nearly as well in elucidating the vocally complex or erratic.

The fact is, of course, that we have not done much worse in dealing with oscillatory misbehavior than most of the broader sciences of which we are a part. All have been impeded by a paucity of scientific tools for describing disorder, modeling instability, and characterizing capriciousness.

The outlook improved dramatically about 20 years ago with the recognition of the pivotal importance, broad applicability, and enormous explanatory power of a radically different way of considering natural phenomena. The new discipline is formally known as the *theory of nonlinear dynamics*, but it is more popularly called *chaos theory*. It offers a different way of looking at life functions[16-18] that has begun to have a signif-

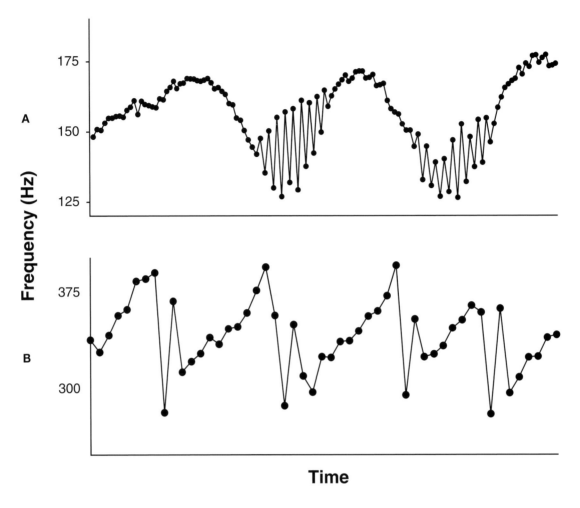

Fig 15–1. Fundamental frequency of successive periods during sustained vowels. **A.** An aged spasmodic dysphonic woman, showing subharmonic oscillation during the low parts of a tremor cycle; **B.** very complex patterns of F_0 change in the voice of a dysphonic patient.

icant impact in the biomedical world. Cochlear function,[19] abnormal motor behavior,[20] cardiac electrical instability,[21-25] Cheyne-Stokes respiration,[26] cerebral electrophysiology,[27] and even menopausal hot flashes[28] have been explored with the new tools—both qualitative and quantitative—that it provides. The application of chaos theory to voice production is now well under way.[29-45] It holds the promise of important breakthroughs in understanding those erratic phenomena of voice, normal and disordered, that have thus far proved so intractable.

The purpose of this chapter is to consider a few of the most basic concepts of chaos theory, and to show how they might profitably be applied to problems of vocal dysfunction. The theory itself is intensely mathematical, and the mathematics can be quite difficult and counterintuitive. It is, therefore, useful to take a very informal concept-oriented approach even though doing so greatly circumscribes the extent to which important areas can be developed. The purpose is not to provide a tutorial introduction to applied chaos theory so much as to suggest something of the flavor of this relatively new branch of the sciences and to suggest why it holds such promise. To do this, some conjectures will be proposed that might explain the sudden appearance of phonatory anomalies that are so characteristic of disordered voices. Insofar as possible, we will proceed in a completely non-mathematical (and consequently nonrigorous) way, because it seems likely that doing so will meet the needs of most readers who would like to understand the general tenor of what is involved, but who are unlikely to want to tackle nonlinear dynamical analyses themselves (at least not yet).

Numerophiles and those who wish really to explore the area should consult a good general text.*

Chaos Defined

The very term "chaos" has become trendy, a fashionable buzzword that is too often dropped into discussions as a synonym for "erratic," "unpredictable," or "very complex." But the word *chaos* has, in fact, a very specific definition. If it is to be a useful concept, it is important to specify exactly what "chaos" really means.

Basically, behavior can be said to be chaotic **if and only if**:

- *It is the product of a deterministic system.* "Deterministic" means that the observed behavior is governed by a rule. We may not understand what that rule is but we must know that it does, in fact, exist and that it is controlling the system. *The fact that there is a governing nonlinear rule is the sine qua non of a chaotic system.*

- *The system is nonlinear.* In the simplest sense, a linear system is one whose function can be plotted as a straight line on a graph. Figure 15–2A is an example. All other things being equal, it shows that airflow through the vocal tract is directly and *linearly* proportional to the pressure in the lungs. A *nonlinear* function, on the other hand, is represented by a curved line (which can be quite complex). Figure 15–2B is illustrative. It shows the relationship that has been observed[60] between subglottal pressure and the intensity of the vocal signal.

- Despite the determinism (rule-based operation) of the generating system, the *output is nonetheless unpredictable.* This requirement needs to be understood carefully. It does, of course, imply that the behavior might be random-looking. But it also allows, for example, for the system to produce a number of different *patterns of response* (within each of which a succession of output states might be completely predictable). If one is not able to specify, to any arbitrarily specified level of precision, which pattern will be produced at any given time, the sys-

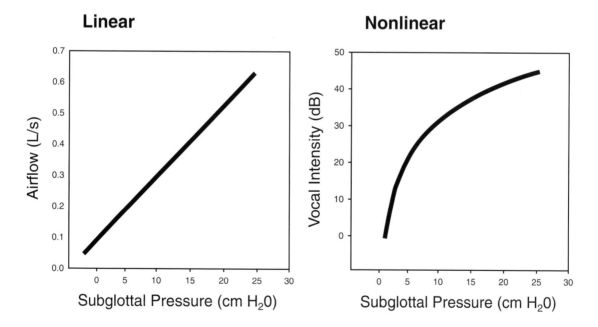

Fig 15–2. Linear and nonlinear functions.

*The classic source of understanding for numerophobes is Gleick (1987),[46] a volume that appeared for many weeks on the best-seller lists. A very brief nontechnical presentation is Crutchfield, Farmer, et al (1986)[47] For those who can tolerate a minimal mathematical exposition, Abraham and Shaw[48-51] offer an excellent—and lighthearted—starting point that calls for no background at all. More mathematically rigorous introductions are provided by Rasband,[52] Baker and Golub,[53] Moon,[54] and Thompson and Stewart.[55] Eubank and Farmer (1990)[56] is a classic, and is surprisingly approachable. A good overview of chaos in several scientific disciplines is available in Cvitanovic (1984),[57] while Glass and Mackey[58] explore nonlinear dynamics of various biological systems, and West[59] concisely reviews nonlinear dynamics considered in pathophysiology.

tem may validly be described as chaotic (provided, of course, that the other requirements are met).

- The system must have a relatively small number of parameters. That is, it must be controlled by only a few factors. Put another way, a chaotic system, however much it behaves in complex ways, must nonetheless be a fairly simple system. For reasons that will shortly become clear, it is described as a "low dimensional" system.

- *Finally, the behavior of the system must be "exquisitely sensitive to initial conditions."* What this means is that extremely small differences in some controlling parameter can have dramatically large effects on the qualitative aspects of the system's behavior. Note, in Figure 15–3, how changing the coefficient a

in the function $x_{n+1} = ax_n(1-x_n)$ by a mere 0.005, from $a = 3.855$ to $a = 3.860$, alters the qualitative nature of the output dramatically.[**]

In fact, radical shifts in the output of a chaotic system can be produced by changes that are *infinitesimally* small. "Infinitesimal" is used here in its literal, mathematical sense. Therefore, we can never have enough decimal places in our specification of the controlling variable to be able to predict the resultant behavior of the system with absolute certainty. Furthermore, an infinitesimally small difference is, from a practical point of view, a difference of zero. This implies that a chaotic system can change its behavior for no measurable reason at all.

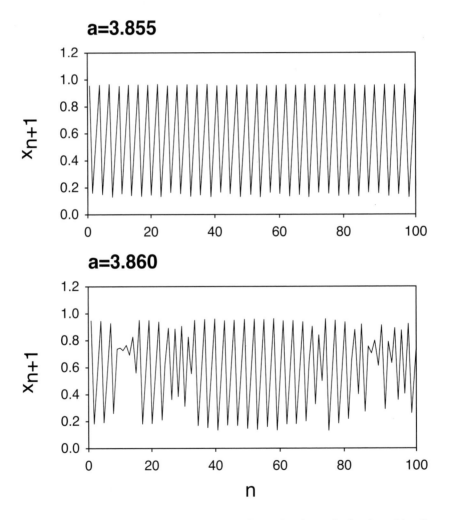

Fig 15–3. Output of the "logistic equation" can be dramatically altered by tiny changes of its coefficient "a."

[**]Known as the "logistic equation" this is a favorite example of a chaotic generator. Despite its extreme simplicity, its output can be astoundingly complex. Any of the texts cited in the previous footnote will provide more information about this "simple" system.

Dynamics of a System

It is vital to understand that one cannot tell if a system is behaving in a chaotic manner just by looking at its output. Consider the two data sets plotted in Figure 15–4. One was produced by a chaotic system (that is, by a system that has the defining characteristics just discussed). The other, as best one can tell, is simply random. Which is the chaotic one? There are often ways to find out, but looking is not one of them. Not everything that looks random is chaotic.

Trajectories in State Space

How can one describe the dynamics (the behavior) of a system? One of the best ways is to plot its behavior in *state space* (often called *phase space*). It is easier to understand what this means from an example than from a definition, and the example will prove useful in developing some further concepts.

Consider a pendulum—like one that hangs from a clock, illustrated in Figure 15–5. Give it, for the sake of our example, the rather special property that it is not subject to friction, so that once started, it swings forever. It turns out that the dynamics of this extraordinarily simple (linear) system can be fully described in terms of the position and velocity of the pendulum. We can show their relationship graphically, as in Figure 15–6. The position of the pendulum (in degrees, θ) to the left or right of midline is plotted on the horizontal axis, while its speed (in degrees per second, toward the left or right) is plotted on the vertical axis. The (two-dimensional) space that these axes create is one example of a *state space* (also called a *phase space*). The ellipse that results is a *trajectory* that passes through all the points in this space that are possible for a simple pen-

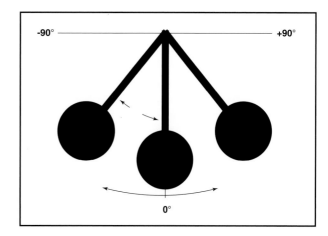

Fig 15–5. Simple pendulum, swinging through an angle θ.

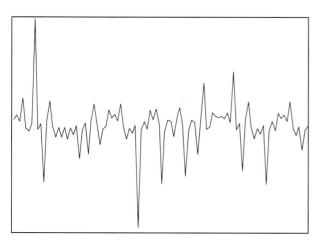

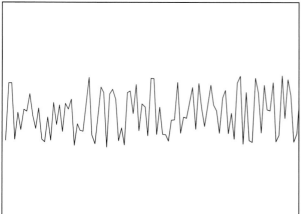

Fig 15–4. Only one of these patterns was produced by a chaotic system. Which one?

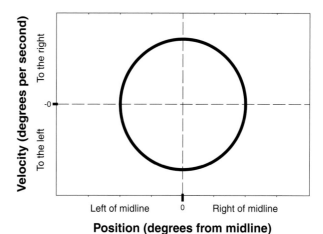

Fig 15–6. Relationship of the position and velocity of the pendulum of Figure 15–5. The plane of the graph is the "state space" of the pendulum system.

dulum. It, therefore, demarcates all the combinations of position and speed that this uncomplicated dynamic system can have. As it happens, the pendulum is so simple that a two-variable state space is enough to define its dynamics *completely*. That is, there is nothing else that we need to know (or would have to derive) about this system to understand all its operation.

If the pendulum were free to swing not only from side to side, but also front to back (so that its motion described not an arc, but a circle) then we would need another axis to describe its motion in this direction, as in Figure 15–7. Adding an axis creates a three-dimensional space, which is the minimum necessary to describe this system. Hence, it could be called a three-dimensional dynamical system. "Dimension" is the way in which we specify the number of axes, each representing an independent variable, that is necessary to describe the dynamics of a system.

Attractors

Real pendulums, of course, are subject to friction. With each oscillation a little energy is lost and the width of the swing decreases, until finally the pendulum hangs at rest. To counter this, pendulum clocks have a mechanism that gives the pendulum a little "kick" when it passes a certain position in its swing cycle, adding back the energy that it lost during the previous oscilla-

tion. Because of the kick the trajectory of the pendulum system in state space has a little "glitch" in it, as in Figure 15–8.

Now, the amount of energy added by each kick is constant, and is just enough to keep the pendulum's arc at a given width. Suppose, therefore, that the pendulum is started by pulling it very far from the midline—to a position much further out than it would normally swing. Remembering that the once-per-cycle kick only provides enough energy for a swing of moderate width, it is clear that the amount of energy lost to friction on the initial huge swing will not be fully made up by the kick. Therefore, the next swing will be a little less energetic, and a little less wide. In fact, more energy is lost during each wider-than-normal swing than is restored by the kick, and so the swings will constantly become less wide until the arc is just the right size—the size at which the energy lost is exactly made up by the energy that the kick adds. Because, at this arc width, the energy loss and addition are exactly balanced, the pendulum will continue to oscillate in an arc of that width forever (or as long as the clock is kept wound up). The situation is illustrated in Figure 15–9A.

A similar situation prevails, in reverse, if we start the pendulum swinging from a position that is not as far out as it usually goes. Each swing, being smaller than usual, loses less energy than the standard-sized once-per-cycle kick delivers, so with each swing there is a net gain of energy, and each oscillation is a bit larg-

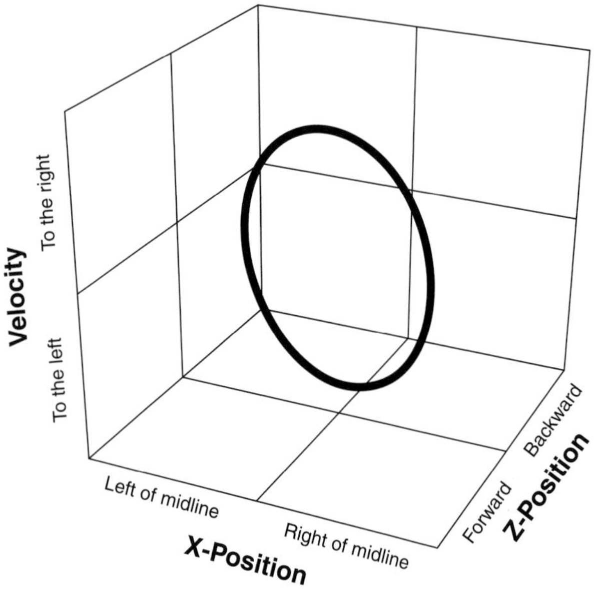

Fig 15–7. A third axis is required to describe the movement of a pendulum that can swing not only side-to-side, but also front-to-back. The state space of such a pendulum is three-dimensional.

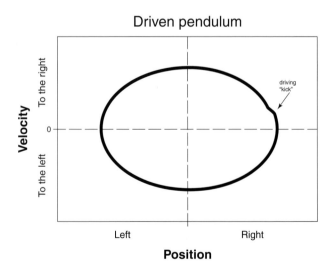

Fig 15–8. A real pendulum needs a small "kick" during each swing to make up for frictional losses. The kick produces a glitch in the trajectory in phase space, but delivers the energy that keeps the system going.

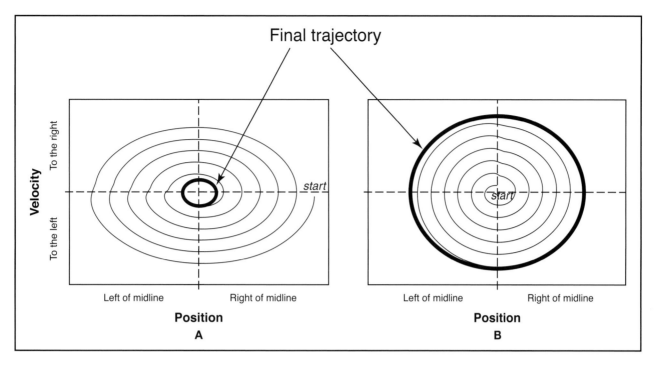

Fig 15–9. The constant-sized kick provides just enough energy to keep the pendulum swinging with an arc of only a certain size—no bigger and no smaller. No matter how the pendulum is started, it will end up swinging with an arc of that certain size. The system is attracted to a special trajectory in state space.

er than the one before (Fig 15–9B). Finally, the swing is large enough that the energy lost equals the energy gained, and thereafter the pendulum follows the same trajectory in phase space "forever."

The final trajectory, then, has an important property. Starting the pendulum from almost anywhere in the state space—with however much displacement from the midline, and with however strong a push one might give it—it will always end up swinging with the same frequency and arc width. All paths seem to be compelled to head for the same final trajectory, which is therefore called an *attractor*.

Model Behavior

The human vocal system is extraordinarily complex and is largely inaccessible to direct observation. Furthermore, there is a very limited number of ways in which one can manipulate it for experimental purposes. One means of getting around these problems is to use a mathematical model of the vocal folds (and sometimes of other elements of the vocal tract as well). A respectable number of models have been developed, each expressing its creator's conceptualization of the nature of the forces driving phonatory oscillation. One of the least complex and best known is the

Ishizaka-Flanagan (1972)[61] model. It simplifies each vocal fold to an upper and a lower mass. They are more or less tightly coupled to each other but each is free to move toward or away from the glottis. The user chooses such important biomechanical and aerodynamic parameters as the size and stiffness of each mass, the length of the glottis, the subglottal pressure, and so on. Despite its very significant simplification of a complex system, it does provide a useful portrayal—validated by comparison to real phonation—of vocal fold oscillation under a wide range of physiologic conditions. Furthermore, its simplicity is ideal for present purposes, because it makes it possible to explore the potential for chaotic behavior in a "phonatory apparatus" that has only a few controlling variables, and hence in a system that should be easily understandable.

Model Phonation

If we set parameters for the two-mass model to some reasonable values—say moderate stiffness and subglottal pressure—and let it run, it oscillates quite well. Typical vibration is shown in Figure 15–10. The shaded area in the plot is the region where this vocal fold moves past the midline, and hence overlaps the opposite fold. Obviously, in real life this cannot happen.

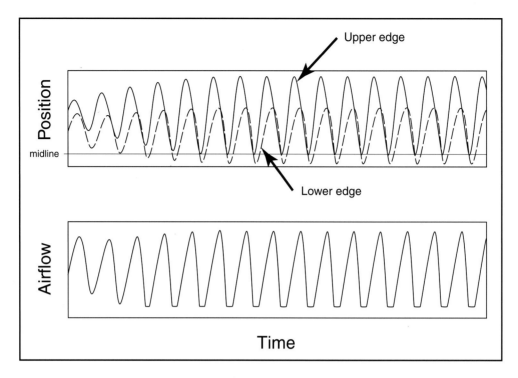

Fig 15–10. Typical oscillation just after onset of the vocal folds in the two-mass model. *Top*: Position of the vocal fold's upper and lower edges. *Bottom*: Transglottal airflow.

Instead, the vocal folds collide and deform each other. However, in the purely mathematical world of the model all things are possible, and the position trace has been allowed to extend into this realm of impossibility to provide some sense of how much deformation there would be.

Note that, as in the living larynx, there is a phase difference between the upper and lower lips of the vocal fold. Also, again as in nature, it takes a few oscillatory cycles for full vibratory amplitude to be achieved. The record of airflow through the modeled glottis shows a regular train of pulses, although their shape is not a precise representation of that of real voice.

One way to show the dynamics of the model's vocal fold in a state space is to plot the position of the upper mass of the vocal fold against the position of the lower mass, as in Figure 15–10. The trajectory of the system in this state space bears an obvious resemblance to the outward-spiraling trajectory of a simple pendulum shown in Figure 15–9B. That is, driven by the energy boost from the subglottal pressure, the trajectory spirals out from the starting condition until ulti-

mately it reaches and is held by an attractor. The attractor itself is quite different, however. Instead of being a single line in state space, it appears to be "unstable" in that it is a cluster of lines. An enlargement of a small region of the attractor, shown on the right of Figure 15–11, reveals that the lines of the attractor show signs of being "bundled." In fact, although not shown here, each "bundle" of lines could be shown to be itself composed of bundles, and those bundles of still other bundles, and so on, ad infinitum. With a little mathematical trickery—the details of which are beyond our present discussion[†]—it is possible to "cut" across these bundles, something like chopping across a fistful of spaghetti, and then to look at the cut surface. If we do this, as in Figure 15–11B, we find that not only are the lines "bundled," but the bundles are arranged in layers. As it happens, if we were to repeatedly enlarge each layer, we would see that each layer is itself composed of layers—layers within layers, ad infinitum. In short, the appearance of the attractor at every magnification would have very much the appearance of any other magnification. This property

[†]Except, perhaps, to note that the result is termed Poincaré section, and to suggest that the techniques for doing this and for interpreting the results are found in numerous introductory texts in the field of nonlinear dynamical systems theory.

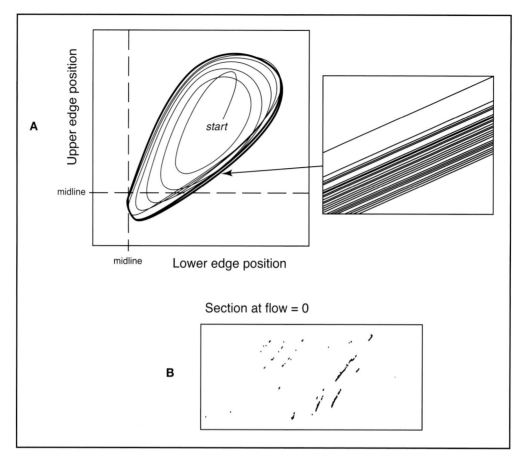

Fig 15–11. Oscillation of the vocal fold of the two-mass model shown in an "upper-edge/lower-edge" state space. **A.** After start-up the system seems to be drawn to an attractor. However, magnifying that attractor shows that it is really a bundle of separate lines. Increasing the magnification would reveal ever-smaller bundles of lines. **B.** Plotting a "cross-section" of the attractor shows that the bundles of lines that compose it are arranged in layers. This is, therefore, a "strange attractor" that has fractal properties.

of any small part being a miniature version of the whole—technically referred to as "self-similarity at all scales"—makes the attractor a "fractal" structure.[‡] An attractor that is fractal is said—in the technical jargon of nonlinear dynamics—to be *strange*. Strange attractors are characteristic of chaotic systems.

The Ishizaka-Flanagan two-mass model, and other simple models of the vocal folds have, in fact, been shown to be chaotic systems,[30,37,64,65] and thus can serve us well in our present exploration of the role of chaos in vocal dysfunction.

A Moment's Consideration of an Important Bias

Although oscillation of the model's vocal folds is governed by an attractor, that attractor, by being fractal, allows each cycle—in fact, it *requires* each cycle—to be slightly different from every other one. That is worth thinking about for a moment, because the oscillation we are dealing with here is generated by an equation. An equation does not change while the model is running. An equation does not involve perturbing fac-

---

[‡]Because fractal shapes are often surprisingly and intriguingly beautiful they have captured the imagination of many in recent years. Accordingly, there are many excellent books for neophytes who would like to learn more about them. The best known is by Mandelbrot (1977),[62] who founded the field of fractal geometry. A somewhat more useful text—complete with computer algorithms for generating fractal images—is Peitgen and Saupe, 1988.[63]

tors—variations in subglottal pressure, small alterations of muscle tension, minuscule shifts of mucus, or shifts of vocal tract posture. Despite this, the output shows observable perturbation.

Our bias is to believe that any effect—such as the radical shifts of F_0 of Figure 15–1—must have a proximate cause which is, in principle, identifiable. That bias accounts for several theories and speculations concerning the origins of, for example, frequency and amplitude perturbation. However, perturbation in the output of a mathematical model is a common observation (for example Wong, Ito, et al, 1991)[64] and can only be an inherent result of the equations that form it. It cannot, in a model, be the product of immediate outside causes. The question naturally arises: How much of the perturbation of the normal (real) vocal signal is caused by small pressure variations, little muscle twitches, and the like. How much is simply inherent in the vocal fold dynamics—as shown by a strange attractor? Similarly, the theory of nonlinear dynamics makes it clear that the behavior of a system can alter in the absence of any external influence. Effects do not necessarily have immediate causes.

Basin of Attraction: The Attractor's Realm

It is worthwhile to look at the dynamics of the pendulum once again. Recall that it gets a little push whenever it passes a given point in its swing, and this little boost is just sufficient to replace the energy lost to friction. Figure 15–12 recapitulates some things that were said about this system earlier. That is, if the pendulum is started from a position either more than or less than its usual displacement, oscillations either diminish or enlarge until their amplitude represents an equilibrium between the energy gain and loss. The final trajectory that represents this equilibrium state is an attractor, because the dynamics of the system seem—in some metaphorical sense—to be drawn to it.

The plane of the state space of Figure 15–12 contains all the possible combinations of position and velocity that, in principle, a pendulum could have. A reasonable question is "Which starting combinations of position and velocity (that is, which starting positions in the state space) will produce a trajectory that ends up on the attractor? Are there any regions (starting combinations of position and velocity) that will *not* lead to the attractor?"

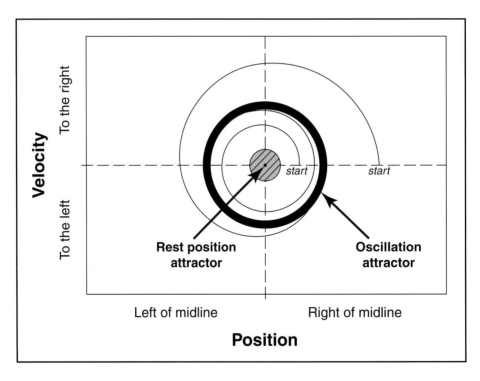

Fig 15–12. The pendulum's state space really has two attractors. One—shown by a heavy line—is an oscillation, but the other—represented by a dot in the middle of the plane—is hanging motionless. Most starting points on the plane lead to the oscillation attractor, but some lead to the motionless condition. There are two "basins of attraction" in the state space.

It might seem that all positions in the space are equally subject to the attractor's lure, but that is *not* the case. The reason is that the pendulum gets its absolutely essential little boost only when it swings past a given position in its arc. If its starting swing is not wide enough to pass this point it gets no push and, therefore, its lost energy will not be returned. Absent the restoration of frictional losses, the pendulum's swing grows ever more feeble. Rather than reach the attractor, it will end up hanging, absolutely still, at the 0 position/0 velocity locus in the state space. In fact, that point is itself a "point attractor" for all position-velocity combinations that do not take the pendulum past the boost-point in its swing. The gray shading marks the starting region from which the trajectory is attracted not to sustained oscillation but to hanging at rest.

The state space of Figure 15–12 is thus composed of two different regions that, so to speak, dictate different outcomes for the dynamics of the system. There is a zone (shaded gray) within which starting points lead to a "point attractor" (the rest position). There is also a zone that occupies all the rest of the plane, and within which all starting points lead ultimately to the oscillatory attractor. Each zone is the *basin of attraction* for its attractor.

Voice specialists have used the concept of a basin of attraction, even if unknowingly, for quite some time. The voice range profile (VRP, Figure 15–13) is considered an important evaluative tool. What it depicts is the region in a vocal intensity—vocal frequency "state space" in which (essentially) periodic oscillation of the vocal folds (that is, voice) is possible.[††] Outside the VRP's polygon, vocal fold motion (if there is any) is not periodic, and, hence, is not phonatory. The VRP polygon can, therefore, be considered to be the boundary of a "phonatory oscillation basin of attraction."

In the case of the pendulum the boundaries of the basins of attraction are neat and well defined. But this is not always—or even commonly—the case in more complex systems. In fact, it is not really the case for the VRP, because if the patient's voice were to be tested at every frequency (instead of at decibel intervals) of the phonatory frequency range, minor variations in maximal and minimal vocal intensity would make the boundary line much more jagged.

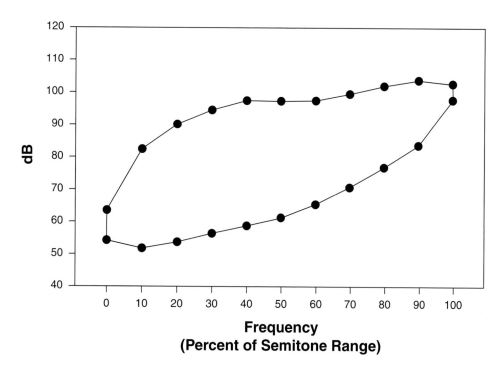

Fig 15–13. A typical voice range profile.

[††]Purists would not be happy with this statement. For one thing, vocal intensity and vocal F_0 are not parameters that govern vocal fold oscillation—they are measures of some aspects of the results of oscillation—and, in fact, are not even independent. For another thing, the VRP boundary includes at least two different kinds of phonatory oscillation (modal and falsetto register, for instance), and each is likely to have its own attractor. Nonetheless, the analogy is a useful one—both from the point of view of theory and from the perspective of clinical interpretation.

The structure of a basin of attraction can be very complex indeed, and its boundary can be exceedingly irregular. Those possibilities will be crucial to our consideration of voice irregularities and will be visited again later.

Vocal Irregularities: The Chaotic Point of View

We are now ready to look at some different kinds of vocal irregularity from a nonlinear dynamics point of view.

Intermittent Aperiodicity: The Case of the Missing Vibration

The voice of the dysphonic patient is often characterized by significant increases of frequency and amplitude perturbation, and very brief failures of vocal fold oscillation are not uncommon. A traditional view of vocal fold physiology would likely hold that instability of muscular tension and/or subglottal air pressure is responsible for the increases in jitter and shimmer, while the transient failures are probably the product of "twitches"—brief alterations of muscle tension.

However, nonlinear dynamics theory offers a different possibility. Figure 15–14 shows the output (glottal flow pulses and state-space representation) when the two-mass model is set for conditions of low vocal fold tension and moderate subglottal pressure. The flow record shows what, at first glance, seems to be completely erratic glottal pulses. Yet, there are short regions of subharmonic oscillation ("diplophonia") and, interestingly enough, two instances (arrows) where phonatory oscillation is momentarily seriously impaired. It is clearly not possible for these aberrations to be the result of instabilities of muscular tension or driving pressure, much less muscle twitches, because the model includes no such phenomena.

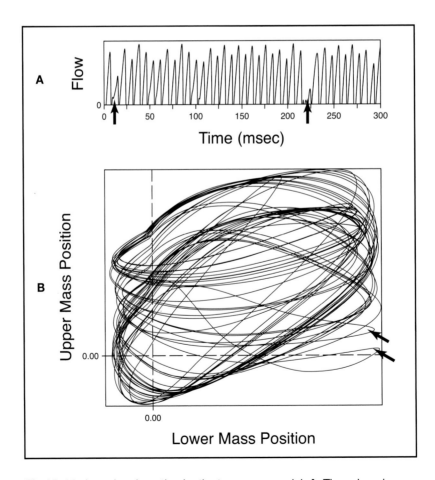

Fig 15–14. Irregular phonation by the two-mass model. **A.** Time-domain representation of airflow. **B.** State-space representation.

The representation of the dynamics in the upper-mass/lower-mass state space shows a very complex attractor[‡‡] that roves over a large area of the plane that it occupies. The situation is similar to that of Figure 15–11, only greatly exaggerated. The complexity of the attractor forces each glottal cycle to be somewhat different from its neighbors and results in the bursts of pattern that are seen. Occasionally the attractor visits relatively extreme positions (arrows). Simultaneous observation of the development of the attractor and the glottal pulse record makes it clear that glottal pulses are "missed" at these instants. What nonlinear dynamics theory says is that vocal irregularities might not have their origins in physiologic instability.

Start-up Problems

Sometimes it is difficult to get the voice going. There may be a transient aphonia (a "frog in the throat," as the saying has it) or a bizarre "glitch" of vocal frequency—bane of the adolescent male. The fault is usually laid to mucus, or to a difficulty of tensional adjustment, or perhaps to poorly controlled vocal fold adduction. However, once again, nonlinear dynamics theory offers another and simpler possibility.

Figure 15–15 shows the glottal pulsing and associated dynamics for a different choice of parameters for the two-mass model. The records of transglottal flow show that oscillation is initially quite unstable but then converts to a more regular pattern. The state-space plots indicate that, for most of the time period shown, the vocal folds are "flopping" erratically, but, ultimately, their behavior is captured by the attractor, and stable phonation ensues. It is worth pointing out once again that no outside influence—such as a change of vocal fold tension, or an alteration of the subglottal pressure—has occurred to stabilize phonatory function. The model's parameters have not changed. Both types of behavior—irregular dysphonic vibration and stable phonatory oscillation—have been produced by the very same physiologic conditions. It has simply taken a while for the dynamics of the situation to find the attractor.

Swirling Around the Basin

It is not unusual for a dysphonic patient to have periods of relatively good voice interrupted by moderate-ly long episodes of altered phonation or aphonia. While these might be the result of changes in the status of the vocal tract, they might also reflect switching of the dynamics of the vocal system from one attractor to another.

To see why this might happen, we return to the concept of the basin of attraction. It was noted earlier that, unlike the smooth basin boundaries of Figures 15–12 and 15–13, the basin boundaries of chaotic attractors are exceedingly irregular. In fact, they are fractal. This means, let us recall, that they exhibit self-similarity at all scales, so that every time a region is magnified more detail appears.

The relevance of this to the problem of sudden shifts of vocal fold oscillation can be explored with Figure 15–16, which shows part of a (computed) basin of attraction and its boundary. Although the data of Figure 15–16 actually have no relationship to voice production,[†††] it will be useful to pretend that the figure shows a vocal-fold tension/subglottal pressure state space. The white region is part of the basin of attraction for the attractor for stable vocal fold vibration; call it the "phonation basin." Tension/pressure combinations in the black zone are outside the phonation basin and will result in erratic (dysphonic or aphonic) behavior of the vocal folds. Call this the "dysphonia zone."

Even when viewed at low magnification (Figure 15–16A), the boundary of the phonation basin looks extremely irregular. Enlarging just the little bit of it in the rectangle shows more detail (Fig 15–16B), and demonstrates that the phonation basin is "invaded" by fine projections of the dysphonia zone that were not observable at the lower magnification. Enlarging a rectangular zone of Fig 15–16B shows even deeper extensions into the phonation basin. If one were to continue the process of enlargement one would discover (because the boundary is fractal) that there are ever-finer incursions of the dysphonia zone into the phonation basin. In fact, continuing the magnification to infinity would reveal that there are extensions that are *infinitesimally* wide.

The numerous and ever-finer projections of the dysphonia region show that the phonation basin (the part of state space in which the dynamics of the system is drawn to a regular-phonation attractor) is, in actuality, infested with dysphonia regions—some of them only infinitesimally large. Those regions, although

---

[‡‡]Running the model for a long time with these parameters produces a trajectory (which, for the sake of clarity, is not reproduced here) that strongly suggests that this is, in fact, an attractor. Note that this level of complexity is not uncommon among strange attractors.

[†††]Those with some prior experience in nonlinear dynamics theory or fractal geometry might recognize that part of the boundary of Mandelbrot set has been pressed into service for this illustration.

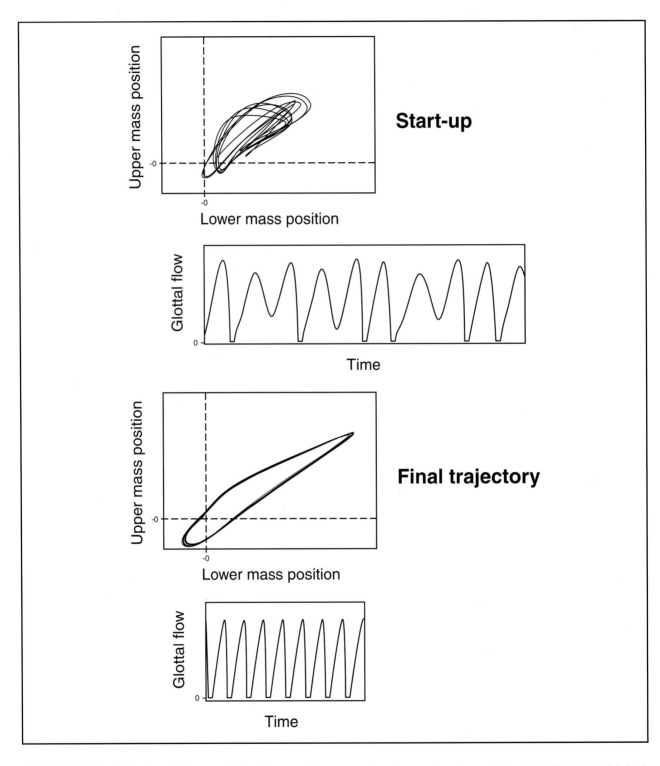

Fig 15–15. When first started, the vocal folds of the model may "flop" irregularly (state-space and time-domain representation at top). Ultimately, however, the system may be captured by an attractor, and regular oscillation established (lower state-space and time-domain plots).

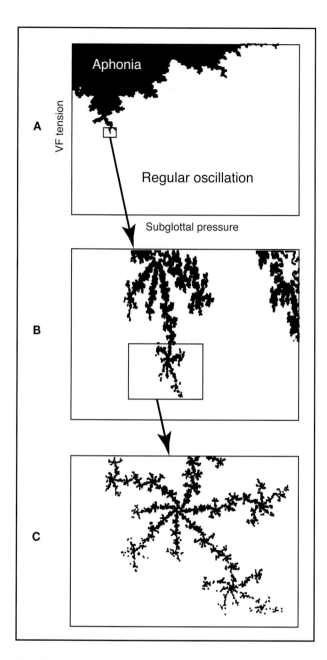

Fig 15–16. A basin of attraction may be deeply penetrated by ever-finer fingers of a different basin. Therefore, what appears to be inside one basin may actually be part of another.

therefore also riddled with tiny regions that will lead to a stable attractor. The contamination of each zone with areas that "belong to" the other grows more severe as one approaches the boundary—which, in the common understanding of the word, is not so much a separation as a fuzzy region.

During oscillation, the subglottal pressure and vocal fold tension are constantly varying. Put another way, the location of the system in the pressure/tension state space is constantly changing. If the state of the system finds itself in one of those regions that belongs to the dysphonia zone it may be attracted away from the stable phonatory attractor, causing regular phonation to end. Similarly, during aphonic behavior, the trajectory may encounter a small region that may cause it to be drawn back to the phonatory attractor, re-establishing regular oscillation. It might seem that this is just a fancy way of saying that shifts of vocal function are caused by alterations of phonatory parameters. However, because the "misplaced" regions (phonation basin in the dysphonia zone; dysphonia zone embedded in phonation basin) may be infinitesimally small, it may require only an unmeasurably tiny alteration of control parameters to drive the dynamics into one of them. An "unmeasurably tiny" variation is, in practice, *no* variation. From the point of view of nonlinear dynamics theory, it is perfectly reasonable that phonation might undergo major qualitative changes in the absence of any observable cause.

The Misbehavior of Intact Systems

Basic concepts of nonlinear dynamics, then, offer alternative explanations for at least some of the aberrant behavior of the vocal system that commonly plague the dysphonic patient. Transient vocal "glitches," problems of voice initiation, and the intrusion of erratic or unusually patterned vibration can all easily be accommodated within the construct of chaos theory. A significant advantage accrues from this point of view: It becomes unnecessary to invoke the causative intervention of antecedent momentary events which have often been at best difficult, and quite commonly impossible, to detect in living patients.

It would be foolish in the extreme to propose that nonlinear dynamics theory is the appropriate explanatory model for all vocal dysfunctions.[###] It could even be argued that it is not optimal for most disorders. However, it is ideally suited to the hitherto-inexplicable and odd phenomena that are frequent conun-

surrounded by the phonation basin, are actually *outside* it. From these minuscule or infinitesimal areas the dynamics is not drawn to the phonation attractor. In exactly the same way, the phonation basin has projections that extend into the dysphonia zone, which is

---

[###]The belief that aspects of the theory not considered here may offer a much better framework for the description of vocal function does not seem too far a stretch.

drums of routine clinical practice. Nonlinear dynamics theory suggests that some dysphonias—and perhaps many—may be the product of an intact *phonatory system*. The possibility is clear that at least some voice problems—and perhaps many—betray not structural or physiologic, but rather *dynamical* disorders.[66-68]

The future may be much more chaotic.

References

1. van den Berg Jw. Subglottic pressures and vibrations of the vocal folds. *Folia Phoniatr.* 1957;9:65–71.
2. van den Berg Jw. Myoelastic-aerodynamic theory of voice production. *J Speech Hear Res.* 1958;1:227–244.
3. van den Berg Jw, Zantema JT, Doornenbal P Jr. On the air resistance and the Bernoulli effect of the human larynx. *J Acoust Soc Am.* 1957;29:626–631.
4. Titze IR. The human vocal cords: a mathematical model. Part I. *Phonetica.* 1973;28:129–170.
5. Titze IR. The human vocal cords: a mathematical model. Part II. *Phonetica.* 1974;29:1–21.
6. Buder EH, Cannito MP, Dressler D, Woodson GE, Murry T. Phonatory analysis of spasmodic dysphonia: modulations, subharmonics, and Botox response. Presented at: Annual Meeting of the American Speech-Language-Hearing Association; 1999; San Antonio, Tex.
7. Baer T. Vocal jitter: a neuromuscular explanation. In: Lawrence V, Weinberg B, eds. *Transcripts of the Eighth Symposium: Care of the Professional Voice.* New York, NY: Voice Foundation; 1980:19–24.
8. Larson CR, Kempster GB, Kistler MK. Changes in voice fundamental frequency following discharge of single motor units in cricothyroid muscles. *J Speech Hear Res.* 1987;30:552–558.
9. Titze IR. A model for neurologic sources of aperiodicity in vocal fold vibration. *J Speech Hear Res.* 1991;34:460–472.
10. Kaiser JF. Some observations on vocal tract operation from a fluid flow point of view. In: Titze IR, Scherer RC, eds. *Vocal Fold Physiology: Biomechanics, Acoustics, and Phonatory Control.* Denver, Colo: Denver Center for the Performing Arts; 1983:359–386.
11. Teager HM, Teager SM. Active fluid dynamic voice production models, or: There is a unicorn in the garden. In: Titze IR, Scherer RC, eds. *Vocal Fold Physiology: Biomechanics, Acoustics, and Phonatory Control.* Denver, Colo: Denver Center for the Performing Arts; 1983:386–401.
12. Liljencrants J. Numerical simulations of glottal flow. In: Gauffin J, Hammarberg B, eds. *Vocal Fold Physiology: Acoustic, Perceptual, and Physiological Aspects of Voice Mechanisms.* San Diego, Calif: Singular Publishing; 1991:98–112.
13. Shadle CH, Barney AM, Thomas DW. An investigation into the acoustics and aerodynamics of the larynx. In: Gauffin J, Hammarberg B, eds. *Vocal Fold Physiology: Acoustic, Perceptual, and Physiological Aspects of Voice Mechanisms.* San Diego, Calif: Singular Publishing; 1991:73–82.
14. Lind J, ed. *Newborn Infant Cry.* Uppsala, Sweden: Almqvist and Wiksells; 1965.
15. Wasz-Höckert O, Lind J, Vuorenkoski V, Partanen T, Valanne E. *The Infant Cry: A Spectrographic and Auditory Analysis.* London, England: Heinemann; 1968.
16. Glass L. Nonlinear dynamics of physiological function and control. *Chaos.* 1991;1:247–250.
17. Goldberger AL, Rigney DR, West BJ. Chaos and fractals in human physiology. *Sci Am.* 1990;262(2):43–49.
18. Pool R. Is it healthy to be chaotic? *Science.* 1989;243:604–607.
19. Teich MC, Lowen SB, Turcott RG. On possible peripheral origins of the fractal auditory neural spike train. In: Lim DJ, ed. *Abstracts of the Fourteenth Midwinter Meeting: Association for Research in Otolaryngology;* 1991:50.
20. Beuter A, Labrie C, Vasilakos K. Transient dynamics in motor control of patients with Parkinson's disease. *Chaos.* 1991;1:279–286.
21. Goldberger AL. Cardiac chaos. *Science.* 1989;243:1419.
22. Sheldon R, Riff K. Changes in heart rate variability during fainting. *Chaos.* 1991;1:257–264.
23. Kaplan DT, Talajic M. Dynamics of heart rate. *Chaos.* 1991;1:251–256.
24. Coumel P, Maison-Blanche P. Complex dynamics of cardiac arhythmias. *Chaos.* 1991;1:335–342.
25. Skinner JE, Goldberger AL, Mayer-Kress G. Chaos in the heart: implications for clinical cardiology. *Biotechnology.* 1990;8:1018–1024.
26. Kryger MH, Millar T. Cheyne-Stokes respiration: stability of interacting systems in heart failure. *Chaos.* 1991;1:265–269.
27. Rapp PE, Bashore TR, Martinerie JM, Albano AM, Zimmerman ID, Mees AI. *Brain Topogr.* 1989;2:99–118.
28. Kroenenberg F. Menopausal hot flashes: randomness or rhythmicity? *Chaos.* 1991;1:271–278.
29. Pickover CA, Khorsani A. Fractal characterization of speech waveform graphs. *Comput Graphics.* 1986;10:51–61.
30. Awrejcewicz J. Bifurcation portrait of the human vocal cord oscillations. *J Sound Vibration.* 1990;136:151–156.
31. Baken RJ. Irregularity of vocal period and amplitude: a first approach to the fractal analysis of voice. *J Voice.* 1990;4:185–197.
32. Mende W, Herzel H, Wermke K. Bifurcations and chaos in newborn cries. *Physics Lett A.* 1990;145:418–424.
33. Herzel H, Steinecke I, Mende W, Wermke K. Chaos and bifurcations in voiced speech. In: Mosekilde E. ed. *Complexity, Chaos, and Biological Evolution.* New York, NY: Plenum Press; 1991.
34. Titze IR, Baken RJ, Herzel H. Evidence of chaos in vocal fold vibration. In: Titze IR, ed. *Vocal Fold Physiology: Frontiers in Basic Science.* San Diego, Calif: Singular Publishing; 1993:143–188.
35. Baken RJ. The aged voice: a new hypothesis. *Voice* (Journal of the British Voice Association). 1994;3:57–73.
36. Kakita Y, Okamoto H. Visualizing the characteristics of vocal fluctuation from the viewpoint of chaos: An attempt toward qualitative quantification. In: Fujimura O, Hirano M, eds. *Vocal Fold Physiology: Voice Quality Control.* San Diego, Calif: Singular Publishing; 1994:235–348.

37. Steinecke I, Herzel H. Bifurcations in an asymmetric vocal-fold model. *J Acoust Soc Am*. 1995;97:1874–1884.

38. Herzel H, Berry D, Titze IR, Steinecke I. Nonlinear dynamics of the voice: signal analysis and biomechanical modeling. *Chaos*. 1995;5:30–34.

39. Berry DA, Herzel H, Titze IR, Story BH. Bifurcations in excised larynx experiments. *J Voice*. 1996:10;129–138.

40. Fletcher, NH. Nonlinearity, complexity, and control in vocal systems: In: Davis PJ, Fletcher NH, eds. *Vocal Fold Physiology: Controlling Complexity and Chaos*. San Diego, Calif: Singular Publishing; 1996:3–16.

41. Herzel H. Possible mechanisms of vocal instabilities. In: Davis PJ, Fletcher NH, eds. *Vocal Fold Physiology: Controlling Complexity and Chaos*. San Diego, Calif: Singular Publishing; 1996:63–75.

42. Kumar A, Mullick SK. Nonlinear dynamical analysis of speech. *J Acoust Soc Am*. 1996;100:615–629.

43. Behrman A, Baken RJ. Correlation dimension of electroglottographic data from healthy and pathologic subjects. *J Acoust Soc Am*. 1997;102:2371–2379.

44. Ouaknine M, Giovanni A, Guelfucci B, Teston B, Triglia JM. Nonlinear behavior of vocal fold vibration in an experimental model of asymmetric larynx: role of coupling between the two folds. *Revue de Laryngologie, Otologie, et Rhinologie*. 1998;119:249–252.

45. Behrman A. Global and local dimensions of vocal dynamics. *J Acoust Soc Am*. 1999;106:432–443.

46. Gleick J. *Chaos: Marking a New Science*. New York, NY: Viking Penguin; 1987.

47. Crutchfield JP, Farmer JD, Packard NH, Shaw RS. Chaos. *Sci Am*. December 1986;255:46–57.

48. Abraham RH, Shaw CD. *Dynamics—The Geometry of Behavior. Part One: Periodic Behavior*. The Visual Mathematics Library: VisMath Vol 1. Santa Cruz, Calif: Aerial Press; 1982.

49. Abraham RH, Shaw, CD. *Dynamics—The Geometry of Behavior. Part Two: Chaotic Behavior*. The Visual Mathematics Library: VisMath Vol 2. Santa Cruz, Calif: Aerial Press; 1983.

50. Abraham RH, Shaw CD. *Dynamics—The Geometry of Behavior. Part Three: Global Behavior*. The Visual Mathematics Library: VisMath Vol 3. Santa Cruz, Calif: Aerial Press; 1985.

51. Abraham RH, Shaw CD. *Dynamics—The Geometry of Behavior. Part Four: Bifurcation Behavior*. The Visual Mathematics Library: VisMath Vol 4. Santa Cruz, Calif: Aerial Press; 1982.

52. Rasband SN. *Chaotic Dynamics of Nonlinear Systems*. New York, NY: Wiley; 1990.

53. Baker GL, Golub JP. *Chaotic Dynamics: An Introduction*. New York, NY: Cambridge University Press; 1990.

54. Moon FC. *Chaotic Vibrations: An Introduction for Applied Scientists and Engineers*. New York, NY: Wiley; 1987.

55. Thompson JMT, Stewart HB. *Nonlinear Dynamics and Chaos: Geometrical Methods for Engineers and Scientists*. New York, NY: Wiley; 1986.

56. Eubank S, Farmer D. *An Introduction to Chaos and Randomness*. Boston, Mass: Addison-Wesley; 1990.

57. Cvitanovic P, ed. *Universality in Chaos*. 2nd ed. New York, NY: Adam Hilger (IOP Publishing, Ltd.); 1984.

58. Glass L, Mackey MC. *From Clocks to Chaos*. Princeton, NJ: Princeton University Press; 1988.

59. West BJ. *Fractal Physiology and Chaos in Medicine*. Singapore: World Scientific; 1990.

60. Isshiki N. Regulatory mechanism of voice intensity variation. *J Speech Hear Res*. 1964;7:17–29.

61. Ishizaka K, Flanagan JL. Synthesis of voiced sounds from a two-mass model of the vocal cords. *Bell Sys Tech J*. 1972;51:1233–1268.

62. Mandelbrot BB. *The Fractal Geometry of Nature*. New York, NY: Freeman; 1977.

63. Peitgen H-O, Saupe D, eds. *The Science of Fractal Images*. New York, NY: Springer-Verlag; 1988.

64. Wong D, Ito M, Cox NB, Titze IR. Observation of perturbations in a lumped-element model of the vocal folds with application to some pathological cases. *J Acoust Soc Am*. 1991;89:383–394.

65. Lucero JC. Dynamics of the two-mass model of the vocal folds: Equilibria, bifurcations, and oscillation region. *J Acoust Soc Am*. 1993;94:3104–3111.

66. Mackey MC, Glass L. Oscillations and chaos in physiological control systems. *Science*. 1977;197:287–289.

67. Goldberger AL, West BJ. Chaos in physiology: Health or disease. In: Holton A, Olsen LF, eds. *Chaos in Biological Systems*. New York, NY: Plenum Press; 1987:1–5.

68. Mackey MC, Milton JC. Dynamical diseases. *Ann NY Acad Sci*. 1987;504:16–32.

16

Voice and Forensics

Harry F. Hollien

Although many practitioners in clinical areas carry out research that is both timely and sophisticated, much of the knowledge basic to their speciality is provided by individuals who are primarily scholars and/or scientists. Thus, otologists and audiologists are supported (in part, anyway) by psychoacousticians and auditory physiologists. So too are speech pathologists and laryngologists consumers of much of the material produced by phoneticians (specialists, who are often referred to, in this part of the world anyway, as voice and/or speech scientists). As you might expect, the latter group (the phonetic scientists) interfaces with yet other groups of professionals (ie, engineers, linguists, psychiatrists, specialists in diving, etc); they do so for a variety of practical and scientific reasons. In turn, they learn from these other specialists—about problems, about behaviors, about methods—just as they do from the clinical speech and hearing professionals. This cross-fertilization can be both rich and valuable.

The focus of this chapter is about one of these relationships, one where phonetic scientists have been challenged by the needs and problems of several groups of interrelated practitioners and have been able to respond by drawing on their talents, training, and experience. The area(s) to which I am referring are the forensic sciences. The practitioners in question are primarily law enforcement and/or intelligence personnel, attorneys, and jurists. Phoneticians interface with these professionals in much the same manner as they have with laryngologists, speech/voice pathologists, and voice teachers. In fact, the relationship between phonetics and forensics has grown so much over the past 20 to 30 years that there is now a subspecialty within the phonetic sciences called forensic phonetics. Recently, I described this area in a book, *The Acoustics of Crime*, [1] as well as in a number of articles

and chapters.[2-5] Moreover, this specialty now has its own society; it is called the International Association of Forensic Phonetics (IAFP). We publish a journal in collaboration with forensic linguists (they started their society before we did); it is called *Forensic Linguistics: The International Journal of Speech, Language and the Law* and it is published by the University of Birmingham (Edgbaston, Birmingham B15, 2TT, UK). The current IAFP officers also can be contacted at that address.

But what is forensic phonetics and what does it do for those specialties cited above? First, it serves them in traditional ways by providing information and testing relationships; it also provides support just as it does for the clinical areas of speech and voice. In any event, forensic phonetics can be defined as a professional specialty based on the utilization of current knowledge about the communicative processes—including the development of specialized techniques and procedures—for the purpose of meeting certain of the needs of legal groups and law enforcement agencies. Although many of these developments and approaches also can be used to assist military, industrial, and security organizations, the forensic phonetics interface is primarily with the criminal justice and judicial systems. As such, it constitutes one of the practical applications of the phonetic sciences; and, as stated, it also has led to the development of specialized techniques, equipment, and approaches in support of their needs.

Forensic phonetics consists of two general areas. One involves the electroacoustical analysis of speech and voice signals that have been transmitted and stored; the other involves the analysis (both physical and perceptual) of communicative behaviors. The first area is focused on problems such as the proper transmission and storage of spoken exchanges, the authentication of tape recordings, the enhancement of speech on tape recordings, speech decoding, legal transcripts, and similar problems. The second major area involves issues such as the identification of speakers, the process of obtaining information relative to the physical and/or psychological states of a talker (stress, psychosis, intoxication, are examples), and the analysis of speech for evidence of deception or authorship. This chapter will not cover all of these areas—much less still others that are associated with this specialty but on a secondary basis (for listings, see Hollien[1]). Rather, the focus here will be on just three of the content areas: (1) the accurate processing and decoding of speech/voice (for forensic purposes, of course), (2) the identification of speakers from voice, and (3) the detection of (certain) behavioral states by analysis of speech/voice.

Although the reasons for such activities should become obvious after the cited areas are reviewed, it might be useful to briefly describe some of the extant problems. First, it should be noted that a surprisingly large percentage of all human (oral) discourse occurs in situations other than those that are "face-to-face" in nature. For example, in Western Europe, and especially in North America, a significant proportion of the total number of spoken messages will occur over telephone links, radio, television, or the Internet. Moreover, much of this speech—plus a percentage of the face-to-face exchanges—is tape-recorded or electronically stored by some other technique. To illustrate, a large number of organizations systematically record all or most of their incoming telephone calls (plus many of those outgoing); and this practice is being adopted by many other groups (ie, by security agencies, industry, schools, hospitals, and so on). Of yet greater importance: (1) the extent (and sophistication) of electronic surveillance is expanding, (2) many legal and law enforcement interviews are captured by multiple recording systems, and (3) most (acoustic) activities in courtrooms are being recorded. Note also that many of the procedures already developed by forensic phoneticians can be utilized to enhance these activities and also to aid in the solution of crimes (already committed); prevent crimes that are being planned; ensure the accuracy of legal records; assist decision makers during trials; and so on. It would now appear timely to consider the selected issues, and their current solutions, in some detail.

Problems with Speech Fidelity

Without a doubt, intelligible, accurate speech (whether "live" or stored) is important to many groups; included in this long list are law enforcement agencies, other units within the criminal justice system, and the courts. For example, the effectiveness of many detectives would be sharply reduced if suddenly they could no longer utilize tape recordings for surveillance, during interrogation, and/or for record keeping. Indeed, it is possible that analysis of signals stored on tape recordings ranks among the more powerful of the tools that investigators currently have at their disposal. On the other hand, any degradation of the intelligibility and/or quality of these signals (by distortion, noise, interference, etc) can create problems (sometimes severe) with the aforementioned surveillance, interrogations, investigations, and so on. With specialized knowledge about the problems, plus effective processing procedures, the amount of information captured and utilized can be substantial.

Sources of Difficulty

The tape recordings generated for legal and law enforcement purposes are rarely high fidelity; indeed, they often (very often it seems) are of rather limited quality. The two main sources of this difficulty are distortion and noise. Both result primarily from use of inadequate equipment, poor recording techniques, or events occurring in the acoustic environment within which the tape recordings were made[1,6-8] The degradation of speech intelligibility by and within equipment can result from: (1) reduction of signal bandwidth, (2) harmonic distortion, (3) system noise, and (4) intermittent masking/reduction/elimination of the target sounds. The equipment employed in the field is rarely laboratory quality but rather consists of body bugs, telephones, line taps, suction cup pickups, and so on. Although most of the transducers and systems employed provide for the adequate transfer of speech (the frequency band necessary for good speech intelligibility rarely exceeds 200–4000 Hz), degradation will develop rapidly if these conditions are combined. For example, when noise is added to target speech recorded with inexpensive or very small tape recorders, the end result is speech that is not intelligible enough for easy decoding or, perhaps, any decoding at all. Poorly maintained, or inappropriately used, equipment often can lead to problems of this type. Finally, although very slow recording speeds permit a great deal of information to be captured on small reels of tape, intelligibility will be degraded; because too much material is crowded into very small areas of magnetic space; even small distortions, when added, can result in sharply debased messages.

Noise, even by itself, can be a culprit also; and it takes many forms.[1,8] One such source is "forensic noise" (ie, competing speech, music, and so on). However, the more common types of noise can be: (1) broadband or narrow band, (2) that with a natural frequency or frequencies (60 Hz hum for example), or (3) steady-state or intermittent. It can result from friction sources (ie, the wind, clothing movement, fans/blowers), radio transmission, vehicle operation, explosions, and so on. Some of the effects of noise can be mitigated by the elimination of the part of its spectrum that exists outside of the functional speech range (ie, below 350 Hz and above 3500 Hz). So too can noises, which have "natural frequencies," be countered as often their "narrow frequency band" effect can be eliminated or reduced even if it is located within the speech range. Intermittent or impact noise—street noise, gunshots, video games, bells, horns, explosions, doors closing, and so on—can obscure speech but usually only on an intermittent basis. Because these impact noises (as well as their sources) are extremely variable, it is virtually impossible to list them all.

Finally, although it is not practical to describe all of the potential problems that can reduce speech intelligibility, suffice to say they are legion. But, even so, can speech be enhanced for listening and/or decoded for forensic purposes? In many cases, it can.

Remedies

First, it should be acknowledged that a number of scientists and engineers have been developing fairly sophisticated machine techniques designed to reconstruct degraded speech. They employ approaches such as bandwidth compression, cross-channel correlation, mean least squares analysis, all-pole models, group delay functions, linear adaptive filtering, linear predictive coefficients, cepstrum techniques, deconvolution, and so on.[9-14] However, many of these techniques, at this time, do not appear to be functionally easy to apply in the forensic milieu; most are complex, time consuming, and costly. In any case, they will not be reviewed to any great extent in this chapter; rather the procedures to be described will include some of the more practical and easily applied approaches currently in use.[1,6-8,15]

A General Procedure

Reasonably good techniques are available to upgrade tape recordings for decoding purposes. The initial step is to protect the "original" tape recording by making a good quality copy. This approach will reduce deterioration due to tape breakage, accidental erasure, stretching, and twisting or friction wear to the recording oxide. Imagine the problems that would be encountered if important evidence in a criminal case was thus compromised.

Second, the examiner will listen to the tape recording one or more times before attempting to process it.

This procedure permits development of a good working knowledge of its contents as well as of the types of interference and degradation that exist. By this process, strategies can be designed to counter the problems found.

It often will be necessary to apply frequency biasing and filtering techniques. They may be understood by observation of the hardware systems found in Figure 16–1. It will be noted that, even if digital in nature, the filtering often will be conducted in stages rather than in a single pass. Moreover, the phased approach will avoid the need to cascade a large number of filters into a single equipment array; because when filters are used in series, signal reduction can be severe; and they must be isolated from each other to avoid interaction effects.

Another issue, just how acoustic energy patterns affect human hearing (and ultimately that of the decoders) also is important. It has long been known that energy at lower frequencies will tend to mask that at higher frequencies, whereas energy at higher frequencies will not affect lower ones but rather will act as a distraction. Thus, frequencies occurring below the speech band will mask it to the greatest extent. Fortunately, this low-frequency noise often can be removed (to some extent) by good filtering techniques. Finally, even though its presence can be quite annoying, noise above 3000 Hz will not tend to mask speech very much; however, the irritation it creates can be reduced either by analog or digital filtering.

Filtering Techniques

A brief consideration of how filtering is accomplished might prove useful (see again Fig 16–1). As is well known, analog filtering is the easiest to use. In its simplest form, it can be referred to as biasing or equalization; and such circuits often are found on tape recorders, amplifiers, or home audio systems. However, comb and notch filters are more powerful. For example, if spectral analysis shows that a noise source is producing a relatively narrow band of high energy at or around a specific frequency, a notch filter centering on that frequency may be employed to reduce its debilitating effect. Notch filters with a center frequency around 60 Hz are particularly helpful in reducing the speech-masking effects of AC "hum." Comb filters consist of a series of separately controllable notch filters arrayed in a systematic sequence from low frequencies to high. They can be used to continuously modify the spectrum of a signal by selectively attenuating undesirable frequency bands. For example, they can be operated simultaneously as a bandpass filter (350–3500 Hz) and one or more notch filters; or it can

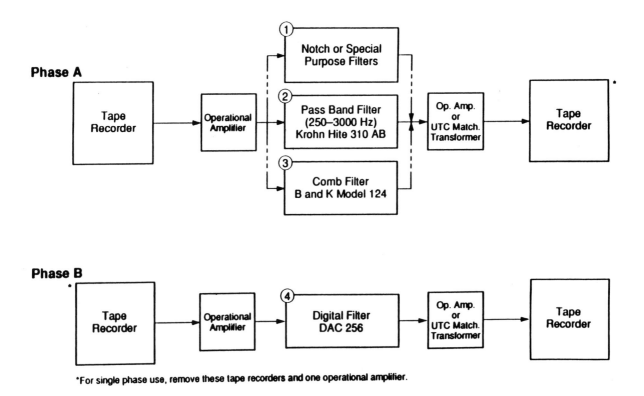

Fig 16–1. This block diagram demonstrates how analog and/or digital filtering can be accomplished. The three analog filters (1-3) can be used singly or cascaded; however, they would not be employed in parallel (as shown). A typical configuration would be to place a comb filter and a digital filter (both isolated) in a series.

be cascaded with other units to increase the filtering effects of the total system.

An important class of filters is digital in nature. Basically, these filters digitize the signal a set number of times each second (say, 20 K). They then determine the energy bands throughout the spectrum and remove the unwanted frequencies. Of course, this process is somewhat more complicated than just described. One example should suffice. A common unit provides two modes of automatic operation. It employs a 256th order filter that rapidly designs its own characteristics to remove unwanted noise by adaptive predictive deconvolution. It works best for linear noise (many noise signals are predictable) but can process nonlinear signals by "short-time correlation." The second (more powerful) mode feeds the noise to one of the unit's channels as a reference and the same noise plus the target speech to the other. The process then becomes one of adaptive noise cancellation. Incidentally, all of the digital filtering techniques can be carried out either by appropriate hardware or by computer software. In practice, digital filtering can be very helpful, especially when analog filters fail to remove enough of the unwanted interference. On the other hand, digital approaches can create problems also (ie, the resulting signal can be distorted or add what sounds like an echo). It must be remembered, also, that filtering techniques may not work all that well if the noise exists *within* the speech frequency band. In such cases, other techniques plus skilled human decoders must be applied.

Variable-Speed Tape Recorders

Variable-speed tape recorders sometimes can be useful in upgrading speech intelligibility; the process can be accomplished by means of hardware or computer software. Approaches of this type exist in two classes: (1) where only a simple (often manual) increase or decrease in recorder speed is possible and (2) where expansion and compression circuits have been added so that the tape speed can be altered with minimal disruption of the speech spectra. The first procedure is especially useful when the speed of the original tape recorder has been varied for some reason. In the second instance, the perceived pitch of the talker's voice is altered but his or her articulatory characteristics change but little. Manipulations of both of these systems can be especially effective when they are combined with filtering.

In Summary

Many techniques can be used to enhance the speech stored on tape recordings. The preceding paragraphs sketched out only a few. Suffice it to say that they must be applied robustly if messages are to be decoded and transcribed. The second stage is the actual decoding.

Speech Decoding and Transcripts

The subsequent phase in the extraction of utterances and messages from distorted tapes involves speech decoding. Although these procedures are well established, some of the situations wherein problems are encountered will be discussed briefly. As stated earlier, difficulties often result from: (1) tape recordings being made under less than optimal conditions, (2) recordings that are the product of electronic surveillance, (3) dialogue or utterances that were recorded under less than ideal conditions, and (4) material inadvertently added to a tape recording that was being made for other purposes. Although the relevant speech in these cases *may* be comprehendible, such is not always the case (even after enhancement). In those instances, formal decoding will have to be applied with trained personnel attempting to accurately reproduce the recorded speech in written form.[16,17] It must be added that the decoders will face not only the channel or system distortions described above but also speaker-related problems. Difficulties of this type can result from a number of intended and inadvertent behaviors by the talker or talkers. They include: (a) disguise (almost always intentional), (b) dialects and foreign languages, (c) variation in speech rate (often unintended), (d) effects of stress or fear, (e) effects of alcohol/drugs/health states, and (f) additional speakers, and/or interruptions by other speakers. Although the existence of these conditions may not be a problem, any of them can increase degradation of speech intelligibility and make decoding more difficult. As with system distortions, these factors should be identified early and dealt with individually. For example, the use of specialized decoders for foreign language dialects sometimes is warranted. Note also that efficient and accurate decoding requires that the cited professionals be exposed to formal training primarily in phonetics and linguistics.

Noise and Masking

It must be assumed, of course, that the masking effects of noise already have been mitigated insofar as is possible; the residue, thus, may or may not create problems for the decoder. For one thing, the effects of noise may not always be as debilitating as might be expected; and speech often can be understood even in the presence of rather intense nonspeech signals. This phenomenon is due largely to the internal redundancy of language and the structure of an utterance. Thus, if the competing noise (especially if broadband) is *only* twice as intense as the speech, the spoken message often will remain intelligible or nearly so. Even more surprising, the intensity of the interference signal sometimes can reach a level as much as four times greater than that of the speech (depending on the type of noise, of course) before it completely destroys intelligibility. Thus, the problem often is that noise is more of a distraction than a block to comprehension; and it may not prevent efficient decoding especially if the transcriber is well trained.

An issue closely related to noise and masking involves human capabilities for sensory processing of an auditory nature. Of these, three factors are of particular importance; they are (1) foreground-background processing, (2) binaural listening, and (3) auditory illusions (especially those related to speech). Foreground-background processing is best illustrated by the picture where a white vase can be observed in the middle of a figure (foreground) and that silhouettes of two (identical) people facing each other can be seen at the sides. In audition, the parallel process involves a person's ability to attend selectively to particular elements within a heard stimulus (the so-called "cocktail party" effect). In the case of speech in noise, the human auditor often can focus on the speech and relegate the noise to the background—at least to some extent. As would be expected, much of this processing occurs at the cortical level; it is aided by binaural listening and directional hearing. It also is one of the reasons humans tend to make better speech decoders than do machines.

Binaural listening simply means that the auditor hears the signal simultaneously in both ears (it does not have to be stereophonic also). All that is necessary to appreciate this procedure is to alternately listen to some speech first through a single earphone and then through two. It often is surprising how much recorded conversations will be enhanced when a switch is made to good quality binaural earphones.

Speech decoders also are aided by auditory "illusions." Indeed, no special training is necessary here as most people have learned naturally to process distorted or partly heard speech. Although much of the relevant processing of this type takes place at the cortical level, the nonlinearities in the hearing modality also contribute. One thing that happens is that listeners intuitively learn to fill in those parts of speech that are distorted or missing; they do so by attending to coarticulation and the characteristics of the linguistic environment in which utterances are heard. For example, a vowel and its transitions alone often can provide enough information to permit a decoder to correctly "hear" missing consonants (and, hence, the entire word); certain speech sounds within a word can be obliterated (or replaced by noise) and still be understood; and a talker's fundamental frequency is perceived even though it has not been passed to the listener because of limited frequency response (of a telephone, say). Actually, there is no mystery about these auditory illusions[18] as their nature is lawful; they depend partly on the neurophysiological structure of the listener's ear, partly on training, and partly on his or her experience. In any case, they serve to aid an individual involved in a difficult speech decoding task.

Linguistic Elements

Basic knowledge about the segmentals (vowels, consonants) and other speech elements is a fundamental part of the decoder's repertoire. Indeed, comprehension of phoneme place and manner will provide the decoder with many useful insights. And, to be effective, decoders also must be familiar with both word structure and the characteristics of word boundaries.[19,20] As you know, linguistic rules exist for word structure (just as they do for sentence structure); and these rules provide important information about what a word might be (or should be) when it cannot be heard clearly. Moreover, knowledge about word boundaries is important; it bears especially on spectrography when utilized to provide a visual picture of an utterance. A solid understanding of word and phoneme boundaries/characteristics is especially important when the decoding task is particularly challenging.

Second, analysis of the linguistic stress patterns exhibited by a speaker also can be helpful in the preparation of accurate transcripts. The many nonlinguistic gestures a person uses to enhance the meaning of a message are well known.[21,22] Speakers employ suprasegmentals (or paralinguistic elements) to create emphasis; included are variation in speaking fundamental frequency, phoneme/syllable/word duration, vocal intensity, and so on. Familiarity with these features and how they affect speech can provide important clues when transferring heard discourse into written form. Finally, knowledge about the nature and characteristics of dialects,[23-25] either foreign or regional, also can be important. For example, recognition of a specific dialect can provide an assist when it is necessary to correctly link each of the speakers heard on a tape to the messages they produce.

Coarticulation refers to the production of oral speech; it describes how each speech sound uttered affects those near it. Specifically, it can be said that, when an individual moves from one speech sound to another, the position of the articulators for the first sound, modifies the placement precision of the articulators for the second sound. So too does the position the articulators take for the second phoneme affect the first; and these modifications extend out to several phonemes—and in both directions. However, the greater the distance between the speech sounds, the smaller the effect. As would be expected, these differences in articulatory movements also change the acoustic characteristics of a phoneme. Thus, the vowel /u/ is slightly different acoustically if it is preceded by a /d/ than if it is led by an /m/. In turn, the /m/ is modified if succeeded by an /i/ rather than the /u/. In any event, these relationships can be exploited to enhance decoding efficiency.

The Mechanics of Decoding

To understand how the speech found on degraded tape recordings is decoded and turned into a written transcript, it also is necessary to understand something about the mechanics of the decoding process itself. First of all, if the method utilized by the decoder does not involve thorough and structured techniques—or if he or she is not properly trained—the product probably will be inadequate or worse. In short, it is important to employ a thorough and systematic approach to decoding if the transcript is to be reasonably accurate and essentially unchallengeable.

Because the techniques associated with good decoding are rather extensive, only a very brief review will be provided. First, the decoder will listen to the entire tape recording on good quality equipment. This approach involves more than simple familiarization; it also permits a log to be initiated, difficult material to be identified, proper names to be learned, and any idiosyncratic characteristic of the recording noted. This listening process then is repeated as the decoders begin transcript development. As you might expect, the decoder simply starts at the beginning and reproduces the heard utterances in sequence. Codes are used to indicate (1) where questions exist, (2) where decoding may be possible but is questionable, and (3) when words are inaudible or unintelligible. It is necessary to continue (and replicate) this process until no further improvement in the written transcript can be made.

The most common approach to the decoding task is simply to have a trained, experienced individual carry it out. However, a somewhat more efficient approach is to have one decoder develop the transcript and then have a second review and refine it. Perhaps the best approach of all is to have two different decoders complete the task independently and then have yet a third verify the work and/or resolve any disagreements. Although this (third) approach is a little cumbersome and expensive, it is sometimes necessary when the challenge presented is severe and an accurate transcript is critical. An example involves recordings associated with aircraft disasters (CVR or cockpit tapes). Instances that are less critical but still of some importance are when the speech captured involves "street talk," foreign languages, or dialects; if the material is highly technical; or if it contains language not familiar to ordinary decoders.

Once the listening procedure is complete and a reasonable transcript has been developed, it is necessary to apply the cited codes in order to identify the talkers, problem portions of the transcript, and other events. Also, the decoder should identify each talker by number (or by name, if possible) and by sex. Specialized systems of this type have been developed[17]; their use is mandatory if the transcript is to clearly describe all of the events contained on the tape recording. Finally, as has been implied, proper names are often quite difficult to decode. That is, although speech and language are internally redundant—and markedly affected by text and coarticulation, there is little-to-no external information inherently associated with a proper name. However, information external to the material on the tape recording may provide an assist here.

Once the decoding process has been completed and the confusions resolved, the entire document should be structured in final form and carefully evaluated for errors. The potency of the written word, as applied to the criminal justice system, is not to be underestimated. Juries, for example, can be powerfully influenced by a transcript. Thus, the messages and information found on a tape recording must be established as accurately and fairly as possible.

Finally, it must be noted that the efficient decoding of distorted or masked speech involves not only the tasks described above. It also demands a good understanding of the law enforcement milieu and the criminal justice system.

Speaker Identification

Almost every adult who enjoys normal hearing has had the experience of recognizing some unseen speaker (usually, but not always, someone familiar to them) solely from listening to his or her voice. It probably was from this common, everyday experience that the concept of speaker identification was born. However, references to it in novels, comic strips, movies, and especially television have resulted in distortion of its basic nature. Indeed, many people believe that: (1) law enforcement can identify a talker from his voice and do so both easily and infallibly, (2) "voiceprints" are the direct equivalent of fingerprints, and so on. But what is the reality here? Well, it now should be clear that, although many of the cited opinions are gross exaggerations, there is *some* basis for them. A short review follows.

Definitions

Speaker identification is one of two different types of speaker recognition, the other being speaker verification. Specifically, it is defined as the task of identifying an unknown speaker from samples of his or her voice. This process can be a rather difficult one, primarily because it often must be accomplished in the face of system distortions (reduced bandpass, noise, distortion, etc) and/or speaker distortions (stress, disguise, impairments, etc). Worse yet, the talker usually is uncooperative—especially if there is a crime involved. In other instances, a match is not possible at all, either because the unknown talker is not among the suspects or the tape recordings of the unknown voice are simply too poor to be of any use.

Speaker verification, on the other hand, involves subjects who want to be recognized. Here, high quality equipment and sophisticated processing techniques can be used; and many reference samples of the talker's speech are available or can be obtained. Speaker verification is employed to permit a person access to secure areas, to bank by telephone, to communicate with (verifiable) personnel in space capsules or other remote locations, and so on. As is obvious, speaker verification poses a much less formidable challenge than does speaker identification. As a matter of fact, the verification problem would be solved if valid speaker identification were to become possible.

Problems

The first problem is a basic one. Anyone who attempts to develop speaker identification will discover that it is not yet known if the speech/voice of each individual is so unique that it will always be different from that of any other person. Nor, has it been unassailably established that *intersubject* speaker variability will always be greater than *intrasubject* variability. Fortunately, these problems are not controlling, because there already are ways to accomplish reasonably good identification, especially within the boundaries offered by the forensic environment.

As you probably noted from the introduction, the operational problems faced can be sorted into two categories: (1) system distortions and (2) difficulties with speakers. System distortion occurs as a result of occurrences such as reduced frequency response (eg, telephone transmissions), noise, distortions, interruptions, and so on. In these cases, some of the information about the talker can be lost or is masked; and, just as in speech decoding, such reductions increase the difficulty of achieving correct identification.

Second, difficulties with speakers also can be debilitating. As would be expected, many criminals experience fear, anxiety, or some sort of stresslike emotions when they commit a crime. The usual consequence is a change in one or more of their speaking characteristics. The effects of ingested drugs, alcohol, or health states (such as a bad cold) also can interfere with the identification process. Worst of all, the unknown talker may attempt voice disguise.

On the other hand, there are conditions or events which suggest that identification/differentiation among voices is possible. For one thing, it has been postulated[1,26-31] that a given individual's speech signal contains features that are sufficiently unique and consistent to that person that, at least, some successful identifications can be carried out. Indeed, both available data and logic permit the assumption that certain elements within a talker's speech tend to be relatively idiosyncratic as a result of that person's anatomy, physiology, and motor control plus the habituated speech patterns they employ. Further, social, economic, geographic, and educational factors as well as maturation level, psychological/physical states, sex, and intelligence also tend to affect speech in relevant ways. Obviously, when these factors are combined, they can create a fairly unique cluster of features. In turn, it has been established that, if a number of these features are measured, it will be possible (in many instances anyway) to successfully discriminate among talkers on the basis of the resulting composite analysis or (structured) profile. Thus, although there may be no single attribute within a person's speech that is of sufficient strength and uniqueness to permit differentiation, the use of a group of features can permit successful recognition.

Some History

Primitive efforts in the area of voice recognition probably antedate recorded history, and such attempts have been continued down through the millennia.

There was a relevant trial in an English court several hundred years ago, and speaker identification admissibility in the United States may be traced as far back as 1904 (Mack vs Florida[32]). Even so, the issue is a complex one for, as it turns out, it matters who is testifying and in what court. For example, some courts will permit witnesses to "identify" a speaker (from voice judgments) only if they can satisfy the presiding jurist that they really know that person. This approach is a reasonable one; as it is consistent with relevant research. That is, if a witness has been in close contact with a speaker for a long period of time, he or she probably can recognize the speaker's voice—and be fairly accurate in doing so. Moreover, many courts also permit a qualified specialist to render an opinion after comparing a sample of the unknown talker's speech (usually from an evidence tape) to an appropriate exemplar recording. Here, the professional conducts an examination and then decides if two talkers are involved or only one. But, before either of these approaches is described, yet a third type of aural-perceptual speaker identification should be considered; it involves *earwitness* lineups or "voice parades."

Earwitness Identification

An earwitness lineup (or a voice parade) usually involves a person who has heard, but has not seen, another individual who is otherwise not known to him. Later (usually, very much later), he or she is asked to remember what that person sounded like and attempt to identify a suspect as the individual involved in the original confrontation. Ordinarily, this type of lineup is conducted by law enforcement agents. What happens is that an administrator inserts an exemplar (provided by the suspect) into a group of 3 to 6 recorded speech samples obtained from other people. The witness is then required to listen to all of the samples and make a choice among them as to which one was the perpetrator. However, this approach has come under some fire in the past,[1,33,34] because it exhibits several problems. For example, sometimes the suspect's exemplar is compared to speech uttered by individuals who speak in quite a different manner than he does; in other instances, ambient cues exist on the tape. Either of these occurrences can result in false positives. Second, some administrators attempt to base their procedures on those drawn from eyewitness identification, a procedure that parallels earwitness lineups in some ways but is quite different in others. Problems with witness memory/emotions and/or with conditions existing at the time of the confrontation are numerous and can add to the complexity of the process. Extensive reviews of these and related issues are available.[33,35-37]

Moreover, research in this area is continuing and additional information is being generated[35,38-41]; so too are guidelines as to how valid auditory lineups may be structured.[7,36] Finally, the operational criteria to follow have been developed to mitigate the cited difficulties; a fairly detailed description of them is found in Hollien.[27]

An appropriate structuring of earwitness lineups may be best understood by consideration of the following outline:

Definition: An earwitness lineup is a procedure where a witness who has heard, but not seen, a suspect attempts to pick his or her voice from a field of voices.

Parity: The procedure must be conducted in a manner that is scrupulously fair to both the earwitness(es) and the suspect(s). Accurate records must be kept of all phases of the procedure.

Validity: The witness must demonstrate that he or she has adequate hearing and that he or she attended to the speaker's voice at a level that would permit identification. Witnesses should be told that the suspect may or may not be present in the lineup and that only one suspect will be evaluated at a time.

Procedure: All samples should be recorded with as good acoustic fidelity as is possible; they should be presented in an identical manner. The same or similar speech should be used, samples should be of equal length, ambient background should be parallel for all samples, and so on. Utterances should be of neutral material. Between five and eight foils or distractor speakers should be used. Each of them should be similar to the suspect with respect to age and dialect plus social, economic, and educational status. The suspect's voice can be described to the foil talkers, but they must not have heard it. Once a tape recorded "lineup" has been developed, a series of 2 to 3 mock trials should be carried out with 4 to 6 dispassionate individuals as listeners. If they consistently identify the suspect as the target (even though they have never heard his voice), the lineup tape must be restructured.

Presentation: The witness(es) should then listen to the tape and be asked to identify (or not identify) one of the samples as the person they originally heard. However, they should be reassured that it is not *necessary* to make a selection. Two appropriate approaches are available for presentation purposes.

The first is referred to as the "serial" approach. Here, the suspect's speech sample is embedded among several other samples (produced by the foil or distractor talkers). The samples are played in sequence and the witness makes a judgment. The entire tape may be replayed as structured or with the order of the individual samples rearranged. This procedure may be applied either to assist the witness in making a decision or to establish the reliability of the witness' judgments.

The second of the two procedures has been named the "sequential" approach; it is best understood by consideration of Figure 16–2. In this case, two small rooms are used with the first containing the witness (A), the administrator (D), and a video camera (E); the second is the site of a TV monitor (F) and observers (G). Each of the samples is recorded on its own tape (C), and these tapes are provided to the witness one at a time (in any order). Once all of them have been played, the witness may request—and play—any or all of them, and in any order desired.

Reasonably good judgments are possible using either procedure, but the second appears to be the most powerful.

The Aural-Perceptual Approach

This section will focus on the aural-perceptual approach to speaker identification; it also will feature the forensic phonetician rather than the lay listener who either attempts to identify familiar speakers or participates in an earwitness lineup. Also briefly reviewed are what is, or is not, considered possible; the strengths and weaknesses of several approaches and how the forensic phonetician can develop appropriate skills. But, first, what research can be used in support of the aural-perceptual approach to speaker identification?

The first of the modern studies[42] in this area is a classic. In this case, a psychologist (McGehee) became interested in the subject from her observations of Charles Lindbergh's voice identification of Bruno Hauptmann (the man who was convicted of kidnaping the Lindbergh baby). Her procedures paralleled what Lindbergh did; that is, she had her auditors listen to an individual and then attempt to identify him within a group of other talkers of the same sex and do so at various latencies (1 day to 5 months). McGehee reported that the percentage of correct identifications was quite high initially but that falloff in accuracy was gradual but steady—from 83% correct identification the day after exposure to only 13% after about 5 months. To a great extent, contemporary research substantiates McGehee's general findings; that is, it appears that untrained individuals can make fairly good aur-

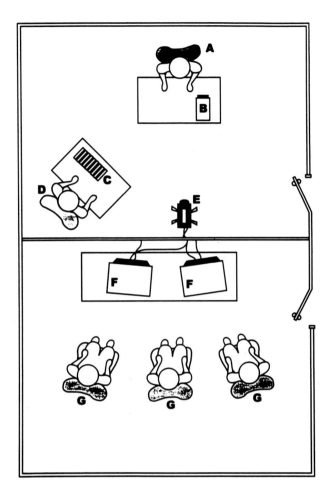

Fig 16–2. A graphic display of the "sequential" approach to earwitness identification. A is the witness, B = a tape recorder, C = the tape recordings, D is the administrator, E = the videocam, F = the TV monitors, and G shows observers.

relationships apparently interfere even with identification of even known speakers.[1,27,44-46] It also has been reported that speaker disguise, presence of dialects, subjects who sound alike, and high noise levels can operate to reduce identification accuracy[1,26,27,30,47-54]—as can (possibly anyway) the presence of stress and other emotions.

On the other hand, it has been demonstrated that there are many elements within the speech signal, which serve to permit accurate identifications. Indeed, people use processing of this type to make the many day-to-day identifications they do, and the accuracy of the techniques they use has been confirmed by research. What they do is attend to those features or events that consistently occur within any utterance. The processing of these natural speech characteristics (most of them are suprasegmentals) also forms the basis of most of the formal aural-perceptual (and some machine) approaches used to identify speakers. What are some of these features? One is speaking fundamental frequency level or SFF[1,27,55-58]; perceptually this attribute is heard as pitch level and variability. A second includes vowel formant frequencies, ratios, and transitions.[27,58-60] Third, attempts have been made[55,58] to compare the relative importance of the source (voice) and vocal tract (articulators) for these purposes; it was found that both of them contribute—and do so additively. In addition, phonemic effects on the identification task have been investigated. It has been reported that, although the level of correct perceptual identification varies as a function of the vowel produced, consonant-vowel transitions, vocal tract turbulence, and inflections, these elements, nonetheless, can be used to identify speakers.[30,59,61] Finally, voice quality, speech prosody/timing, and other features all appear to interrelate with the identification process. In short, quite a number of natural speech features can be used to support the aural-perceptual speaker identification process. They are particularly effective when used in groups (ie, in the development of profiles).

The summation that follows is based on—and complements—the relationships cited above, especially those that are positively associated with the perceptual identification task. First, speakers known to the listener are the easiest to identify by voice; and accuracy here can be quite high. Second, if the listener's familiarity with a talker's speech is reinforced occasionally, levels of correct identification can be sustained. Third, larger and better speech samples lead to more accurate aural-perceptual identifications. Fourth, good quality samples aid in the identification process. Fifth, although listeners can be variable in their ability to make accurate judgments, some are naturally quite good at it. Sixth, listeners appear to be successful in using a num-

al-perceptual identifications initially but this level cannot be sustained.

Although the answers to all potential questions are not available even today, a number of key studies have been carried out; hence some models can be constructed. Early examples include Bricker and Pruzansky[43] who reported high levels of correct identification when they used *sentences* as stimuli. Thus, it appears that, although identification accuracy is possible, it is correlated with sample size and duration. It also has been established that the identification task can be degraded by such things as increasing the number of speakers to be identified, substituting whispered for normal speech, recording the sample under degraded speaking conditions, varying speech materials, and so on. When these conditions exist, a listener's performance tends to deteriorate somewhat. Either that or they need very long speech samples. Moreover, these ber of the natural features that are found within speech/voice. And finally, phonetic training appears to aid in successful identifications, especially if the practioner is a trained/experienced forensic phonetician.

As was suggested in the preceding paragraph and especially by item six above, a number of natural speech features can be employed for identification purposes. They are formalized as follows.

Speaking Fundamental Frequency or Heard Pitch. The parameters here are general pitch level (high, medium, low) as well as the variability and patterning of pitch usage. Many individuals exhibit habituated pitch patterns that can aid the listener in the identification task.

Articulation. The focus in this instance is (especially) on idiosyncratic phoneme production. The controlling word here is idiosyncratic; because, to be useful in identification, an individual's phoneme production must be, in some manner, a little different from that of other speakers.

General Voice Quality. There is little doubt that the general quality of a sound-producing mechanism aids in its identification. Many aspects of voice quality are useful here (eg, the use of vocal fry is an example).

Prosody. This parameter set involves how an individual's speech timing, or temporal patterning, affects the ability to identify him or her from voice. It is well known that auditors listen to how slow, or fast, a person talks; how smooth or choppy the presentation is; and so on. Thus, speech timing and melody provide cues about identity.

Vocal Intensity. Although limited data are available on vocal intensity, its usage is thought to be a viable recognition feature. However, in practice, it is difficult to assess absolute intensity; because even small environmental changes can result in marked variations in energy level. Nevertheless, it is theorized that evaluation of variability patterns can be useful.

General Speech. Several general speech features also are important. Although the main focus here is on segmentals; they also include attributes such as (1) dialect, (2) unusual use of linguistic stress, (3) idiosyncratic language patterns, (4) speech impediments, and (5) idiosyncratic pronunciations. These features extend beyond the simple articulatory or prosody considerations discussed above and can provide robust cues for the recognition of speakers.

All of the above vectors will be used as the basis of a structural approach to aural-perceptual speaker identification; it will be described later in this chapter.

Applied Research

A substantial corpus of applied research is available; it also is relevant to this discussion. Most of it is based on the fact that people who identify each other by voice do so only after carrying out auditory and cognitive processing of the heard signal. Questions can be asked then if people exist who can organize and effectively use these processes (it appears that forensic phoneticians can do so) and what are some of the elements in the forensic milieu that can affect it.

One study carried in response to these questions was conducted by Shirt[62] who studied the ability of general phoneticians (not specialists) to make identification judgments. She developed a test based on 74 recorded voices provided her by the British Home Office; she then asked 20 phoneticians and an equal number of untrained controls to carry out three fairly difficult identification tasks. She found that, although the best control did as well as the phoneticians, the phoneticians (overall) were fairly accurate and did a rather better job than the untrained subjects. Moreover, neither of the groups was permitted to utilize any kind of structured analysis procedure; and the phoneticians were not trained in the forensic sciences.

Koester[63] also reported that his (general) phoneticians did very much better than his untrained controls in several experiments where they attempted to identify people they knew; again unstructured procedures were used. Not one of Koester's phoneticians made even a single error in the entire experiment. These studies, plus field evidence, suggest that phoneticians can meet the identification challenge rather effectively even when not allowed more than a brief exposure to a voice. It also appears that they can do even better if they are familiar with forensics, trained to task, and operate in a structured manner.

Many of the issues reviewed above have been challenged (especially in the legal setting). Accordingly, we carried out a series of studies to test several of the criticisms. In the first,[48] we attempted to estimate listeners' ability to resist the effects of talker disguise and stress and assess the importance of listeners being acquainted with the talkers. Speakers were 10 adult males who had recorded speech samples under normal conditions as well as those of stress (electric shock) and free disguise. The three classes of listeners were individuals who knew the talkers very well, did not know them but were trained to recognize their voices, and neither knew the talkers nor understood

English (they also received training, however). The identification task itself was a very difficult one. As may be seen in Figure 16–3, listeners who knew the talkers performed best and the non-English-speaking auditors did the worst. Moreover, it was found that the normal and stress conditions were not very different from each other; whereas the disguised productions resulted in significantly fewer correct identifications. Thus, although it appears possible that listeners who know speakers can identify them even under very difficult conditions, it is sometimes possible to

fool them (ie, by means of disguise). We also found it was possible to train lay listeners (at least some of them) to recognize talkers at a reasonable level of accuracy.

In another experiment, we studied the effects of stress and/or arousal on speaker identification.[64] The question asked here was: Will the victims of a crime perform better than people who are not stressed by such events? In this instance, young women were prescreened for potential sensitivity to stressors and sorted into two groups: the 20 most susceptible to stress and the 20 least likely to be threatened (controls). The "stress" group was presented 10 minutes of violent video stimuli (attacks on women, rape scenes, death of children) while a male voice read a threatening commentary; the controls saw a pastoral video sequence while hearing a male voice read neutral to supportive material. Their arousal (or lack of it) during the experiment was verified by a standard polygraph technique. Later, speaker recognition (of the male voice) was carried out. The aroused women did better at identifying the talker than did the controls. Thus, it appears that fear/stress/arousal can upgrade a person's ability to correctly identify speakers from their voices.

In a third investigation, we studied speaker identification primarily by contrasting earwitness and eyewitness identification.[65] Specifically, visual and aural-perceptual identifications were made of a simulated crime from sets of photographic and tape-recorded exemplars. Auditors were law school students divided into groups who attempted identifications at various times after a simulated crime took place. The results demonstrated that visual identifications can be quite accurate, less so for speaker identification. Among the other findings were those that supported the position that earwitness testimony should be viewed by judges and juries with some caution. On the other hand, current research[35] demonstrates that witnesses often can apply specific sensory processes to make reasonably good judgments.

The Use of Specialists

Let us return to consideration of the forensic phonetician. Although it has been suggested that even untrained individuals can sometimes carry out speaker identification (if they have natural talent and conditions are favorable), many others cannot do so at any reasonable level of effectiveness. Thus, it would appear hazardous to rely on such individuals. Rather, it would appear that identification tasks should be directed to specialists (ie, people who have extensive and relevant training and experience in their area). Indeed,

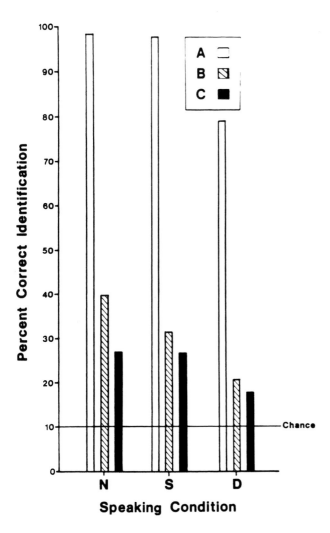

Fig 16–3. The mean (correct) identification of 10 talkers speaking under the conditions of: N = normal, S = stress, and D = disguise. Three listener groups consisted of: A = individuals who knew the talkers very well, B = listeners who did not know the talkers but who were trained to recognize them, and C = those who were trained similarly but did not know either English nor the talkers. The task was to name each speaker for all six of his presentations out of a total of 60.

forensic phoneticians have demonstrated the ability to conduct effective speaker identification even when their judgments are based only on heard stimuli. They can do so if adequate speech samples are available and they employ structured analysis techniques. However, to be considered competent, the specialist also should be able to specify his or her identification rates, demonstrate extensive graduate training in the phonetic sciences (especially in forensic phonetics), have some experience, and provide defensible identification procedures and strategies. What are some of the approaches employed by these particular professionals?

Many phoneticians attempt to determine if the suspect is or is not the perpetrator by aural-perceptually contrasting their speech segmentals (ie, the speech sounds they make, how they use phonemes to construct spoken words, dialects, etc). Such approaches are successful in many instances, especially if the practitioner establishes robust evaluation criteria and can demonstrate the attributes listed in the preceding paragraph. On the other hand, this approach is quite subjective; and its elements tend to be difficult to quantify. A superior approach is to place these techniques in a role that supports more sophisticated methods — such as one based on the suprasegmentals (ie, the natural speech features described both above and, yet again, below. A procedure of this type follows.

An Approach

Of course, the manner in which any identification approach is conducted (ie, just how the speech samples are judged for a match or a nonmatch and how the responses are quantified) is of greatest importance. Accordingly, a suggested procedure (see also Hollien and Hollien[66]) follows. As you might expect, its focus is on the suprasegmentals (ie, the assessment of voice, prosody, frequency patterns, vocal intensity, voice quality, and others); and they, in turn, are supplemented by segmental analysis. The approach permits reasonable quantification and rigor to be achieved, because its application is based on a structured evaluation system. Approaches of this type have been shown to be reasonably successful; the especially useful ones permit confidence level estimates to be generated.

The first step in the process is to obtain multiple speech samples of the unknown (evidence tape) and known (exemplar) speakers and place them in pairs on an evaluation tape. The pairs are played repeatedly, and comparisons are made of one speech parameter at a time. As may be seen from consideration of Figure 16–4, up to 20 parameters may be compared. To reiterate, one parameter at a time is assessed (eg, pitch

patterns); and the process is continued until a judgment can be made. The next parameter is then assessed, and the process replicated until all possible (parameter) comparisons have been completed. At that time, an overall judgment is made. Subsequently, the entire process is independently repeated a number of times.

As can be seen from consideration of Figure 16–4, judgments are made on a 10-point scale; and the likelihood that the two samples are produced by the same speaker can be assessed on the basis of the individual parameter judgments and, especially, by the overall mean. If the collected scores fall between 0 and 3, a match cannot be made; and it may be said that the samples undoubtedly were produced by two different people (see Fig 16–5). If the overall mean scores fall between 7 and 10, a reasonably robust match has been made (Fig 16–6). Scores between 4 and 6 are generally considered neutral but actually are a little on the positive side. For example, if the mean score for 14 sets of evaluations (carried out 3 times overall for a total of 42 assessments) proves to be 5.8 (or 58%), a low-level match has been made; it is one that is not particularly compelling but, nevertheless, is on the positive side. Moreover, it would hardly permit the argument to be made that the samples were produced by two different people. Incidentally, if foil talkers are used, the confidence level can be raised substantially, especially if the mean scores are polarized (ie, 0–3 or 7–10).

In summary, data are now available about people's ability to make aural-perceptual speaker identifications and much of it is positive. For example, it has been demonstrated that (1) most auditors use strategies involving natural speech features for this purpose, (2) specialized training will aid in task success, and (3) some people are better at it than are others. It also is known that elements such as noise, distortion, very short speech samples, and large groups of talkers can degrade the effectiveness of the process. In any case, even though aural-perceptual approaches to speaker identification have some limitations, fairly good results can be expected if the task is highly structured and if the auditors are well-trained professionals who are able to demonstrate reasonably good competency.

The "Voiceprint" Problem

The procedure referred to as "voiceprints" has been pretty much discredited; hence, description of this so-called "method" of speaker identification will not be included in this chapter. If the reader is interested in learning the history of this approach, the controversies surrounding it, and its demise, he or she can consult

```
FORENSIC COMMUNICATION ASSOCIATES
Case Name:                                              FCA REF:


            Aural-perceptual Approach to Speaker Identification
            Score Sheet  -- 0 = U-K least alike; 10 = U-K most alike

                                                            SCORE  RANGE
1. PITCH
      a. Level              0 . . . . 5 . . . . 10

      b. Variability        0 . . . . 5 . . . . 10

      c. Patterns           0 . . . . 5 . . . . 10

2. VOICE QUALITY
      a. General            0 . . . . 5 . . . . 10

      b. Vocal Fry          0 . . . . 5 . . . . 10

      c. Other              0 . . . . 5 . . . . 10

3. INTENSITY
      a. Variability        0 . . . . 5 . . . . 10

4. DIALECT
      a. Regional           0 . . . . 5 . . . . 10

      b. Foreign            0 . . . . 5 . . . . 10

      c. Idiolect           0 . . . . 5 . . . . 10

5. ARTICULATION
      a. Vowels             0 . . . . 5 . . . . 10

      b. Consonants         0 . . . . 5 . . . . 10

      c. Misarticulations   0 . . . . 5 . . . . 10

      d. Nasality           0 . . . . 5 . . . . 10

      e. Other              0 . . . . 5 . . . . 10

6. PROSODY
      a. Rate               0 . . . . 5 . . . . 10

      b. Speech Bursts      0 . . . . 5 . . . . 10

      c. Other              0 . . . . 5 . . . . 10

7. OTHER
      a. Nonfluencies       0 . . . . 5 . . . . 10

      b. Speech Disorders   0 . . . . 5 . . . . 10
         MEAN                                       ___  _____
```

Fig 16–4. A copy of the form developed for use with the suprasegmental speaker identification approach being described.[45,51]

the relevant chapter in either of the author's books on forensic phonetics.[1,27] Large bibliographies of original sources are listed there also.

Machine/Computer Approaches

The speaker recognition issue changes radically when efforts are made to apply modern technology to the problem. Indeed, with the seeming limitless power of electronic hardware and computers, it would seem that solutions should be but a step away. Yet such is not actually the case. For one thing, authors such as Hecker[26] insist that no machines are both as sensitive and as powerful (for these purposes) as is the human ear. What Hecker means by "the ear" is, of course, the entire auditory (sensory) system coupled to the brain with all its sophisticated memory and cognitive functions. On the other side of the issue are

```
                    FORENSIC COMMUNICATION ASSOCIATES
    Case Name: State vs. Jane Doe                          FCA REF: 1491

              Aural-perceptual Approach to Speaker Identification
              Score Sheet  -- 0 = U-K least alike; 10 = U-K most alike

                                                              SCORE  RANGE
    1. PITCH
         a. Level         0  X=====X    .   5  .  .  .  . 10    2    1-3

         b. Variability   0  .  .  X  .  5  .  .  .  . 10       3     3

         c. Patterns      0  .  X==X  .  5  .  .  .  . 10       2    2-3

    2. VOICE QUALITY
         a. General       0  .  .  X======X  .  .  .  . 10      4    3-5

         b. Vocal Fry     0  .  .  .  .  5  X  .  .  . 10       6     6

         c. Other         0  .  .  .  .  5  .  .  .  . 10      NA    NA

    3. INTENSITY
         a. Variability   0  .  X==X  .  5  .  .  .  . 10       3    2-3

    4. DIALECT
         a. Regional      0  X==X  .  .  5  .  .  .  . 10       1    1-2*
        *IMPORTANT
         b. Foreign       0  .  .  .  .  5  .  .  .  . 10      NA    NA

         c. Idiolect      0  .  .  .  .  5  .  .  .  . 10      NA    NA

    5. ARTICULATION
         a. Vowels        0  .  .  .  .  X==X  .  .  . 10       5    5-6

         b. Consonants    0  .  X======X  5  .  .  .  . 10      3    2-4

         c. Misarticulations  0  X  .  .  .  5  .  .  .  . 10   1     1*
        U shows a /d/ for /th/ substitution
         d. Nasality      0  .  .  .  .  X==X  .  .  . 10       6    5-6

         e. Other         0  .  .  .  .  5  .  .  .  . 10      NA    NA

    6. PROSODY
         a. Rate          0  .  .  .  .  X 5  .  .  .  . 10     4     4

         b. Speech Bursts 0  .  .  X==X  .  5  .  .  .  . 10    3    3-4

         c. Staccato (K only)  0  X=====X  .  5  .  .  .  . 10  2    1-3

    7. OTHER
         a. Nonfluencies  0  .  .  .  .  5  .  .  .  . 10      NA    NA

         b. Speech Disorders
            MEAN          0  .  .  .  .  5  .  .  .  . 10      NA    NA

        *Double Weight    Mean of three runs; no foils.      29%   25-35%
```

Fig 16–5. Display of the evaluation of a woman who, as it turns out, was not the criminal.

scientists who argue that, due to burgeoning technology, machines/computers can be made to operate just as efficiently. They probably can, but the task is not an easy one.

First some perspectives. As you might expect, the best way to develop a machine-based speaker identification method is to establish some type of system and test it. For example, a group of vectors or relationships might be chosen and then researched on the basis of the model found in Figure 16–7. As may be seen, the first step is to formulate a vector; the second is to test its ability to discriminate a particular talker from among a fairly large group of talkers. If successful, the work could then proceed; if not, changes would have to be made to the vector's parameters (or parts) and the initial evaluation process replicated. The next stage would be to experiment with the vector where distortions, such as limited bandpass, noise, and/or

FORENSIC COMMUNICATION ASSOCIATES

Case Name: State vs. John Doe   FCA REF: 1475

Aural-perceptual Approach to Speaker Identification

Score Sheet -- 0 = U-K least alike; 10 = U-K most alike

	SCORE	RANGE
1. PITCH		
a. Level 0 . . . . . 5 . X=====X 10	8	7-9
b. Variability 0 . . . . 5 X==X . . 10	7	6-7
c. Patterns 0 . . . . 5 . X==X . 10	7	7-8
2. VOICE QUALITY		
a. General 0 . . . . 5 . X=====X 10	8	7-9
b. Vocal Fry 0 . . X=====X 10	4	3-5
Slightly more fry by U		
c. Other 0 . . . . 5 10	NA	NA
3. INTENSITY		
a. Variability 0 . . . . . 5 X======X 10	7	6-9
4. DIALECT		
a. Regional 0 . . . . 5 . X=====X 10	8	7-9
b. Foreign 0 . . . . 5 10	NA	NA
c. Idiolect 0 . . . . 5 . . X==X 10	9	8-9
Both "Lilt"		
5. ARTICULATION		
a. Vowels 0 . . . . . 5 X=====X . 10	7	6-8
b. Consonants 0 . . . . . 5 X=====X . 10	7	6-8
c. Misarticulations 0 . . . . 5 . . . X 10	9	9
BOTH		
d. Nasality 0 . . . X=======X . . 10	6	4-7
e. Other 0 . . . . 5 10	NA	NA
6. PROSODY		
a. Rate 0 . . . . 5 . X=====X 10	8	7-9
RELATIVELY FAST		
b. Speech Bursts 0 . . . . 5 X==X . . 10	6	6-7
c. CHOPPY 0 . . . . 5 . . X . 10	8	8
7. OTHER		
a. Nonfluencies 0 . . . . 5 . . . X 10	9	9
Show similar articulation problems		
b. Speech Disorders 0 . . . . 5 10	NA	NA
MEAN Neither of two foils matched U or K.	74%	66-81%

Fig 16–6. Assessment of a male suspect who was the perpetrator in question.

talker variation, are present. A fourth phase would be to attempt to increase the power of the system by combining the vectors with each other. The research now would become much more complex, because it would be necessary to compare all potential combinations of vectors and then repeat the procedures for the various types of distortions. And, this process would have to be replicated each time the system was upgraded.

The final phase would be to test the procedure in the field. In this instance, either one of two approaches could be utilized. The first involves the solution of simulated crimes generated under fieldlike conditions and the second application of the system to real-life cases. Either approach should provide useful information about the validity and efficiency of the method, but both have their limitations. For example, even well-designed (simulated) cases are a little artificial and only roughly parallel real-life situations. On the other hand, the use of actual investigations permits only nonscientific confirmation of the results (ie, confessions, convictions, etc); and observations such as these cannot really be substituted for scientific data.

Summary of Approach to the Problem

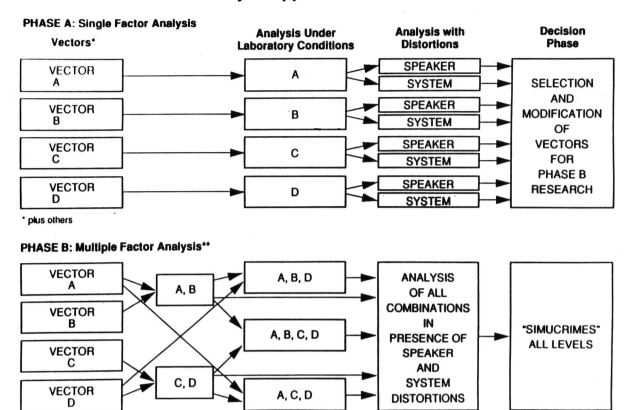

Fig 16–7. Model providing the basis for comprehensive development of a semiautomatic speaker identification system (SAUSI).

Nevertheless, the data obtained can be used to demonstrate if the procedure is of merit or if it is lacking. Finally, although there may be no single parameter or vector that is so robust, or so all-encompassing, that it permits efficient identifications to be made under any and all conditions, a profile approach (ie, one involving a group of vectors) should counter this problem.

Research on Machine Methods

It should be remembered that the focus of this discussion is on speaker identification not speaker verification. The verification task, while formidable, is relatively straightforward in nature. Unless an imposter is present, the talkers are cooperative; and the speech samples are both highly controlled and can be continually updated. Thus, few of the problems associated with the identification task are encountered in the verification domain. Unfortunately, most of the research carried out has been on verification; and this situation is probably due to the fact that it presents the lesser

challenge of the two and that such a system (if valid and effective) would be wildly rewarding (ie, financially). The irony is that, if the speaker identification problem can be met, the speaker verification task would be immediately solved also. Nevertheless, relatively few scientists work in the identification area even though it is of high social consequence.

A number of potentially useful research programs in speaker identification have been initiated by researchers who employed relatively large groups of vectors or factors.[29,67-74] These approaches have included linear prediction, recognition by synthesis, (signal) axis crossings, cross correlation, probability density estimations, cepstrum methods, neural nets, and so on. A number of them were, at least, partly successful; others showed high potential for success if upgrades or modified procedures had been introduced. Unfortunately, very few of these research programs were sustained (note that most of them occurred before the 1990s). A more extensive review of these approaches—plus detailed description of two that were (ie, those of Wojciech Majewski and Robert Rodman) can be found in the author's book *Forensic Voice Identification*.[27]

What happened subsequently was that the general thrust shifted toward verification. An exception to the trend is a program being carried out at the University of Florida.[1,27,56,57,60,75-82] The subject of this program is called SAUSI or Semiautomatic Speaker Identification; it is among the very few efforts that are both extensive and long-term. It should provide a good example as to how the standards cited above can be applied to research of this nature. Also provided will be details of an operational approach to speaker identification.

Natural Speech Vectors

The first step in the development of SAUSI was to identify and evaluate a number of parameters found within the speech signal, ones that had the potential of being effective identification cues. It was determined very early that traditional approaches to signal processing were lacking (due to the many distortions associated with forensics); hence, the "natural" features cited above were adopted. This decision was stimulated by the results from early experiments, the aural-perceptual literature, and the realization that people routinely process heard speech using just such features.

The Profile Concept

A second perspective emerged early in system development. It had been noted that no single vector (applied by itself) seemed able to provide a high level of correct identification for all of the many types of degraded speech encountered in the forensic milieu. In response, those being studied at that particular time were combined into a single test. However, it also was discovered that adding too many features sometimes resulted in a reduction in success. This situation is caused by the process wherein a developing system will improve as relevant parameters are added until it reaches asymptote. At that point, further additions result in movement onto the negative slope of the curve and, as stated, an ultimate reduction in success occurs. This problem was confounded by yet a second one—that of targets being sought in multidimensional space—and it too proved to be a formidable one. We responded by normalizing the data and then using two-dimensional profiles (ie, where all vectors were represented but on an equal basis). The normalization process helped materially by preventing the dominance of a particular vector simply because its calculated values were greater than those of the others; and the profile approach proved robust because it allowed the simultaneous evaluation of many relationships. It also permitted internal validation and "rotations";

that is, we were able to test samples of the unknown speaker, the target talker (the "known"), and a group of foils or controls against the basic reference sample of the "unknown" and do so all at the same time. We used this approach; because, to be valid, a method must show that the unknown talker's test sample is the best match for his (or her) own reference set. Finally, we could use the procedure to carry out multiple replications (rotations) and combine them to provide the basis for a final decision.

The SAUSI Vectors

The natural speech vectors tested, and ultimately adopted, were suggested by our research and that of Stevens.[30] A full description of these vectors may be found in *The Acoustics of Crime*[1] and *Forensic Voice Identification*,[27] and they will be briefly reviewed here.

Long-Term Speech Spectra (LTS). Power spectra have been utilized extensively as speaker identification cues.[1,11,27,52,58,75-78,81,83-87] They appear to provide an effective index of general voice quality. Moreover, it has been found that this vector is resistant to the effects of speaker stress and to limited pass band conditions; however, it does not function particularly well when talkers disguise their voices. LTS analysis involves determining the energy levels for all frequencies throughout the spectrum as a function of time. By this means, the influence of individual phonemes is removed; and general voice quality is reflected. The analysis procedure employs Euclidean distance comparisons for all subjects at multiple points along the frequency curve. The data are then normalized and assessed both directly and as a part of the profile.

Speaking Fundamental Frequency (SFF). As with aural-perceptual approaches, the perception of the fundamental frequency of voice (F_0 or SFF) has been shown to be a fairly good cue for speaker recognition.[1,27,56,72,77,84,88,89] The robustness of SFF appears to have been yet further upgraded by use of a 30-parameter SFF vector (ie, for SAUSI). To be specific, the parameters making up this vector include SFF geometric mean and standard deviation plus the number frequencies in each of 30 semitone intervals (or "bins"). When normalized, these parameters make up a vector, which is used to compare speaking fundamental frequency level, variability, and patterns across subjects in much the same manner as does LTS.[57,79]

Vowel Formant Tracking (VFT). Much use has been made of vowel formant center frequencies, bandwidths, and transitions by individuals using time-frequency-amplitude spectrographic techniques in speaker identification.[1,27,30,31,44,46,47,77,90,91] While that approach was not a particularly sophisticated one (especially when used alone as in "voiceprints"), interpretation of the relevant research suggests that vowel formants definitely are important speaker identification cues (especially when obtained by modern methods). In any case, the VFT parameter is based on the measurement of the center frequencies of the first three formants of several long vowels and calculation of the ratios among them. It now appears that F_1 and F_2 are especially good indicators of speaker identity and appear to be resistant to many kinds of distortion. The software approach utilized consists of preprogrammed vowel formant windows and a vector of 28 parameters. As with the others, VFT is first evaluated separately and then as part of the SAUSI profile.

Temporal Analysis (TED). Relatively little speaker identification research has focused on any of the temporal parameters that can be extracted from the speech wave; there are but few exceptions.[27,57,60,75,76,80,82,92] Nevertheless, strong logic suggests that certain speaker-related prosodic elements can be extracted and used for recognition purposes. For example, given the hypothesis that talkers differ with respect to the temporal factors of speech (ie, in syllables, words, phrases, sentences), it is possible that the time a person takes to produce a specific amount of connected discourse will be useful in the identification task. The approach here involves an energy detection and assessment computer program. The speech energy bursts (and related) are identified and timed as a function of the amount of energy present. The several resulting parameters are merged into a vector and processing/analysis proceeds as with the others.

These vectors (plus several others) have been tested individually and in combination a large number of times in the laboratory and in the field—where attempts were made to "solve" simulated, but structured, crimes. Many experiments—both successful and unsuccessful—were carried out; and most of the basic information about SAUSI has been generated by these 40 to 50 studies. Moreover, the uniqueness of the features was tested differentially under normal and distorted speaking conditions. Finally, when a vector (or cluster of vectors) began to show potential, the research effort was shifted to the field. At that time, the forensic model was invoked and the profile approach applied. It should be remembered that the SAUSI approach addresses the very severe limitations imposed on the identification task by the forensic model (ie, one referent; one test sample within a field of competing samples). This rather harsh research design forces matches (or nonmatches) to be made from a fairly large collection of voices (6–25 in number) on the basis of either the bioequivalence[93] or nearest neighbor statistical procedure. To compensate for this challenge, the rotation approach referred to above is applied; that is, each profile is generated (using the same speakers but different samples) several times and the analyses replicated. The final continuum usually consists of the data from 3 to 5 rotations and includes a summation of all vectors. Hence, any decision is based on several million individual comparisons (factors, parameters, vectors, rotations).

Application

As more and more research was completed, it became increasingly apparent that the mass of data generated by a SAUSI analysis needed to be organized for better interpretation. The first step was to display it as seen in Figure 16–8. This approach assisted the operator in coping with the differential robustness of the vectors

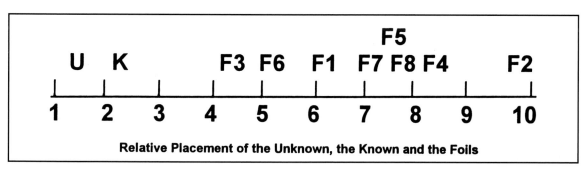

Fig 16–8. Printout of a single SAUSI trial (with F = 8). Note that the unknown-vs-unknown comparison validated the run and that K = U.

as a function of the type of degradation to the signal. As can be seen, the relationships among the unknown talker and the foils are presented for each normalized vector and for the combined vectors. This approach proved satisfactory for system analysis; it also facilitated the decision-making identification process.

The way speakers are evaluated further may be best understood by observation of Figures 16–9 and 16–10. In the first case, the identification of the unknown (U) is sought within a field that also consists of a known talker and controls (foils). The data seen actually are based on several cases where our four mul-

```
Unknown Reference   C:\SAUSI\E3
Unknown Test        C:\SAUSI\E3
Known               C:\SAUSI\E3
Foil  1             C:\SAUSI\E3
Foil  2             C:\SAUSI\E3
Foil  3             C:\SAUSI\E3
Foil  4             C:\SAUSI\E3
Foil  5             C:\SAUSI\E3
Foil  6             C:\SAUSI\E3
Foil  7             C:\SAUSI\E3
Foil  8             C:\SAUSI\E3
Foil  9             C:\SAUSI\E3
Foil 10             C:\SAUSI\E3
Foil 11             C:\SAUSI\E3
```

	LTS	TED	SFF	VFT	SUM
Unknown test	1.0000	1.4818	1.0000	1.0000	1.0000
Known	1.5323	1.0000	1.2836	1.2292	1.1686
Foil 1	3.8862	7.8851	3.9469	2.6166	5.1448
Foil 2	6.1144	4.4177	9.5805	3.1202	6.6102
Foil 3	9.1714	5.4474	5.2633	3.4391	6.6367
Foil 4	9.0549	5.5074	10.0000	10.0000	10.0000
Foil 5	5.9006	3.4713	7.0671	2.0996	5.2058
Foil 6	6.1824	10.0000	9.5805	4.6620	8.7621
Foil 7	9.7969	3.5349	9.5805	3.6224	7.5982
Foil 8	7.6665	8.2456	7.4505	4.4635	7.9845
Foil 9	10.0000	5.4801	9.5805	4.7024	8.5640
Foil 10	8.6318	7.4416	5.8762	4.4418	7.5553
Foil 11	4.0598	4.7911	6.3774	2.7540	5.0393

Fig 16–9. A continuum providing normalized data for the unknown, the known, and 11 foil speakers.

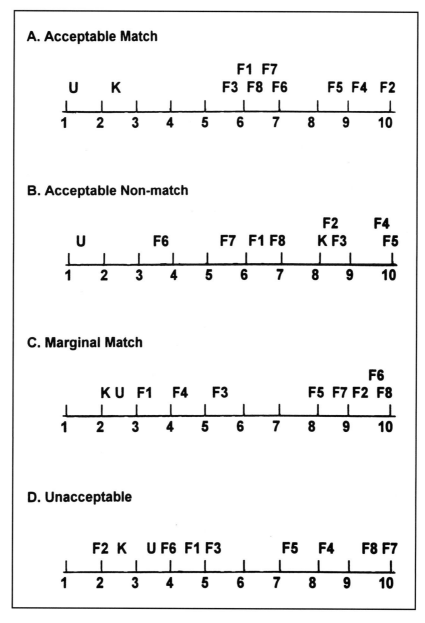

Fig 16–10. Four continua demonstrating degrees of SAUSI acceptable matches to acceptable nonmatches.

tidimensional vectors were normalized and then plotted on a two-dimensional continuum. As may be seen in Figure 16–9, the unknown was chosen as himself and then clearly identified as the known talker. Note also, the data shown in Figure 16–10. Here, a number of matches and nonmatches are contrasted.

At present, the SAUSI system operates fairly well and does so even in most forensic situations. Nevertheless, presentation of data from a recent series of experiments would appear useful; they may be found in

Figure 16–11. The first of these experiments, done in 1988, involved a large number of subjects but only laboratory samples (ie, high fidelity). Note that none of the individual vectors provided 100% correct identification. The second part of this project (not shown) was designed to test the proposition that SAUSI would eliminate a known speaker if he was not also the unknown; it did so and at a level of 100% correct elimination. The second set of experiments done in 1993 also involved a large number of subjects; but this

Conditions and Study	Vectors				
	TED	LTS	SFF	VFT	SUM
A. High Fidelity					
Hollien	62	88	68	85	90
Hollien et al	63	100	100	100	100
Jiang	82	100	80	100	100
B. Noise					
Hollien et al	64	90	77	92	100
Jiang	76	94	76	96	100
C. Telephone Passband					
Hollien et al	55	92	90	88	98
Jiang	58	100	90	96	100

Fig 16–11. Summary data from three major projects evaluating the SAUSI vectors under three environmental conditions. Values are percent correct identification of 25 or more adult male speakers; all samples were subjected to three complete rotations.

time, separate replications were carried out for high fidelity, noise, and telephone passband (Hollien et al[80] and unpublished). As can be seen, this 1993 upgrading of the vectors resulted in marked improvement for all conditions.

In 1995, Jiang[60] further upgraded the SAUSI vectors and then ran a replication of the 1993 experiment. As can be seen from consideration of Figure 16–11, correct identifications were strikingly higher for all conditions; and the correct identification level reached 100% for the summed rotations; it did so even for the two degraded conditions. The overall improvement reported is judged to be due to (1) the upgrading of vector design, (2) better equipment and processing procedures, and (3) insights from both research and field experience.

In summary, virtually all of the research carried out on SAUSI was designed to reflect the forensic model; thus, the system has been tested under rather stringent conditions. The overall results indicate that the strength of an individual vector varies somewhat from situation to situation. Indeed, although no one vector has individ-ually provided consistently high levels of correct identification under any and all conditions, they appeared to compensate for one another, especially when rotated and combined into a normalized two-dimensional profile.

Detecting Stress, Intoxication, and Other Behaviors

Many attempts have been made to detect behavioral states from voice (ie, those resulting from emotions, stress, psychosis, intoxicants, deception, fatigue, and so on). Much of that effort has lacked scientific rigor; and some of it has not even been legitimate. Nonetheless, honest inquiry focused on the several cited conditions has resulted in some useful information. However, to review all of these issues would require a chapter (each); and attempts to condense all of them into this section just might be counterproductive. Accordingly, the only areas to be considered here will be stress and intoxication—plus their effect on speech and voice. They are nicely illustrative; but if you wish to investigate the nature and effects of the other conditions, you should consult the basic literature.

Psychological Stress in Voice

To understand how a person is feeling just from hearing his or her voice is not very easy to do. Yet, there are times when an individual has little else to go on to determine the talker's state and what action he might be intending. Unfortunately, although it can be said that at least some of the relationships between vocal behaviors and psychological stress are known or suspected, many of them are rather tenuous. But is the determination of stress in voice important anyway? Yes, it undoubtedly is, especially with respect to certain types of direct interaction among people. For one thing, it often is important to monitor the potential for stress in personnel who are physically separated from a base or control site (ie, pilots, astronauts, aquanauts, police officers, and others) irrespective of the message content of the spoken interchange. It also can be desirable for a worker at a crisis control center to be able to tell if the caller actually plans to commit suicide or merely wants to talk about it. Are there vocal cues that will aid a patrolman in quickly determining if the perpetrator is about to attack—or others that will warn him of a specific danger during a household disturbance? In short, there are many instances wherein speaker-based information about the stress states of an individual would be quite helpful; and the needs of legal and law enforcement personnel rank high in this regard.

Perspectives

First, it should be noted that the term stress denotes a negative psychological state rather than one that reflects emotions in general. Although it may be just as important to determine when a person is happy as it is to know if he or she is angry, anxious, or fearful, the "reading" of negative emotions is more appropriate in the forensic situation. Moreover, much of the research that has been carried out in these areas has been either on stress or psychosis.

What is psychological stress? Is it fear; is it anger; is it anxiety? Scherer[94,95] suggests that, in general, this problem appears to result from "the lack of a precise specification and description of the emotional state underlying the vocal expression, independent of whether it is induced, posed, or studied naturalistically." This is a fair statement indeed, and one that suggests the scope of the definition problem. Of course, in

laboratory experiments, stress often is identified in terms of the applied stressor. This type of definition is not particularly useful in the real world, however; because, even though the stimuli are described, the emotion(s) or the stress being felt tends to be unknown. Moreover, when various emotions are specifically identified for research purposes, they often are simulated by actors,[1,96,97] an approach that is used primarily because it is rarely possible to record a person's speech while he or she is experiencing full blown stress states and then again under normal speaking conditions.

A third problem, and one which is perhaps more serious than the first two, relates directly to the level of stress. The question is not just "is stress present," but also what is its severity? Thus, no matter how research on stress is approached, both its presence and level should be included. Only detection is ordinarily studied, and virtually all of the research findings to date have omitted level. Moreover, most investigations have been conducted without the application of rigorous controls. It is little wonder, then, that many contradictions and substantial variability appear among the reported data.

Definitions

Back to definitions. The first step in understanding stress is to define it and to do so at a *level* of specificity beyond those suggested above. A reasonable definition, then, would be as follows. Stress, when experienced, reflects some sort of psychological state—especially one that constitutes a response to a threat.[97-99] On the other hand, stress may be induced either internally or externally with "adaptive or coping behavior required"[95,101]; or it may not be "imposed" at all but rather constitute a state where an individual "responds" to stressful conditions. In any event, we define stress as a "psychological state which results as a response to a perceived threat and is accompanied by the specific emotions of fear and anxiety."[1,97,102-104]

When the restrictions implied by this definition are considered, it might seem that the materials to follow would be of somewhat limited use in the forensic milieu. To illustrate, before it is possible to tell if a person's voice is exhibiting stress, it might be necessary to learn something about how he or she sounds under ordinary circumstances. Moreover, the need to make a judgment may come and go so quickly that formal analysis would fall in the difficult-to-impossible category. Yet, it often *is* possible to establish reasonable insights about the stress being experienced by another person and do so by assessment of their vocal characteristics. How is this possible?

The Speaking Correlates of Stress

It has long been accepted that listeners can, indeed, identify some emotions (including stress) from speech samples alone and do so at reasonably high levels of accuracy.[95-97,101,103,105-108] For example, several authors[96,105] have reported that identifications can fall in the 80 to 90% correct range. Of course, most of this research was carried out on "emotions" as portrayed (vocally) by actors, and it may be possible that they created some sort of artificial stereotypes. However, data have been reported,[104,109,110] which can be used to argue that it also is possible to specify the emotions that actually are being experienced. More importantly, if it is possible to discover felt emotions simply by listening to a talker's voice, it also should be possible to identify the relevant acoustical and temporal parameters (within the voice signal) that correlate with these percepts. Indeed, several such features have been identified.

Speaking Fundamental Frequency

Changes in heard pitch or speaking fundamental frequency (SFF or F_0) appear to correlate with psychological stress when it is being experienced. For example, years ago when Fairbanks and Pronovost[96] carried out research with actors, they found that the SFF level was raised for the emotions of fear and anger but not so for others; this relationship tends to be supported by most current studies.[94,106,108,111] Other researchers[108,110] have analyzed the real-life emotions of pilots when in danger and control tower operators under pressure. These talkers also have exhibited a rise in SFF as a function of increased stress. On the other hand, not all authors support this relationship; some[96] found only slight increases in SFF/F_0 as a function of stress, and others[112,113] report mixed results. However, it does appear that moderate to substantial increases in F_0 level usually correlate with the presence of psychological stress. To be useful, however, baseline data ordinarily should be compared to that resulting from the stressful situation. Fundamental frequency variability appears to be a much poorer predictor of stress than does SFF level. Data in this regard are not very orderly; indeed almost any position can be argued—that SFF variability may increase; may decrease, may not change, or may vary from speaker to speaker.[95-97,101,108,111] Thus, a metric of this type probably would not be useful for legal or law enforcement groups (at this stage anyway)

The Intensity of Voice

Vocal intensity is another acoustic parameter that, at least to some extent, correlates with the presence of psychological stress. However, only one group[97] has reported measurements of "absolute" intensity. They found positive correlations, and other investigators[94,108,114] pretty much agree even though they used relative measures. Thus, while inconsistencies occur, the best evidence is that vocal intensity often is increased as a function of stress.

Speech Timing

Identification of the prosodic speaking characteristics related to stress has proven to be a fairly complex process. For example, although some authors indicate that fear and anger appear typified by rapid speaking rates, as well as by short phonatory pauses,[94] others[97,108] tend not to agree. On the other hand, there is a temporal pattern shift that appears to correlate with rise in stress and does so on a fairly universal basis. It is that fewer speech bursts occur when a person speaks while experiencing that emotion. Hence, angry or fearful individuals appear to speak in longer utterances (bursts) than they would ordinarily. Finally, a rather important finding reported in this area is that nonfluencies correlate positively with stress states.

A Model

The above discussion focused on stress rather than on emotions in general. This approach was taken because psychological stress is of primary interest to law enforcement and related agencies. In any event, appropriate data have been combined into a predictive model of the vocal correlates of psychological stress, which is found in Figure 16–12. The patterns seen can be used to (potentially) determine what happens when most people speak under conditions of psychological stress. Specifically, the several shifts that can be expected include the following: (1) speaking fundamental frequency will be raised, (2) nonfluencies will increase, (3) vocal intensity will rise moderately, (4) speech rate will increase slightly, and (5) the number of speech bursts will be reduced. However, it should be remembered that, although this pattern will occur for most people, some individuals will not exhibit it (ie, the cited shifts). Moreover, because the observed characteristics take place as change from neutral speaking characteristics, information of this type will be of greatest value in the criminal justice setting when contrasts can be made to reference profiles.

Detection of Deception

This area (ie, the detection of behavioral states from speech analysis) cannot be concluded without at least a

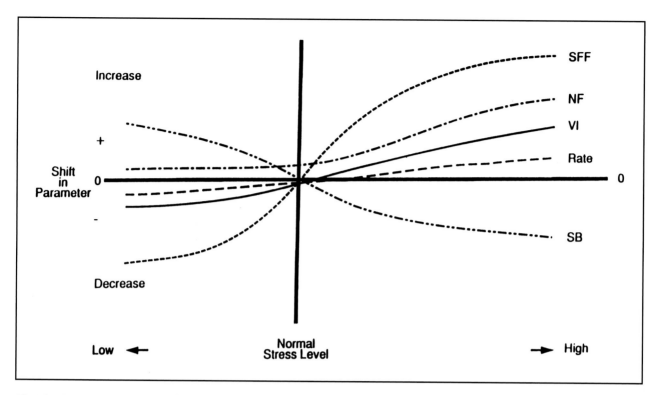

Fig 16–12. A model of the most common shifts in the voice and speech of a person who is experiencing psychological stress. SFF refers to speaking fundamental frequency, NF refers to noninfluencies, VI refers to vocal intensity, and SB refers to the number of speech bursts per unit of time.

passing reference to the so-called "psychological stress evaluators." It is claimed that these devices can be used to detect both stress and lying from voice assessment. I will not develop this issue to any great extent, but a couple of comments would appear germane.

First, if one is going to use a machine to detect lying, there must be a human lie response (ie, a measurable physiological or psychological event that always occurs when a person lies). Lykken says there is no such animal[115] but then so would simple logic. Second, individuals who market "systems" or devices that they purport are able to detect lying from elements within the voice indicate that they utilize the microtremors (or subsonic frequencies) of a human's vocal muscles for such purposes.[1] Are there any studies to support their claims? Not really; indeed the contrary is true[1,103,116-118] In any event, there is a great deal of mystery about how these devices actually work and whether they can validly perform any of the tasks their proponents claimed possible. Based on the available evidence, it can only be concluded that these systems are of no value in the detection of deception—or even of stress. It might even be concluded that using them constitutes fraudulent behavior. If you are interested in this area, you might find it useful to read the references cited.

Alcohol-Speech Relationships

Almost anyone who is asked to do so probably would describe the speech of an inebriated talker as "slurred," "misarticulated," or "confused." But, do commonly held stereotypes of this type square with the results studies have reported? More importantly, are there data to suggest that it is possible to determine a person's sobriety solely from analysis of his or her speech? Unfortunately, few relevant research projects have been carried out in the past and, hence, not a great deal of research has been reported.[119-125] Worse yet, many of those publications are limited in scope. Recently, however, interest in the area has been increasing. Moreover, although only a few of the early authors provided experimental data (ie, many of their presentations were anecdotal, reviews of other research or somewhat tangential to the issue), current efforts tend to be more rigorous in nature.[85,119-130] Please note that Chin and Pisoni's book[131] provides a good general review of this topic.

Underlying Research

It has been demonstrated that the consumption of even moderate amounts of alcohol can result in fairly substantial changes in human behavior. Cognitive function can be impaired,[132,133] as can sensory-motor performance.[132-136] Because the speech act represents the output of a number of high level integrated systems (sensory, cognitive, motor), it is not anomalous to assume that this process may also be susceptible to the influence of extraneous factors such as alcohol consumption. To be specific, it is well known that the oral production of any language involves the use of multiple sensory modalities, high level cortical functioning, complex cognitive processing, and a whole series of central and peripheral motor acts. Interruptions or insults to any of the links in this chain may result in disruptions of, or impairment in, the flow of speech and language.[137] Moreover, the component elements in this system are lawful in their interactions. For example, the speech- signal contains features that can be utilized to identify the specific physiological processes involved in its production. Further, they can interact with each other in ways that provide information about such features as speaker identity and the emotional states being experienced.[1,27] Thus, it would appear legitimate to assume that alcohol consumption also can be reflected in the voice/speech of the talker.

Specific Speech-Intoxication Relationships

Without question, research on the effects of intoxication on much of human behavior is difficult to conduct; and it now appears that study of the alcohol-speech relationships can be numbered among the more severe of these challenges. Indeed, the investigators who have researched the correlations between motor speech and ethanol consumption have experienced substantial problems in designing and conducting studies that exhibit acceptable precision. However, a few relationships already appear to be emerging from their efforts.

Some investigators have focused on the quality of the speech on an "intoxicated-sober" continuum. For example, when certain of them[120,121] had their subjects speak when sober and intoxicated, they found that articulation was degraded, speech rate slowed, and perception of intoxication states increased. Pisoni and Martin[130] also demonstrated that listeners could identify a talker when drunk or when sober, at least 62 to 74% of the time. Degradations in morphology and/or syntax, have been found to occur[124] as have articulatory problems.[121,122] However, the preeminent focus here (see above plus Johnson et al[85] and Natale et al[120]) appears to have been on the paralinguistic features of speech. Prior to our work (see below), various authors predicted that speaking fundamental frequency level, although variable, often is lowered and SFF variabili-

ty can be increased; speaking rate often is slowed; the number and length of pauses is often increased; and amplitude or intensity levels are sometimes reduced. Our research (plus that of the Pisoni group[130]) has validated some of these reports, clarified others, and added to the relevant database. We found that some of the confusions that occurred early on appear related to difficulties in procedure.

Application Difficulties

The basic problem with virtually all of the data reported in the older literature is that they were quite variable. Yet, Klingholz et al[119] appear to believe that they can account for many of these inconsistencies on the basis of inadequate and/or differing research designs. They indicate that the substantial variation observed probably is due to nonobjective measurements of blood alcohol level (BAL), too high a BAL, the use of too few (intoxicated) subjects, and/or analyses that were only qualitative. Most of these observations undoubtedly are correct. But, even after completing their own research, these authors point out that "intoxicated individuals can be falsely classified as sober" (and vice versa) on the basis of the "acoustic analysis" of speech. Moreover, they did not list all of the problems found in the research they reviewed; that is, few if any of the investigators controlled for drinking habits, intoxication level, increasing versus decreasing BAL, or effort. Nor did they employ blind controls who ingested placebos or contrast the effects of alcohol with those resulting from other physiological or psychological states.[125-128] Specifically, any number of (other) behavioral states—stress, fatigue, depression, effort, emotions, and speech/voice disorders—could complicate attempts to determine intoxication level from speech analysis. Further, it may not be possible to make valid judgments unless the target utterances can be compared with a profile of that person's speech when sober.

Our Research Program

Recognizing the confusions and contradictions associated with the intoxication-speech dilemma, we have developed a research program that attempts to resolve some of the conflicts and/or hopefully provide remedies.[126-128] Although currently ongoing, our efforts already have led to solutions for at least some of the problems.

First, the methodological approach we utilized was designed to upgrade the precision of the traditional procedures used to induce acute alcohol intoxication. Instead of administering heavy doses of ethanol—

based on body weight, sex, and so on—our subjects received lighter doses (80-proof rum or vodka) mixed with a soft drink (orange juice, cola) plus Gatorade. The subjects drank at their own pace but breath concentration levels (BrAC) were measured at 10- to 15-minute intervals throughout the experiment. Efficiency was increased by this approach with nausea and discomfort sharply reduced; further, serial measurements were permitted and intoxication level could be highly controlled. Relatively large groups of subjects were studied and all subjects participated in all procedures (ie, all of those in their particular experiment). Figure 16–13 graphically portrays how the intoxication level was tracked for one of the subjects. The "windows" or intoxication levels (ascending or descending) at which speech was studied included (among others) BrAC 0.00 (sober), BrAC 0.04-0.05 (mild), BrAC 0.08-0.09 (legal), and BrAC 0.12-0.13 (severe).

Subjects were carefully selected on the basis of 27 behavioral and medical criteria. After training, they were required to repeatedly produce four types of speech under a variety of conditions and intoxication levels; included were a standard 98-word oral reading passage, articulation test sentences, a set of diadochokinetic gestures, and extemporaneous speech. Standard "drinking practice" evaluations were applied to classify subjects as light, moderate, or heavy drinkers. As may be deduced from the above descriptions, our procedures were very carefully carried out for all conditions and at all levels. Analysis included auditory processing by listeners (drunk-sober, intoxication level, etc), acoustic analysis of the signal, and various classification/sorting (behavioral) tests.

Current Findings

A number of relationships already have emerged from this program of research. First, it appears that auditors of all types are able to detect the presence of intoxication from listening to the talkers' speech and voice; and they can do so at rather high levels of accuracy. On the other hand, they are not so facile at determining the level of intoxication. Although they were able to discriminate among the levels, they tended to overestimate speaker impairment for individuals who were only mildly (to moderately) intoxicated and underestimate the level of involvement for those more severely involved[126] (see also Fig 16–14). Second, it appears possible to accurately simulate rather severe levels of intoxication and even reduce the percept of intoxication if the individual attempts (while inebriated) to sound sober.[125] Moreover (and surprisingly), there seem to be only minor gender differences and few-to-

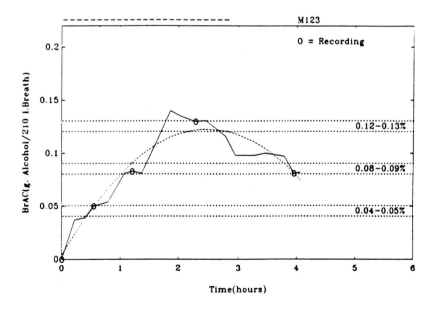

Fig 16–13. A plot of changes in intoxication level as a function of ingesting ethanol. The curve demonstrates a subject's progress relative to increasing levels of intoxication from the beginning to the completion of the experimental portion of a trial (BrAC was not always recorded after the primary run). Note that the speech samples were recorded while the speaker was in each of the windows. The smooth curve is a second order polynomial.

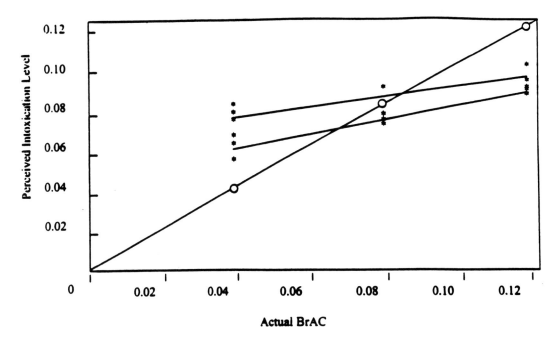

Fig 16–14. Perceived intoxication levels contrasted with the physiologically measured levels (45-degree line with circles) from sober to severely intoxicated (BrAC 0.12-0.13). Four studies are combined for the top set (35 speakers, 85 listeners) and two for the lower set (36 speakers, 52 listeners). Note the overreaction to the speech of people who are mildly intoxicated and the underrating of those who were seriously inebriated.

none for drinking level (light, moderate, heavy). Perhaps the most powerful data to date are those obtained from large groups of subjects in the "primary" investigations (see Figure 16–15). As can be seen, they show at least some shifts for all of the speaking characteristics measured excepting vocal intensity. First, note that speaking fundamental frequency (heard pitch) is raised (not lowered) with increases in intoxication level; this is a relationship suggested by clinicians but not by previous researchers.[138] Most notable of all is the nearly universal slowing down of speech as intoxication increases and the sharp rise of the number of nonfluencies for the same conditions. Perhaps the most striking relationship of all is this last one (see again, Fig 16–15). The correlation here is a very powerful one, and the pattern seen in the figure has been confirmed by several of our more recent studies. In short, patterns are emerging that permit the prediction of the speech/voice behaviors in a large proportion of those individuals who become intoxicated from ingesting ethanol. Finally, we also have broken some new ground as we have discovered that a small group of subjects account for virtually all of the departures from main patterns (we are now studying these deviations also). Finally, although the impact of these findings on the forensic milieu is not yet clear, it very well could prove to be a useful one.

Conclusion

Attempts have been made to describe several of the elements that make up a fairly new and still developing discipline of forensic phonetics. Some areas central to the field are well established; others still operate to create somewhat fuzzy boundaries. Among the topics clearly within the scope of forensic phonetics are (1) the enhancement and decoding of speech on tape recordings, (2) the authentication of tape recordings, (3) speaker identification (if not verification), and (4) the detection of a number of behavioral states from voice/speech analysis. Other elements may or may not be relevant also; only time will tell. In any event, just as with all relatively new fields, much is to be learned about what can and cannot be accomplished by application of the methods and procedures proposed and in use. Fortunately, appropriate baseline materials have been established by relevant practitioners and scientists situated both in America and Europe. These concepts and procedures are being upgraded and extended.

Acknowledgments The research described in this chapter was supported primarily by the National Institutes of Health, the Office of Naval Research, the US Army Research Office, the Justice Department, the Dreyfus Foundation,

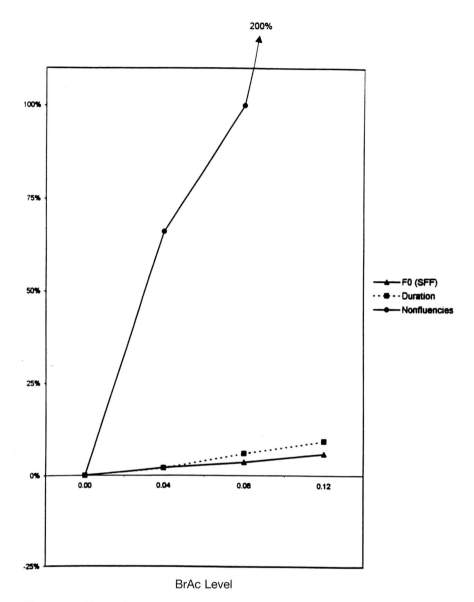

Fig 16–15. The shifts in several parameters as a function of increasing intoxication. The increase in F_0 and reduction in speaking rate (increased duration) are statistically significant. However, they are dwarfed by the dramatic shift in nonfluencies.

and the University of Florida. Grateful thanks is extended to all of them.

References

1. Hollien H. *The Acoustics of Crime.* New York, NY: Plenum; 1990.
2. Hollien H. Forensic phonetics: a new dimension to the phonetic sciences. In: *Festchrift fur Otto von Essen.* Hamburg, Germany: Phonetische Beitrage; 25:157–190.
3. Hollien H. Forensic communication: an emerging specialty. *Criminal Defense.* 1983;10:22–29.
4. Hollien H. The phonetician as a speech detective. In: Casagrande J, ed. *The Linguistic Connection.* New York, NY: University Press of America; 1983:101–132.
5. Hollien H. Forensic phonetics. In: Siegal JA, ed. *Encyclopedia of Forensic Sciences.* San Diego, Calif: Academic Press; 2000:1243–1254.
6. Dean JD. The work of the Home Office tape laboratory. *Police Res Bull.* 1980:35:25–27.
7. Hollien H. Noisy tape recordings in forensics. *ESCA Proceedings, Speech Processing in Adverse Conditions* (Nice, France). 1992:167–170.
8. Hollien H., Fitzgerald JT. Speech enhancement techniques for crime lab use. *Proceedings of the International*

Conference Crime Countermeasures (Oxford, UK). 1977:21–29.

9. Bloch SC, Lyons PW, Ritterman SI. Enhancement of speech intelligibility by "blind" deconvolution. *Proceedings of the Carnahan Conference on Crime Countermeasures (Lexington, Ky).* 1977:167–174.

10. Le Bouquin-Jeannes R. Enhancement of speech degraded by coherent and incoherent noise using a cross-spectral estimator. *IEEE Trans Speech Audio Processing.* 1997;5:404–420.

11. Lee KY. Speech enhancement based on neutral predictive hidden Markov models. *Signal Processing.* 1998;65:373–381.

12. Lim JS, Oppenheimer AV. Enhancement and bandwidth comprehension of noisy speech. *Proc IEEE.* 1979;67:1586–1604.

13. Paul JE, Reames JB, Woods RC. Real-time digital laboratory enhancement of tape recordings. *Proceedings of the Institute of Acoustics. Part I: Police Applications Speech and Tape Recording Analysis.* 1984;6:1–11.

14. Wan EA. Removal of noise from speech using the dual EKF algorithm. *Proceedings of the International Conference on Acoustics, Speech, and Signal Processing, ICASSP, Piscataway, NY,* 1998:181:384.

15. Blain BJ. Tape recording enhancement. *Police Res Bull.* (London, UK Home Office), 1980;35:22–24.

16. Hollien PA. Utilization of blind decoders in phonetics. In: Cohen A, Broecke M, eds. *Tenth International Congress of Phonetic Sciences.* Dordrecht, Holland: Foris Publications; 1983:532.

17. Hollien PA. An update on speech decoding. *Proceedings of the Institute of Acoustics. Part I: Police Applications of Speech and Tape Recording Analysis.* 1984:33–40.

18. Warren RM, Warren PR. Auditory illusions and confusions. *Sci Am.* 1970;223:30–36.

19. Osberger MJ. A comparison between procedures used to locate speech segment boundaries. *J Acoust Soc Amer.* 1979;50:225–228.

20. Peterson GE, Lehiste I. Duration of syllable nuclei in English. *J Acoust Soc Am.* 1960;32:693–703.

21. Aull AM, Zue VW. Lexical stress determination and its application to large vocabulary speech recognition. *IEEE Proc. ICASSP.* 1985;CH218:1549–1552.

22. Cutler A, Foss DJ. On the role of sentence stress in sentence processing. *Lang Speech.* 1977;20:1–10.

23. Bolinger D, Sears DA. *Aspects of Language.* 3rd ed. New York, NY: Harcourt Brace Jovanovich; 1981.

24. Taylor DS. Non-native speakers and the rhythm of English. *Int Rev Appl Ling Lang Teach.* 1981;19:219–226.

25. van Coestsem F, Hendricks R, McCormick S. Accent typology and sound change. *Lingua.* 1981;53:293–315.

26. Hecker MHL. Speaker Recognition: *An Interpretative Survey of the Literature.* ASHA Monograph No 16. Washington, DC: ASHA; 1971.

27. Holien H. *Forensic Voice Identification.* London, UK: Academic Press; 2002.

28. Kuenzel HJ. *Spechererkennung.* Heidelberg, Germany: Kriminalistik; 1987.

29. Nolan JF. *The Phonetic Basis of Speaker Recognition.* Cambridge, UK: Oxford University Press; 1983.

30. Stevens KN. Sources of inter- and intra-speaker variability in the acoustic properties of speech sounds. *Proceedings of the Seventh International Congress of Phonetic Sciences.* Montreal, Canada; 1971:206–232.

31. Tosi O. *Voice Identification: Theory and Legal Applications.* Baltimore, Md: University Park Press; 1979.

32. Mack vs State of Florida. 54 Fla. 55, 44 So. 706 (1907), citing 5, *Howell's State Trials,* 1186.

33. Broeders APA. Earwitness identification: common ground, disputed territory and uncharted areas. *Forensic Linguistics.* 1996;3:1–13.

34. Michel JF. Use of a voice lineup. Presented at the Annual Meeting of the American Academy of Forensic Sciences; Feb 1980; New Orleans, La. Abstract 937(A).

35. DeJong G. Earwitness characteristics and speaker identification accuracy. Unpublished Ph.D. dissertation, University of Florida, Gainesville, Fla.

36. Hollien H, Huntley R, Kuenzel H, Hollien PA. Proposal for earwitness lineups. *Forensic Linguistics.* 1995;2:143–154.

37. Yarmi AD. Earwitness speaker identification. *Psychol Publ Policy Law.* 1995;1:792–816.

38. Bull R, Clifford BR. Earwitness voice recognition accuracy. In: Wells GL, Loftus E, eds. *Earwitness Testimony: Psychological Perspectives.* Cambridge, UK: Cambridge University Press; 1984.

39. Clifford BR. Memory for voices: the feasibility and quality of earwitness evidence. In: Bostock L, ed. *Evaluating Witness Evidence.* Clifford, NY: John Wiley and Sons; 1984.

40. Kuenzel H. On the problem of speaker identification by victims and witnesses. *Forensic Linguistics.* 1994;1:45–58.

41. Yarmey AD. Verbal, visual, and voice identification of rape suspect under different levels of illumination. *J Appl Psychol.* 1986;71:363–370.

42. McGehee F. The reliability of the identification of the human voice. *J Gen Psychology.* 1937;17:249–271.

43. Bricker P, Pruzansky S. Effects of stimulus content and duration on talker identification. *J Acoust Soc Am.* 1966; 40:1441–1450.

44. Carbonell JR, Stevens KN, Williams CE, Woods B. Speaker identification by a matching-from-samples technique. *J Acoust Soc Am.* 1965;40:1205–1206.

45. Huntley RA. Listener skill in voice identification. Presented at the American Academy of Forensic Sciences; February 1992; New Orleans, La. Abstract 105(A).

46. Stevens KN, Williams CE, Carbonell JR, Woods D. Speaker authentication and identification: a comparison of spectrographic and auditory presentation of speech materials. *J Acoust Soc Am.* 1968:44:1596–1607.

47. Endres W, Bambach W, Flosser G. Voice spectrograms as a function of age, voice disguise, and voice imitation. *J Acoust Soc Am.* 1971;49:1842–1848.

48. Hollien H, Majewski W, Doherty ET. Perceptual identification of voices under normal, stressed, and disguised speaking conditions, *J Phonetics.* 1982;10:139–148.

49. Hollien H, Schwartz R. Speaker identification utilizing noncontemporary speech. *J Forensic Sci.* 2001;46:63–67.

50. Houlihan K. The effects of disguise on speaker identification from sound spectrograms. In: Hollien H, Hollien P, eds. *Current Issues in the Phonetic Sciences: Proceedings of the IPS-77 Congress*; Miami Beach, Florida; 17–19 December 1977. Amsterdam, The Netherlands: J Benjamins; 1979:811–820.

51. Kuenzel HJ. Field procedures in forensic speaker identification. *Proceedings of the 12th International Congress of Phonetic Sciences.* Aix-en-Provence, France: Université de Provence; 1991.

52. McGlone RE, Hollien PA, Hollien H. Accoustic analysis of voice disguise related to voice identification. *Proceedings of the International Conference on Crime Countermeasures.* Oxford, UK; July 25–27, 1977:31–35.

53. Pollack I, Pickett JM, Sumby WH. On the identification of speakers by voice. *J Acoust Soc Am.* 1989;26:403–412.

54. Reich AR, Duke JE. Effects of selected vocal disguise upon speaker identification by listening. *J Acoust Soc Am.* 1979;66:1023–1028.

55. Compton AJ. Effects of filtering and vocal duration upon the identification of speakers aurally. *J Acoust Soc Am.* 1963;35L1748–1752.

56. Hollien H, Majewski W, Hollien PA. Analysis of F_0 as a speaker identification technique. *Proceedings of Eighth International Congress of Phonetic Sciences.* Abstract of Papers. 1975:337.

57. Jiang M. Fundamental frequency vector for a speaker identification system. *Forensic Ling.* 1996;1:45–58.

58. LaRiviere CL. Contributions of fundamental frequency and formant frequencies to speaker identification. *Phonetica.* 1975;31:185–197.

59. Iles M. Speaker identification as a function of fundamental frequency and resonant frequencies, Unpublished doctoral dissertation, University of Florida. Gainesville, Fla.

60. Jiang M. Experiments on a speaker identification system. Unpublished doctoral dissertation, University of Florida, Gainesville, Fla.

61. Kuenzel HJ, Koester JP. Measuring vocal jitter in forensic speaker identification. Presented at the American Academy of Forensic Sciences; 1992; New Orleans, La. Abstract 113–114(A).

62. Shirt M. An auditory speaker recognition experiment. *Proceedings of the Institute of Acoustics. Part 1, Police Applications of Speech, Tape Recording Analysis.* London, UK: Documenta Acustica; 1984:71–74.

63. Koester JP. Auditive Spechererkennung bei Experten und Naiven. In *Festschrift Wangler.* Hamburg, Germany: Helmut Buske, AG; 1981;52:171–180.

64. Atwood W, Hollien H. Stress monitoring by polygraph for research purposes. *Polygraph.* 1986;15:47–56.

65. Hollien H, Bennet GT, Gelfer MP. Criminal identification comparison: aural vs. visual identifications resulting from a simulated crime. *J Forensic Sci.* 1983;28:208–221

66. Hollien H, Hollien PA. Improving aural-perceptual speaker identification techniques. In: Braum A, Koester JP, eds. *Studies in Forensic Phonetics.* Trier, Germany, Wissenschaftlicher Verlag; 1995;64:87–64.

67. Atal BS. Effectiveness of linear prediction characteristics of the speech wave for automatic speaker identification and verification. *J Acoust Soc Am.* 1974;55:1304–1312.

68. Bakis R, Dixon NR. Toward speaker-independent recognition-by-synthesis. *IEEE Proc, ICASSP.* 1982:566–569.

69. Basztura CS, Majewski W. The application of long-term analysis of the zero-crossing of a speech signal in automatic speaker identification. *Arch Acoust.* 1978;3:3–15.

70. Broderick PK, Paul JE, Rennick RE. Semi-automatic speaker identification system. In: *Proceedings of the 1975 Carnahan Conference on Crime Countermeasures;* Lexington, Ky; 1975:37–45.

71. Bunge E. Automatic speaker recognition system auros for security systems and forensic voice identification. *Proceedings of the International Conference on Crime Countermeasures;* Oxford, UK; 1977:1–8.

72. Edie J, Sebestyen GS. Voice identification general criteria. Report RADC-TDR-62-278. New York, NY: Rome Air Development Centre, Air Force Systems Command, Griffiss AFB; 1972.

73. Fredouille C, Bonastre JF. Use of dynamic information and second order statistical methods in speaker identification. *RLA2C.* Avignon, France. 1998;3:50–54.

74. Schwartz R, Roncos S, Berouti M. The application of probability density estimation to text-independent speaker identification. *Proceedings of the ICASSP.* 1982:1649–1652.

75. Doherty ET. An evaluation of selected acoustic parameters for use in speaker identification. *J Phonetics.* 1976;4:321–326.

76. Doherty ET, Hollien H. Multiple factor speaker identification of normal and distorted speech. *J Phonetics.* 1978;6:1–8.

77. Hollien H. The profile approach to speaker identification. *Proceedings of the 12th International Congress on Phonetic Sciences (ICPhS);* Aix en Provence, France; 1991:396(A).

78. Hollien H. The future of speaker identification: a model (Plenary). *Proceedings of the 13th International Congress on Phonetic Sciences (ICPhS).* vol 3, 138–145. Stockholm, Sweden; August 1995.

79. Hollien H, Jiang M, The challenge of effective speaker identification (Keynote). *Proceedings RLA2C.* Avignon, France; 1998:2–9.

80. Hollien H, Jiang M, Kuenzel H. Upgrading the SAUSI Prosody (TED) Vector, In: Braun A, Koester J-P, eds. *Studies in Forensic Phonetics.* Trier, Germany, Wissenschaftlicher Verlag; 1993;64:98–108.

81. Hollien H, Majewski W. Speaker identification by long-term spectra under normal and distorted speech conditions. *J Acoust Soc Amer.* 1977;62:975–980.

82. Johnson CC, Hollien H, Hicks JW Jr. Speaker identification utilizing selected temporal speech features. *J Phonetics.* 1984;12:319–327.

83. Hollien H. Consideration of guidelines for earwitness lineups. *Forensic Linguistics.* 1996;3:14–23.

84. Hollien H, Gelfer MP, Huntley R. The neutral speech vector concept in speaker identification. In: Borowski

VA, Koester JP, eds. *Neue Tendenzen in der Anger-wandten Phonetik*. Hamburg, Germany: Helmut Buske Verlag; 1990;62:71–87.

85. Johnson K, Pisoni D, Bernacki R. Do voice recordings reveal whether a person is intoxicated? *Phonetica*. 1990;47:215–237.

86. Zalewski J, Mejewski W, Hollien H. Cross-correlation between long-term speech spectra as a criterion for speaker identification. *Acustica*. 1975;34:20–24.

87. Hollien H, Hicks JW Jr, Oliver LH. A semiautomatic system for speaker identification. *Neue Tendenzen in der angerwandten Phonetik*. Hamburg, Germany: Helmut Buske Verlag; 1990:62:89–106.

88. Jassem W, Steffen-Batog M, Czajka S. Statistical characteristics of short-term average F_0 distribution as personal voice features. In: Jassem W, ed. *Speech Analysis and Synthesis*. vol 3. Warsaw, Poland: Pa'nstwowe Wydawn; 1973:209–228.

89. Wolf JJ. Efficient acoustic parameters for speaker recognition. *J Acoust Soc Am*. 1972;51:2044–2055.

90. Koval S, Krynov S. Practice of usage of spectral analysis for forensic speaker identification. *Proceedings of the Workshop Reconassaince du Locuteur et Ses Spplications Commerciale et Criminalistique (RLA2C)*; Avignon, France; April 20–23, 1998:136–140.

91. Paoloni A, Pierucci P, Ragazzini S. Improving automatic formant tracking for speaker identification. *RLA2C*; Avignon, France; 1998;1:24–27.

92. Onellet P, Tadj C, Dumouchel J-P. Dialog and prosodic models for text-independent speaker identification. *RLA2C*; Avignon, France. 1998;2:41–44.

93. Hsu JC, Hwang J, H-K, Ruberg S. Confidence intervals associated with tests of bioequivalence. *Biometrika*. 1994;81:103–114.

94. Scherer KR. Vocal affect expression: a review and a model for future research. *Psychol Bull*. 1985;99:143–165.

95. Scherer KR. Voice, stress and emotion. In: Appley H, Trumbull R, eds. *Dynamics of Stress: Physiological, Psychological, and Social Perspectives*. New York, NY: Plenum Press; 1986:157–179.

96. Fairbanks G, Provovost W. An experimental study of the pitch characteristics of the voice during the expression of emotion. *Speech Monogr*. 1939;6:87–104.

97. Hicks JW Jr, Hollien H. The reflection of stress in voice-1: understanding the basic correlates. *Proceedings of the Carnahan Conference on Crime Countermeasures; Lexington, Ky*; 1981:189–194.

98. Appley MH, Trumbull R. On the concept of psychological stress. In: Appley MH, Trumbull R, eds. *Psychological Stress: Issues in Research*. New York, NY: Meredith Publishing Co; 1967.

99. Howard R. Neurophysiological studies of stress, arousal and anxiety. In: Spielberger CD, Sarason IG, eds. *Stress and Anxiety*. 1991;13:178–191.

100. Murray IR, Arnott JL. Toward the simulation of emotion in synthetic speech: a review of the literature on the human emotion. *J Acoust Soc Am*. 1993;93:1097–1108.

101. Scherer KR. Vocal indicators of stress. In: Darby J, ed. *Speech Evaluation in Psychiatry*. New York, NY: Grune & Stratton; 1981:171–187.

102. Hollien H. Vocal indicators of psychological stress. In: Wright F, Bahn C, Rieber RW, eds. *Forensic Psychology and Psychiatry*. New York, NY: New York Academy of Sciences; 1980:47–72.

103. Hollien H, Geisson L, Hicks JW Jr. Voice stress evaluators and lie detection. *J Forensic Sci*. 1987; 32:405–418.

104. Hollien H, Saletto JA, Miller SK. Psychological stress in voice: a new approach. *Studia Phonetica Posnaniensia*. 1993;4:5–17.

105. Liberman P, Michaels SB. Some aspects of fundamental frequency and envelope amplitude as related to emotional content of speech. *J Acoust Soc Am*. 1962;34: 922–927.

106. Scherer KR. Personalities markers in speech. In: Scherer KR, Giles H, eds. *Social Markets in Speech*. Cambridge, UK: Cambridge University Press; 1979:147–209.

107. Stepffen-Batog M, Madelska L, Katulska K. The role of voice timbre, duration, speech melody and dynamics in the perception of the emotional coloring of utterances. *Studia Phonetika Posnaniensia*. 1993;4:73–92.

108. Williams CE, Stevens KN. Emotions and speech: some acoustical correlates. *J Acoust Soc Am*. 1972;2:1238–1250.

109. Kuroda I, Fujiwara O, Okamura N, Utsuki N. Method for determining pilot stress through analysis of voice communication. *Aviat Space Environ Med*. 1976;47:528–533.

110. Williams CE, Stevens KN. On determining the emotional state of pilots during flight: an exploratory study. *Aerospace Med*. 1969;40:1369–1372.

111. Cummings K, Clements M. Analysis of glottal waveforms across stress styles. *Proc IEEE, ICASSP*. CH 2847: 369–372.

112. Asparoukhov O, Boyanov B. Computer analysis of speech patients under preoperative stress. *Acustica*. 1994; 80:412–414.

113. Hecker MHL, Stevens KN, von Bismarck G, Williams CE. Manifestations of task-induced stress in the acoustic speech signal. *J Acoust Soc Am*. 1968;44:993–1001.

114. Friedhoff AJ, Alpert M, Kurtzberg RL. An electro-acoustic analysis of the effects of stress on voice, *J Cardiovasc Nurs*. 1964;11:266–272.

115. Lykken DT. *A Tremor in the Blood: Uses and Abuses of the Lie Detector*. New York, NY: McGraw-Hill, Inc; 1981.

116. Kubis J. *Comparison of Voice Analysis and Polygraph as Lie Detection Procedures*. Aberdeen Proving Ground, Md: US Army Land Warfare Laboratory; 1973.

117. McGlone RE. Tests of the psychological stress evaluator (PSE) as a lie and stress detector. *Proceedings of the International Conference on Crime Countermeasures*; Lexington, Ky; 1975:83–86.

118. McGlone RE, Hollien H. Partial analysis of the acoustic signal of stressed and unstressed speech. *Proceedings of the Carnahan Conference on Crime Countermeasures*; Lexington, Ky; 1976:19–21.

119. Klingholz F, Penning R, Liebhardt E. Recognition of low-level of alcohol intoxication from speech signal. *J Acoust Soc Am*. 1988;84:929–935.

120. Natale M, Kanzler M, Jaffe J. Acute effects of alcohol on defensive and primary-process language. *J Addict.* 1980;15:1055–1067.

121. Sobell L, Sobell M. Effects of alcohol on the speech of alcoholics, *J Speech Hear Res.* 1972;15:861–868.

122. Sobell L, Sobel M, Coleman R. Alcohol-induced dysfluency in nonalcoholics, *Folia Phoniatr* (Basel). 1982;34:316–323.

123. Trojan F, Kryspin-Exner K. The decay of articulation under the influence of alcohol and paraldehyde. *Folia Phoniatr.* 1968;20:217–238.

124. Chin SB, Large N, Pisoni D. Effects of alcohol on the production of words in context: a first report. Report 21. Bloomington, Ind: Speech Research Laboratory, Indiana University.

125. Hollien H, DeJong G, Martin CA. Production of intoxication states by actors: perception by lay listeners. *J Forensic Sci.* 1998;43:1153–1162.

126. Hollien H, DeJong G, Martin CA, Schwartz R, Liljegren K. Effects of ethanol intoxication on speech suprasegmentals. *J Acoust Soc Am.* 2001;110:3198–3206.

127. Hollien H, Martin CA. Conducting research on the effects of intoxication on speech. *Forensic Linguistics.* 1996;3:101–127.

128. Hollien H, Liljegren K, Martin CA, DeTong G. Production of intoxication states by actors: acoustic and temporal characteristics. *J Forensic Sci.* 2001;46:68–73.

129. Pisoni DB, Hathaway SN, Yuchtman M. Effects of alcohol on the acoustic-phonetic properties of speech. In: *Alcohol, Accidents and Injuries.* Pittsburgh, Pa: Society of Automotive Engineers; 1986:131–150.

130. Pisoni, DB, Martin CS. Effects of alcohol on the acoustics-phonetic properties of speech: perceptual and acoustic analyses. *Alcohol Clin Exp Res.* 1989;13:577–587.

131. Chin SB, Pisoni D. *Alcohol and Speech.* San Diego, Calif: Academic Press; 1997.

132. Arbuckle T, Chaikelson J, Gold D. Social drinking and cognitive function revisited. *J Stud Alcohol.* 1994;55:352–361.

133. Hindmarch I, Kerr JS, Sherwood N. The effects of alcohol and other drugs on psychomotor performance and cognitive function, *Alcohol Alcohol.* 1991;26:71–79.

134. Connors GJ, Maisto SA. Effects of alcohol, instructions and consumption rate on motor performance. *J Stud Alcohol.* 1980;41:509–517.

135. Moskowitz H, Burns M. Effects of rate of drinking on human performance. *J Stud Alcohol.* 1976;37:598–605.

136. Oei T, Kerschbaumer DM. Peer attitudes, sex, and the effects of alcohol on simulated driving performance, *Am J Drug Alcohol Abuse.* 1990;16:135–146.

137. Netsell R. Speech motor control: theoretical issues with clinical impact. In: Berry WR, ed. *Clinical Dysarthria.* San Diego, Calif: College-Hill Press; 1983:1–19.

138. Cooney O, McGuigan K, Murphy P, Conroy R. Acoustic analysis of the effects of alcohol on the human voice. *J Acoust Soc Am.* 1998; 103:2895.

Glossary

This glossary has been developed from the author's experience and also from a review of glossaries developed by Johan Sundberg (personal communication, June 1995), Ingo Titze (*Principles of Voice Production*, Englewood, NJ: Prentice-Hall, 1994:330–338), and other sources. It is difficult to credit appropriately contributions to glossaries or dictionaries of general terms, as each new glossary builds on prior works. The author is indebted to colleagues whose previous efforts have contributed to the compilation of this glossary.

AAO–HNS: American Academy of Otolaryngology-Head and Neck Surgery

AIDS: Acquired Immune Deficiency Syndrome

abduct: To move apart, separate

abduction quotient: The ratio of the glottal half-width at the vocal processes to the amplitude of vibration of the vocal fold

abscess: Collection of pus

absolute jitter (Jita): A discrete measure of very short term (cycle-to-cycle) variation of the pitch periods expressed in microseconds. This parameter is dependent on the fundamental frequency of the voicing sample. Therefore, normative data differs significantly for men and women. Higher pitch results in lower Jita

absolute voice rest: Total silence of the phonatory system

acceleration: The rate of change of velocity with respect to time (measured in millimeters per square second mm/s^2)

acoustic power: The physical measure of the amount of energy produced and radiated into the air per second (measured in watts)

acoustical zero decibels: 0.0002 microbar

actin: A protein molecule that reacts with myosin to form actinomysin, the contractile part of a myofilament in muscle

acting-voice trainer: (1) *See* **Voice Coach**; (2) A professional with specialized training who may work with injured voices as part of a medical voice team in an effort to optimize speaking voice performance

Adam's apple: Prominence of the thyroid cartilage, primarily in males

adduct: To bring together, approximate

affricate: Combination of plosive and fricative consonants such as /dʒ/

allergy: Bodily response to foreign substances or organisms

alto: (*See* **Contralto**)

alveolar ridge: The bony ridge of the gum into which the teeth insert

AMA: American Medical Association

amplitude: Maximum excursion of an undulating signal from the equilibrium; the amplitude of a sound wave is related to the perceived loudness; mostly it is expressed as a logarithmic, comparative level measure using the decibel (dB) unit

amplitude perturbation quotient (APQ): A relative evaluation of short term (cycle-to-cycle) variation of peak-to-peak amplitude expressed in percent. This measure uses a smoothing factor of 11 periods

amplitude spectrum: A display of relative amplitude versus frequency of the sinusoidal components of a waveform

amplitude to length ratio: The ratio of vibrational amplitude at the center of the vocal fold to the length of the vocal fold

amplitude tremor: Regular (periodic) long-term amplitude variation (an element of vibrato)

amplitude tremor frequency (Fatr): This measure is expressed in Hz and shows the frequency of the most intensive low-frequency amplitude-modulating component in the specified amplitude-tremor analysis range

amplitude tremor intensity index (ATRI): The average ratio of the amplitude of the most intensive low-frequency amplitude modulating component (amplitude tremor) to the total amplitude of the analyzed sample. The algorithm for tremor analysis determines the strongest periodic amplitude modulation of the voice. This measure is expressed in percent

anabolic steroids: Primarily male hormones, increase muscle mass and may cause irreversible, masculinization of the voice. Anabolic steroids help cells convert simple substances into more complex substances, especially into living matter

anisotropic: Property of a material that produces different strains when identical stresses are applied in different directions

antagonist (muscle): An opposing muscle

anterior: Toward the front

anterior commissure: The junction of the vocal folds in the front of the larynx

antibiotic: Drug used to combat infection (bodily invasion by a living organism such as a bacteria or virus). Most antibiotics have action specifically against bacteria

anticoagulant: Blood thinner; agent that impairs blood clotting

antinodes: The "peaks" in a standing wave pattern

antihistamine: Drug to combat allergic response

aperiodic: Irregular behavior that has no definite period; is usually either chaotic or random

aperiodicity: The absence of periodicity; no portion of the waveform repeats exactly

aphonia: The absence of vocal fold vibration; this term is commonly used to describe people who have "lost their voice" after vocal fold injury. In most cases, such patients have very poor vibration, rather than no vibration; and they typically have a harsh, nearly whispered voice

appendix of the ventricle of Morgagni: A cecal pouch of mucous membrane connected by a narrow opening with the anterior aspect of the ventricle. It sits between the ventricular fold in the inner surface of the thyroid cartilage. In some cases, it may extend as far as the cranial border of the thyroid cartilage, or higher. It contains the openings of 60 to 70 mucous glands, and it is enclosed in a fibrous capsule, which is continuous with the ventricular ligament. Also called *appendix ventriculi laryngis*, and *laryngeal saccule*

aria: Song, especially in the context of an opera

arthritis: Inflammation of joints in the body

articulation: Shaping of vocal tract by positioning of its mobile walls such as lips, lower jaw, tongue body and tip, velum, epiglottis, pharyngeal sidewalls, and larynx

articulators: The structures of the vocal tract that are used to create the sounds of language. They include the lips, teeth, tongue, soft palate, and hard palate

arytenoid cartilages: Paired, ladle-shaped cartilages to which the vocal folds are attached

arytenoid dislocation: A condition frequently causing vocal fold immobility or hypomobility due to separation of the arytenoid cartilage from its joint and normal position atop the cricoid cartilage

ASHA: American Speech-Language-Hearing Association

aspirate: Speech sound characterized by breathiness

aspirate attack: Initiation of phonation preceded by air, producing /h/

aspiration: (1) In speech, the sound made by turbulent airflow preceding or following vocal fold vibration, as in /hɑ/. (2) In medicine, refers to breathing into the lungs substances that do not belong there such as food, water, or stomach contents following reflux. Aspiration may lead to infections such as pneumonia, commonly referred to as *aspiration pneumonia*

asthma: Obstructive pulmonary (lung) disease associated with bronchospasm, and difficulty expiring air

atmospheric pressure: The absolute pressure exerted by the atmosphere, usually measured in millimeters of mercury (mmHg)

atresia: Failure of development. In the case of the larynx, this may result in fusion or congenital webbing of the vocal folds, or failure of development of the trachea

atrophy: Loss or wasting of tissue. Muscle atrophy occurs, for example, in an arm that is immobilized in a cast for many weeks

attractor: A geometric figure in state space to which all trajectories in its vicinity are drawn. The four types of attractors are (1) *point*, (2) *limit cycle*, (3) *toroidal*, and (4) *strange*. A point trajector draws all trajectories to a single point. An example is a pendulum moving toward rest. A limit cycle is characteristic of periodic motion. A toroidal attractor represents quasiperiodic motion (often considered a subset of periodic motion). A strange attractor is associated with chaotic motion

back vowel: A vowel produced by pulling the tongue posteriorly, with relation to its neutral position

bands: Range of adjacent parameter values; a frequency band is an ensemble of adjacent frequencies

band pass filter: Filter that allows frequencies only within a certain frequency range to pass

baritone: The most common male vocal range. Higher than bass and lower than tenor. Singer's formant around 2600 Hz

basement membrane: Anatomic structure immediately beneath the epithelium

bass: (*See* **Basso**)

bass baritone: In between bass and baritone. Not as heavy as basso profundo, but typically with greater flexibility. Must be able to sing at least as high as F_4. Also known as *basso contante* and *basso guisto*. Baritones with bass quality are also called *basse taille*

basso: Lowest male voice. Singer's formant around 2300–2400 Hz

basso profundo: Deep bass. The lowest and heaviest of the bass voices. Can sing at least as low as D_2 with full voice. Singer's formant around 2200–2300 Hz. Also known as *contra-basso*

bel canto: Literally means "beautiful singing." Refers to a method and philosophical approach to singing voice production

benchmark: The standard by which other similar occurrences are judged

benign tumors: Tumors that are not able to metastasize or spread to distant sites

Bernoulli's principle: If the energy in a confined fluid stream is constant, an increase in particle velocity must be accompanied by a decrease in pressure against the wall

bifurcation: A sudden qualitative change in the behavior of a system. In chaos, for example, a small change in the initial parameters of a stable (predominantly linear) system may cause oscillation between two different states as the nonlinear aspects of the system become manifest. This transition is a bifurcation

bilabial covering: Using the lips to constrict the mouth opening and "cover" the sound. This technique is used commonly by young singers in the form of slight vowel distortion to attenuate upper harmonics and make a sound richer and less brash.

bilateral: On both sides

bilateral vocal fold paralysis: Loss of the ability to move both vocal folds caused by neurologic dysfunction

biomechanics: The study of the mechanics of biological tissue

bleat: Fast vibrato, like the bleating of a sheep

body: With regard to the vocal fold, the vocalis muscle

Boyle's law: In a soft-walled enclosure and at a constant temperature, pressure and volume are inversely related

bravura: Brilliant, elaborate, showy execution of musical or dramatic material

break: (*See* **Passagio**)

breathy phonation: Phonation characterized by a lack of vocal fold closure; this causes air leakage (excessive airflow) during the quasi-closed phase, and this produces turbulence that is heard as noise mixed in the voice

bronchitis: Inflammation of the bronchial tubes in the lungs

bronchospasm: Forceful closing of the distal airways in the lungs

bruxism: Grinding of the teeth

bulimia: Self-induced vomiting to control weight

butterfly effect: Refers to the notion that in chaotic (nonlinear dynamics) systems a minuscule change in initial condition may have profound effects on the behavior of the system. For example, a butterfly flapping its wings in Hong Kong may change the weather in New York

cancer: An abnormality in which cells no longer respond to the signals that control replication and growth. This results in uncontrolled growth and tumor formation, and may result in spread of tumor to distant locations (metastasis)

carrier: (1) In physics, a waveform (typically a sinusoid) whose frequency or amplitude is modulated by a signal. (2) In medicine, a person who is colonized by an organism (typically bacteria such as streptococcus or pneumococcus), but who has no symptoms or adverse effects from the presence of the organism.

Nevertheless, that carrier is able to transmit the organism to other people in whom it does cause a symptomatic infection

cartilage: One of the tissues of the skeleton; it is more flexible than bone

cartilage of Wrisberg: Cartilage attached in the mobile portion of each aryepiglottic fold

cartilage of Santorini: Small cartilage flexibly attached near the apex of the arytenoid, in the region of the opening of the esophagus

castrato: Male singer castrated at around age 7 or 8, so as to retain alto or soprano vocal range

category: Voice type classified according to pitch range and voice quality; the most frequently used categories are bass, baritone, tenor, alto, mezzosoprano, and soprano, but many other subdivisions of these exist

caudal: Toward the tail

central vowel: A vowel produced with the tongue at or near neutral position

chaos: A qualitative description of a dynamic system that seems unpredictable, but actually has a "hidden" order. Also a mathematical field that studies fractal geometry and nonlinear dynamics

chaotic behavior: Distinct from random or periodic behavior. A chaotic system *looks* disorganized or random but is actually deterministic, although aperiodic. It has sensitive dependence on initial condition, has definite form, and is bounded to a relatively narrow range (unable to go off into infinity)

chest voice: Heavy registration with excessive resonance in the lower formants

coarticulation: A condition in which one phoneme influences the production of phonemes before and after it, resulting commonly in degradation of the quality and clarity of the surrounding sounds

cochlea: Inner ear organ of hearing

coefficient of amplitude variation (vAm): This measure, expressed in percent, computes the relative standard deviation of the peak-to-peak amplitude. It increases regardless of the type of amplitude variation

coefficient of fundamental frequency variation (vF$_0$): This measure, expressed in percent, computes the relative standard deviation of the fundamental frequency. It is the ratio of the standard deviation of the period-to-period variation to the average fundamental frequency

collagen: The protein substance of the white (collagenous) fibers of cartilage, bone, tendon, skin, and all of the connective tissues. Collagen may be extracted, processed, and injected into the vocal fold to treat various abnormalities

collagenase: An enzyme that catalyzes the degradation of collagen

coloratura: In common usage, refers to the highest of the female voices, with range well above C$_6$. May use more whistle tone than other female voices. In fact, coloratura actually refers to a style of florid, agile, complex singing that may apply to any voice classification. For example, the bass runs in Händel's *Messiah* require coloratura technique

complex periodic vibration: A sound that repeats regularly. A pattern of simultaneously sounding partials

complex sound: A combination of sinusoidal waveforms superimposed upon each other. May be complex periodic sound (such as musical instruments) or complex aperiodic sound (such as random street noise)

complex tone: Tone composed of a series of simultaneously sounding partials

component frequency: mathematically, a sinusoid; perceptually, a pure tone. Also called a *partial*

compression: A deformation of a body that decreases its entire volume. An increase in density

concert pitch: Also known as *international concert pitch*. The standard of tuning A$_4$. Reference pitch has changed substantially over the last 200 to 300 years

condensation: An increase in density

constructive interference: The interference of two or more waves such that enhancement occurs

contact ulcer: A lesion with mucosal disruption most commonly on the vocal processes or medial surfaces of the arytenoids. Caused most commonly by gastroesophageal reflux laryngitis and/or muscular tension dysphonia

contrabasso: (*See* **Basso profundo**)

contraction: A decrease in length

contralto: Lowest of the female voices. Able to sing F$_3$ below middle C, as well as the entire treble staff. Singer's formant at around 2800–2900 Hz

conus elasticus: Fibroelastic membrane extending inferiorly from the vocal folds to the anterior superior border of the cricoid cartilage. Also called the *cricovocal ligament*. Composed primarily of yellow elastic tissue. Anteriorly, it attaches to the minor aspect of the thyroid cartilage. Posteriorly, it attaches to the vocal process of the arytenoids

convergent: With regard to glottal shape, the glottis narrows from bottom to top

corner vowels: (ɑ), (i), and (u); vowels at the corners of a vowel triangle; they necessitate extreme placements of the tongue

corticosteroid: Potent substances produced by the adrenal cortex (excluding sex hormones of adrenal origin) in response to the release of adrenocorticotropic hormone from the pituitary gland, or related substances. Glucocorticoids influence carbohydrate, fat, and protein metabolism. Mineralocorticoids help regular electrolyte and water balance. Some corticosteroids have both effects to varying degrees. Corticosteroids may also be given as medications for various effects, including anti-inflammatory, antineoplastic, immune suppressive, and ACTH secretion suppressive effects, as well as for hormone replacement therapy

countertenor: Male voice that is primarily falsetto, singing in the contralto range. Most countertenors are also able to sing in the baritone or tenor range. Countertenors are also known as *contraltino* or *contratenor*

cover: (1) In medicine, with regard to the vocal fold, the epithelium and superficial layer of lamina propria. (2) In music, an alteration in technique that changes the resonance characteristics of a sung sound, generally darkening the sound

cranial nerves: Twelve paired nerves responsible for smell, taste, eye movement, vision, facial sensation, chewing muscles, facial motion, salivary gland and lacrimal (tear) gland secretions, hearing, balance, pharyngeal and laryngeal sensation, vocal fold motion, gastric acid secretion, shoulder motion, tongue motion, and related functions

creaky voice: The perceptual result of subharmonic or chaotic patterns in the glottal waveform. According to IR Titze, if a subharmonic is below about 70 Hz, creaky voice may be perceived as pulse register (vocal fry)

crescendo: To get gradually louder

cricoid cartilage: A solid ring of cartilage located below and behind the thyroid cartilage

cricothyroid muscle: An intrinsic laryngeal muscle that is used primarily to control pitch (paired)

crossover frequency: The fundamental frequency for which there is an equal probability for perception of two adjacent registers

cycle: One complete set of regularly recurring events

cysts: Fluid-filled lesions

damp: To diminish, or attenuate an oscillation

damped oscillation: Oscillation in which energy is lost during each cycle until oscillation stops

decibel: One tenth of a bel. The decibel is a unit of comparison between a reference and another point. It has no absolute value. Although decibels are used to measure sound, they are also used (with different references) to measure heat, light, and other physical phenomena. For sound pressure, the reference is 0.0002 microbar (millionths of one barometric pressure). In the past, this has also been referred to as 0.0002 dyne/cm^2, and by other terms

decrescendo: (*See* **Diminuendo**)

deformation: The result of stress applied to any surface of a deformable continuous medium. Elongation, compression, contraction, and shear are examples

dehydration: Fluid deprivation. This may alter the amount and viscosity of vocal fold lubrication and the properties of the vocal fold tissues themselves

destructive interference: The interference of two or more waves such that full or partial cancellation occurs

dialect: A variety of a spoken language, usually associated with a distinct geographical, social, or political environment

diaphragm: A large, dome-shaped muscle at the bottom of the rib cage that separates the lungs from the viscera. It is the primary muscle of inspiration and may be co-activated during singing

diminuendo: To get gradually softer

diphthong: Two consecutive vowels occurring in the same syllable

displacement: The distance between two points in space, including the direction from one point to the other

displacement flow: Air in the glottis that is squeezed out when the vocal folds come together

diuretic: A drug to decrease circulating body fluid generally by excretion through the kidneys

divergent: With regard to the vocal folds, the glottis widens from bottom to top

dizziness: A feeling of imbalance

dorsal: Toward the back

down-regulation: Decreased gene expression, compared with baseline

dramatic soprano: Soprano with powerful, rich voice suitable for dramatic, heavily orchestrated, operatic roles. Sings at least to C$_6$

dramatic tenor: Tenor with heavy voice, often with a suggestion of baritone quality. Suitable for dramatic roles that are heavily orchestrated. Also referred to as *tenora robusto*, and *helden tenor*. The term helden tenor (literally "heroic" tenor) is used typically for tenors who sing Wagnerian operatic roles

dynamics: (1) In physics, a branch of mechanics that deals with the study of forces that accelerate object(s). (2) In music, it refers to changes in the loudness of musical performance

dysmenorrhea: Painful menstrual cramps

dyspepsia: Epigastric discomfort, especially following meals; impairment of the power or function of digestion

dysphonia: Abnormal voicing

dysphonia plica ventricularis: Phonation using false vocal fold vibration rather than true vocal fold vibration. Most commonly associated with severe muscular tension dysphonia Occasionally may be an appropriate compensation for profound true vocal fold dysfunction

dystonia: A neurological disorder characterized by involuntary movements, such as unpredictable, spasmodic opening or closing of the vocal folds

edema: Excessive accumulation of fluid in tissues, or "swelling"

elastic recoil pressure: The alveolar pressure derived from extended (strained) tissue in the lungs, rib cage, and the entire thorax after inspiration (measured in Pascals)

electroglottograph (EGG): Recording of electrical conductance of vocal fold contact area versus time; EGG waveforms have been frequently used for the purpose of plotting voice source analysis

electromyograph (EMG): Recording of the electric potentials in a muscle, which are generated by the neural system and which control its degree of contraction; if rectified and smoothed the EMG is closely related to the muscular force exerted by the muscle

elongation: An increase in length

embouchure: The shape of the lips, tongue, and related structures adopted while producing a musical tone, particularly while playing a wind instrument

endocrine: Relating to hormones and the organs that produce them

endometriosis: A disorder in which endometrial tissue is present in abnormal locations. Typically causes excessively painful menstrual periods (dysmenorrhea) and infertility

epiglottis: Cartilage that covers over the larynx during swallowing

epilarynx: A region bordered by the rim of the epiglottis and the glottis synonymous with epiglottal tube. This resonating region is considered by some to be the site of origin of the singer's formant

epithelium: The covering, or most superficial layer, of body surfaces

erythema: Redness

esophagus: Tube leading from the bottom of the pharynx to the stomach; swallowed food is transported through this structure

expansion: A deformation of a body such that the entire volume increases

extrinsic muscles of the larynx: The strap muscles in the neck, responsible for adjusting laryngeal height and for stabilizing the larynx

Fach (German): Literally, job specialty. It is used to indicate voice classification. For example, lyric soprano and dramatic soprano are different Fachs

false vocal folds: Folds of tissue located slightly higher than and parallel to the vocal folds in the larynx

falsetto: High, light register, applied primarily to men's voices singing in the soprano or alto range. Can also be applied to women's voices

fibroblasts: Cells responsible in part for the formation of scar in response to tissue injury

fibrosis: Generally refers to a component of scar caused by cross-linking of fibers during a reactive or a reparative process

flat singing: Usually refers to pitch (frequency) lower than the desirable target frequency. Sometimes also used to refer to a singing style devoid of excitement or emotional expression

flow: The volume of fluid passing through a given cross-section of a tube or duct per second; also called volume velocity (measured in liters per second)

flow glottogram: Recording of the transglottal airflow versus time, ie, of the sound of the voice source. Generally obtained from inverse filtering, FLOGG is the acoustical representation of the voice source

flow phonation: The optimal balance between vocal fold adductory forces and subglottic pressure, producing efficient sound production at the level of the vocal folds

flow resistance: The ratio of pressure to flow

fluid: A substance that is either a liquid or a gas

fluid mechanics: The study of motion or deformation of liquids and gases

flutter: Modulation in the 10–12 Hz range

F_0: Fundamental frequency

F_0–tremor frequency (Fftr): This measure is expressed in Hz and shows the frequency of the most intensive low-frequency F_0 modulating component in the specified F_0 tremor analysis range

F_0–tremor intensity index (FTRI): The average ratio of the frequency magnitude of the most intensive low-frequency modulating component (F_0 tremor) to the total frequency magnitude of the analyzed sample. The algorithm for tremor analysis determines the strongest periodic frequency modulation of the voice. This measure is expressed in percent

focal: Limited to a specific area. For example, spasmodic dysphonia may be focal (limited to the larynx), or part of a group of dystonias that affect other parts of the body such as the facial muscles or muscles involved in chewing

force: A push or pull; the physical quantity imparted to an object to change its momentum

forced oscillation: Oscillation imposed on a system by an external source

formant: Vocal tract resonance; the formant frequencies are tuned by the vocal tract shape and determine much of the vocal quality

formant tuning: A boosting of vocal intensity when F_0 or one if its harmonics coincides exactly with a formant frequency

front vowel: A vowel formed by displacing the tongue anteriorly, with regard to its neutral position

functional residual capacity (FRC): Lung volume at which the elastic inspiratory forces equal the elastic expiratory forces; in spontaneous quiet breathing exhalation stops at FRC

fractal: A geometric figure in which an identical pattern or motif repeats itself over and over on an ever-diminishing scale. Self-similarity is an essential characteristic

fractal dimension: Fractal dimensions are measures of fractal objects that can be used to determine how alike or different the objects are. Box counting algorithms and mass-radius measurement are two common approaches to determining fractal dimension. The fractal dimension represents the way a set of points fills a given area of space. It may be defined as the slope of the function relating the number of points contained in a given radius (or its magnification) to the radius itself. For example, an object can be assessed under many magnifications. The coast of Britain can be measured, for example, with a meter stick or a millimeter stick, but the latter will yield a larger measure. As magnification is increased (smaller measuring sticks), a point will be reached at which small changes in magnification no longer significantly affect length. That is, a plot of coastline length versus magnification reaches a plateau. That plateau corresponds to fractal dimension. The more irregular the figure (eg, coastline), the more complex and the more space it occupies, hence, the higher its fractal dimension. A perfect line has a fractal dimension of 1. A figure that fills a plane has a fractal dimension of 2. Fractal dimension cannot be used alone to determine the presence or absence of chaotic behavior

frequency analysis: Same as spectrum analysis

frequency tremor: A periodic (regular) pitch modulation of the voice (an element of vibrato)

fricative: A speech sound, generally a consonant, produced by a constriction of the vocal tract, particularly by directing the airstream against a hard surface, producing noisy air turbulence. Examples include *s* produced with the teeth, *s* produced with the lower lip and upper incisors, and *th* produced with the tongue tip and upper incisors

frontal (or coronal) plane: An anatomic plane that divides the body into anterior and posterior portions; across the crown of the head

functional voice disorder: An abnormality in voice sound and function in the absence of an anatomic or physiologic organic abnormality

fundamental: Lowest partial of a spectrum, the frequency of which normally corresponds to the pitch perceived.

fundamental frequency (F_0): The lowest frequency in a periodic waveform; also called the first harmonic frequency

gas: A substance that preserves neither shape nor volume when acted upon by forces, but adapts readily to the size and shape of its container

gastric: Pertaining to the stomach

gastric juice: The contents of the stomach, ordinarily including a high concentration of hydrochloric acid.

gastroesophageal reflux (GER): The passage of gastric juice in a retrograde fashion from the stomach into the esophagus. These fluids may reach the level of the larynx or oral cavity, and may be aspirated into the lungs

gastroesophageal reflux disease (GERD): A disorder including symptoms and/or signs caused by reflux of gastric juice into the esophagus and elsewhere. Heartburn is one of the most common symptoms of GERD. (*See* also **Laryngopharyngeal reflux**)

genomics: The study of genes (genetic material) made up of DNA, and located in the chromosomes of the nuclei of cells in an organism.

glide: A written consonant that is produced as a vowel sound in transition to the following vowel. Examples include: /j/ and /w/

glissando: A "slide" including all possible pitches between the initial and final pitch sounded. Similar to portamento and slur

globus: Sensation of a lump in the throat

glottal: At the level of the vocal folds

glottal chink: Opening in the glottis during vocal fold adduction, most commonly posteriorly. It may be a normal variant in some cases

glottal resistance: Ratio between transglottal airflow and subglottal pressure; mainly reflects the degree of glottal adduction

glottal stop (or click): A transient sound caused by the sudden onset or offset of phonation

glottal stroke: A brief event in which air pressure is increased behind the occluded glottis and then released, more gently than following a glottal stop. Glottal strokes are used to separate phonemes in linguistic situations in which running them together might result in misunderstanding of the meaning

glottis: Space between the vocal folds. (*See* also **Rima glottitis**)

glottis respiratoria: The portion of the glottis posteriorly in the region of the cartilaginous portions of the vocal folds

glottis vocalis: The portion of the glottis in the region of the membranous portions of the vocal folds

grace days: Refers to a former contractual arrangement, especially in European Opera Houses, in which women were permitted to refrain from singing during the premenstrual and early menstrual portions of their cycles, at their discretion

granuloma: A raised lesion generally covered with mucosa, most commonly in the region of the vocal

process or medial surface of the arytenoid. Often caused by reflux and/or muscle tension dysphonia

halitosis: Bad breath

harmonic: A frequency that is an integer multiple of a given fundamental. Harmonics of a fundamental are equally spaced in frequency. Partial in a spectrum in which the frequency of each partial equals n times the fundamental frequency, n being the number of the harmonic

harsh glottal attack: Initiating phonation of a word or sound with a glottal plosive

head voice: A vocal quality characterized by flexibility and lightness of tone. In some classifications, it is used to designate a high register of the singing voice

hemorrhage: Rupture of a blood vessel. This may occur in a vocal fold

hertz: Cycles per second (Hz) (named after Gustav Hertz)

high pass filter: Filter which only allows frequencies above a certain cutoff frequency to pass; the cutoff is generally not abrupt but, rather, gentle and is given in terms of a roll-off value, eg, 24 dB/octave

histogram: Graph showing the occurrence of a parameter value; thus, a fundamental frequency histogram shows the occurrence of different fundamental frequency values, eg, in fluent speech or in a song

Hooke's law: Stress in proportion to strain; or, in simpler form, force is proportional to elongation

hormones: Substances produced within the body that affect or control various organs and bodily functions

hyoid bone: A horseshoe-shaped bone known as the "tongue bone." It is attached to muscles of the tongue and related structures, and to the larynx and related structures

hyperfunction: Excessive muscle effort for example, pressed voice, muscle tension dysphonia

hypernasal: Excessive nasal resonance

hypofunction: Low muscular effort, for example, soft breathy voice

hyponasal: Deficient nasal resonance

hypothyroidism: Lower than normal output of thyroid hormone. This condition is referred to commonly as an "underactive thyroid," and often results in malaise, weight gain, temperature intolerance, irregular menses, muffling of the voice, and other symptoms

Hz: (*See* **Hertz**)

impotence: The inability to accomplish penile erection

in vitro: Outside the living body, for example, an excised larynx

in vivo: In the living body

incompressibility: Property of a substance that conserves volume in a deformation

inertia: Sluggishness; a property of resisting a change in momentum

inferior: Below

infertility: The inability to accomplish pregnancy

infraglottic: Below the level of the glottis (space between the vocal folds). This region includes the trachea, thorax, and related structures

infraglottic vocal tract: Below the level of the vocal folds. This region includes the airways and muscles of support (Infraglottic is synonymous with subglottic)

infrahyoid muscle group: A collection of extrinsic muscles including the sternohyoid, sternothyroid, omohyoid, and thyroid muscles

insertion: The point of attachment of a muscle with a bone that can be moved by the muscle

intensity: A measure of power per unit area. With respect to sound, it generally correlates with perceived loudness

interarytenoid muscle: An intrinsic laryngeal muscle that connects the two arytenoid cartilages

intercostal muscles: Muscles between the ribs

interval: The difference between two pitches, expressed in terms of musical scale

intrinsic laryngeal muscles: muscles within the larynx responsible for abduction, adduction, and longitudinal tension of the vocal folds

intrinsic pitch of vowels: Refers to the fact that in normal speech certain vowels tend to be produced with a significantly higher or lower pitch than other vowels

inverse filtering: Method used for recovering the transglottal airflow during phonation; the technique implies that the voice is fed through a computer filter that compensates for the resonance effects of the supraglottic vocal tract, especially the lowest formants

inverse square law: Sound intensity is inversely proportional to the square of the distance from the sound source

IPA: International Phonetic Alphabet (*See* **Appendix I**)

isometric: Constant muscle length during contraction

iteration: In mathematics, the repetitive process of substituting the solution to an equation back into the same equation to obtain the next solution

jitter: Irregularity in the period of time of vocal fold vibrations; cycle-to-cycle variation in fundamental frequency; jitter is often perceived as hoarseness

jitter percent (Jitt): A relative measure of very short term (cycle-to-cycle) variation of the pitch periods expressed in percent. The influence of the average fundamental frequency is significantly reduced. This parameter is very sensitive to pitch variations

juvenile papillomatosis: A disease of children characterized by the clustering of many papillomas (small blisterlike growths) over the vocal folds and elsewhere in the larynx and trachea. Papillomatosis may also occur in adults, in which case the adjective *juvenile* is not used. The disease is caused by human papilloma virus

keratosis: A buildup of keratin (a tough, fibrous protein) on the surface of the vocal folds

kinematics: The study of movement as a consequence of known or assumed forces

kinetic energy: The energy of matter in motion (measured in joules)

klangfarbe: Tone color, referring to vocal quality

labiodental: A consonant produced by bringing the lower lip in contact with the upper front teeth

lag: A difference in time between one point and another

lamina propria: With reference to the larynx, the tissue layers below the epithelium. In adult humans, the lamina propria consists of superficial, intermediate, and deep layers

laminar: Smooth or layered; in fluid mechanics, indicating parallel flow lines

laminar flow: Airflow in smooth layers over a surface (as differentiated from irregular, or turbulent flow)

laryngeal saccule: (*See* **Appendix of the Ventricle of Morgagni**)

laryngeal sinus: (*See* **Ventricle of Morgagni**)

laryngeal ventricle: Cavity formed by the gap between the true and false vocal folds

laryngeal web: An abnormal tissue connection attaching the vocal folds to each other

laryngectomy: Removal of the larynx. It may be total, or it may be a "conservation laryngectomy," in which a portion of the larynx is preserved

laryngitis: Inflammation of laryngeal tissues

laryngitis sicca: Dry voice

laryngocele: A pouch or herniation of the larynx, usually filled with air and sometimes presenting as a neck mass. The pouch usually enlarges with increased laryngeal pressure as may occur from coughing or playing a wind instrument.

laryngologist: Physician specializing in disorders of the larynx and voice, in most countries. In some areas of Europe, the laryngologist is primarily responsible for surgery, while diagnosis is performed by phoniatricians

laryngomalacia: A condition in which the laryngeal cartilages are excessively soft and may collapse in response to inspiratory pressures, obstructing the airway

laryngopharyngeal reflux (LPR): A form of gastroesophageal reflux disease in which gastric juice affects the larynx and adjacent structures. Commonly associated with hoarseness, frequent throat clearing, granulomas, and other laryngeal problems, even in the absence of heartburn

laryngospasm: Sudden, forceful, and abnormal closing of the vocal folds

larynx: The body organ in the neck that includes the vocal folds. The "voice box"

larynx height: Vertical position of the larynx; mostly measured in relation to the rest position

larynx tube: Cavity formed by the vocal folds and the arytenoid, epiglottis, and thyroid cartilages and the structures joining them

laser: An acronym for *light amplification by stimulated emission of radiation*. A surgical tool using light energy to vaporize or cauterize tissue

lateral: Toward the side (away from the center).

lateral cricoarytenoid muscle: Intrinsic laryngeal muscle that adducts the vocal folds through forward rocking and rotation of the arytenoids (paired)

LD50: In determining drug toxicity, the LD50 is the amount of the substance that will cause death in 50% of test specimens (lethal dose for 50%)

lesion: In medicine, a nonspecific term that may be used for nearly any structural abnormality

legato: Smooth, connected

leukoplakia: A white plaque. Typically, this occurs on mucous membranes, including the vocal folds

level: Logarithmic and comparative measure of sound intensity; the unit is normally dB

lied: Song, particularly art song

lift: (*See* **Passagio**)

ligament: Connective tissue between articular regions of bone

linear system: A system in which the relation between input and output varies in a constant, or linear, fashion

lingual: Related to the tongue

linguadental: A consonant produced by bringing the tongue in contact with the teeth

linguapalatal: A consonant produced by bringing the tongue in contact with the hard palate

lip covering: Altering lip shape to make a sound less brash or bright, and "rounder" or more "rich"

liquid: A substance that assumes the shape of its container, but preserves its volume

loft: A suggested term for the highest (loftiest) register; usually referred to as *falsetto voice*

logistic map: A simple quadratic equation that exhibits chaotic behavior under special initial conditions and parameters. It is the simplest chaotic system

Lombard effect: Modification of vocal loudness in response to auditory input. For example, the tendency to speak louder in the presence of background noise

long-term average spectrum (LTAS): Graph showing a long-time average of the sound intensity in various frequency bands; the appearance of an LTAS is strongly dependent on the filters used

longitudinal: Along the length of a structure

longitudinal tension: With reference to the larynx, stretching the vocal folds

loudness: The amount of sound perceived by a listener; a perceptual quantity that can only be assessed with an auditory system. Loudness corresponds to intensity, and to the amplitude of a sound wave

low pass filter: Filter which allows only frequencies below a certain frequency to pass; the cutoff is generally not at all abrupt but gentle and is given in terms of a roll-off value, eg, 24 dB/octave

LTAS: An acronym for long-term-averaged spectrum

lung volume: Volume contained in the subglottic air system; after a maximum inhalation following a maximum exhalation the lung volume equals the vital capacity

lyric soprano: Soprano with flexible, light vocal quality, but one who does not sing as high as a coloratura soprano

lyric tenor: Tenor with a light, high flexible voice

malignant tumor: Tumors that have the potential to metastasize, or spread to different sites. They also have the potential to invade, destroy, and replace adjacent tissues. However, benign tumors may have the capacity for substantial local destruction, as well

Mandelbrot's set: A series of two equations containing real and imaginary components that, when iterated and plotted on a two-dimensional graph, depict a very complex and classic fractal pattern

mandible: Jaw

marcato: Each note accented

marking: Using the voice gently (typically during rehearsals) to avoid injury or fatigue

masque (mask): "Singing in the masque" refers to a frontal tonal placement conceptualized by singers as being associated with vibration of the bones of the face. It is generally regarded as a healthy placement associated with rich resonant characteristics and commonly a strong singer's formant (or "ring")

mechanical equilibrium: The state in which all forces acting on a body cancel each other out, leaving a zero net force in all directions

mechanics: The study of objects in motion and the forces that produce the motion

medial (or mesial): Toward the center (midline or midplane).

melisma: Two or more notes sung on a single syllable

menopause: Cessation of menstrual cycles and menstruation. Associated with physiologic infertility

menstrual cycle: The normal, cyclical variation of hormones in adult females of child-bearing age, and bodily responses caused by those hormonal variations

menstrual period: The first part of the menstrual cycle, associated with endometrial shedding and vaginal bleeding

messa di voce: Traditional exercise in Italian singing tradition consisting of a long prolonged crescendo and diminuendo on a sustained tone

metastasis: Spread of tumor to locations other than the primary tumor site

mezza voce: Literally means "half voice." In practice, means singing softly, but with proper support

mezzo soprano: Literally means "half soprano." This is a common female range, higher than contralto but lower than soprano

middle (or mixed): A mixture of qualities from various voice registers, cultivated in order to allow consistent quality throughout the frequency range

middle C: C_4 on the piano keyboard, with an international concert pitch frequency of 261.6 Hz

millisecond: One thousandth of a second; usually noted ms. or msec

modulation: Periodic variation of a signal property; for example, as vibrato corresponds to a regular variation of fundamental frequency, it can be regarded as a modulation of that signal property

motor: Having to do with motion. For example, motor nerves allow structures to move

motor unit: A group of muscle fibers and the single motor nerve that activates the fibers

mucocele: A benign lesion filled with liquid mucus

mucolytic: A substance that thins mucous secretions

mucosa: The covering of the surfaces of the respiratory tract, including the oral cavity and nasal cavities, as well as the pharynx, larynx, and lower airways. Mucosa also exits elsewhere, such as on the lining of the vagina

mucosal tear: With reference to the vocal folds, disruption of the surface of the vocal fold. Usually caused by trauma

mucosal wave: Undulation along the vocal fold surface traveling in the direction of the airflow

modulation: The systematic change of a cyclic parameter, such as amplitude or frequency

momentum: Mass times velocity; a quantity that determines the potential force that an object can impart to another object by collision

muscle fascicles: Groups of muscle fibers enclosed by a sheath of connective tissue

muscle fibers: A long, thin cell; the basic unit of a muscle that is excited by a nerve ending

muscle tension dysphonia: Also called muscular tension dysphonia. A form of voice abuse characterized by excessive muscular effort, and usually by pressed phonation. A form of voice misuse

mutational dysphonia: A voice disorder. Most typically, it is characterized by persistent falsetto voice after puberty in a male. More generally, it is used to refer to voice with characteristics of the opposite gender

myasthenia gravis: A neuromuscular junction disease associated with fatigue

myoelastic-aerodynamic theory of phonation: The currently accepted mechanism of vocal fold physiology. Compressed air exerts pressure on the undersurface of the closed vocal folds. The pressure overcomes adductory forces, causing the vocal folds to open. The elasticity of the displaced tissues (along with the Bernoulli effect) causes the vocal folds to snap shut, resulting in sound.

myofibril: A subdivision of a muscle fiber; composed of a number of myofilaments

myofilament: A microstructure of periodically arranged actin and myosin molecules; a subdivision of a myofibril

myosin: A protein molecule that reacts with actin to form actinomycin, the contractile part of a myofilament

nasal tract: Air cavity system of the nose

NATS: National Association of Teachers of Singing

natural oscillation: Oscillation without imposed driving forces

neoplasm: Abnormal growth. May be benign or malignant

nervous system: Organs of the body including the brain, spinal cord, and nerves. Responsible for motion, sensation, thought, and control of various other bodily functions

neurotologist: Otolaryngologist specializing in disorders of the ear and ear-brain interface (including the skull base), particularly hearing loss, dizziness, tinnitus, and facial nerve dysfunction

neutral vowel: A vowel produced in the center of the oral cavity.

nodes: The "valleys" in a standing wave pattern

nodules: Benign growths on the surface of the vocal folds. Usually paired and fairly symmetric. They are generally caused by chronic, forceful vocal fold contact (voice abuse)

noise: Unwanted sound

noise-to-harmonic ratio (NHR): A general evaluation of noise percent in the signal and includes jitter, shimmer, and turbulent noise

nonlinear dynamics: (*See also* **Chaos** and **Chaotic Behavior**) The mathematical study of aperiodic, deterministic systems that are not random and cannot be described accurately by linear equations. The study of nonlinear systems whose state changes with time

nonlinear system: Any system in which the output is disproportionate to the input

objective assessment: Demonstrable, reproducible, usually quantifiable evaluation, generally relying on instrumentation or other assessment techniques that do not involve primarily opinion, as opposed to subjective assessment

octave: Interval between two pitches with frequencies in the ratio of 2:1

off-glide: Transition from a vowel of long duration to one of short duration

olfaction: The sense of smell, mediated by the first cranial nerve

on-glide: Transition from a sound of short duration to a vowel of longer duration

onset: The beginning of phonation

open quotient: The ratio of the time the glottis is open to the length of the entire vibratory cycle

oral contraceptive: Birth control pill

organic disorder: A disorder due to structural malfunction, malformation, or injury, as opposed to psychogenic disorders

organic voice disorder: Disorder for which a specific anatomic or physiologic cause can be identified, as opposed to psychogenic or functional voice disorders

origin: The beginning point of a muscle and related soft tissue

oscillation: Repeated movement, back and forth

oscillator: With regard to the larynx, the vibrator that is responsible for the sound source, specifically the vocal folds

ossicle: Middle ear bone

ossify: To become bony

ostium: Opening

otolaryngologist: Ear, nose, and throat physician

otologist: Otolaryngologist specializing in disorders of the ear

overtone: Partial above the fundamental in a spectrum

ovulation: The middle of the menstrual cycle, associated with release of an ovum (egg), and the period of fertility

palatal: Related to the palate (*See* also **Linguapalatal**)

papillomas: Small benign epithelial tumors that may appear randomly or in clusters on the vocal folds, larynx, and trachea and elsewhere in the body. Believed to be caused by various types of human papillomavirus (HPV), some of which are associated with malignancy

parietal pleura: The outermost of two membranes surrounding the lungs

partial: Sinusoid that is part of a complex tone; in voiced sounds, the partials are harmonic implying that the frequency of the nth partial equals n times the fundamental frequency

particle: A finite mass with zero dimensions, located at a single point in space

pascal (Pa): International standard unit of pressure; one newton (N) per meter squared (m^2)

Pascal's law: Pressure is transmitted rapidly and uniformly throughout an enclosed fluid at rest

pass band: A band of frequencies minimally affected by a filter

passaggio (Italian): The break between vocal registers

period: (1) In physics, the time interval between repeating events; shortest pattern repeated in a regular undulation; a graph showing the period is called a waveform. (2) In medicine, the time during the menstrual cycle associated with bleeding and shedding of the endometrial lining

period doubling: One form of bifurcation in which a system that originally had x period states now has 2x periodic states, with a change having occurred in response to a change in parameter or initial condition

period time: In physics, duration of a period

periodic behavior: Repeating over and over again over a finite time interval. Periodic behavior is governed by an underlying deterministic process

peristalsis: Successive contractions of musculature, which cause a bolus of food to pass through the alimentary tract

perturbation: Small disturbances or changes from expected behavior

pharyngocele: A pouch or herniation of part of the pharynx (throat), commonly fills with air in wind players

pharynx: The region above the larynx, below the velum and posterior to the oral cavity

phase: (1) The manner in which molecules are arranged in a material (gas, liquid, or solid); (2) the angular separation between two events on periodic waveforms

phase plane plot: Representation of a dynamic system in state space

phase space: A space created by two or more independent dynamic variables, such as positions and velocities, utilized to plot the trajectory of a moving object

phase spectrum: A display of the relative phases versus frequency of the components of a waveform

phonation: Sound generation by means of vocal fold vibrations

phoneme: A unit of sound within a specific language

phonetics: The study of speech sounds

phonetogram: Recording of highest and lowest sound pressure level versus fundamental frequency that a voice can produce; phonetograms are often used for describing the status of voice function in patients. Also called *voice range profile*

phoniatrician: A physician specializing in diagnosis and nonsurgical treatment of voice disorders. This specialty does not exist in American medical training, where the phoniatrician's activities are accomplished as a team by the laryngologist (responsible for diagnosis and surgical treatment when needed) and speech-language pathologist (responsible for behavioral voice therapy)

phonosurgery: Originally, surgery designed to alter vocal quality or pitch. Now used commonly to refer to all delicate microsurgical procedures of the vocal folds

phonotrauma: Vocal fold injury caused by vocal fold contact during phonation, associated most commonly with voice abuse or misuse

phrenic nerve: The nerve that controls the diaphragm. Responsible for inspiration. Composed primarily of fibers from the third, fourth, and fifth cervical roots

piriform sinus: Pouch or cavity constituting the lower end of the pharynx located to the side and partially to the back of the larynx. There are two, paired pyriform sinuses in the normal individual

pitch: Perceived tone quality corresponding to its fundamental frequency

pitch matching: Experiment in which subjects are asked to produce the pitch of a reference tone

pitch period perturbation quotient (PPQ): A relative evaluation of short term (cycle-to-cycle) variation of the pitch periods expressed in percent

pleural space: The fluid-filled space between the parietal and visceral pleura

plosive: A consonant produced by creating complete blockage of airflow, followed by the buildup of air pressure, which is then suddenly released, producing a consonant sound

Poincaré section: A graphical technique to reveal a discernable pattern in a phase plane plot that does not have an apparent pattern. There are two kinds of Poincaré sections

polyp: A sessile or pedunculated growth. Usually unilateral and benign, but the term is descriptive and does not imply a histological diagnosis

posterior: Toward the back

posterior cricoarytenoid muscle: An intrinsic laryngeal muscle that is the primary abductor of the vocal folds (paired)

power: The rate of delivery (or expenditure) of energy (measured in watts)

power source: The expiratory system including the muscles of the abdomen, back, thorax, and the lungs. Responsible for producing a vector of force that results in efficient creation and control of subglottal pressure

power spectrum: Two-dimensional graphic analysis of sound with frequency on the x axis and amplitude on the y axis

prechaotic behavior: Predictable behavior prior to the onset of chaotic behavior. One example is period doubling

pressed phonation: Type of phonation characterized by small airflow, high adductory force, and high subglottal pressure. Not an efficient form of voice production. Often associated with voice abuse, and common in patients with lesions such as nodules

pressure: Force per unit area

prevoicing: Phonation that occurs briefly before phonation of a stop consonant

prima donna: Literally means "first lady." Refers to the soprano soloist, especially the lead singer in an opera

primo passaggio: "The first passage"; the first register change perceived in a voice as pitch is raised from low to high

proteomics: The study of proteins

psychogenic: Caused by psychological factors, rather than physical dysfunction. Psychogenic disorders may result in physical dysfunction or structural injury

pulmonary system: The breathing apparatus including the lungs and related airways

pulse register: The extreme low end of the phonatory range. Also know as *vocal fry* and *Strohbass*, characterized by a pattern of short glottal waves alternating with larger and longer ones, and with a long closed phase

pure tone: Sinusoid. The simplest tone. Produced electronically. In nature, even pure-sounding tones like bird songs are complex

pyrotechnics: Special effects involving combustion and explosion, used to produce dramatic visual displays (similar to fireworks), indoors or outdoors

pyrosis: Heartburn

quadrangular membrane: Elastic membrane extending from the sides of the epiglottic cartilage to the corniculate and arytenoid cartilages. Mucosa covered. Forms the aryepiglottic fold and the wall between the piriform sinus and larynx

quasiperiodic: A behavior that has at least two frequencies in which the phases are related by an irrational number

radian: The angular measure obtained when the arc along the circumference of the circle is equal to the radius

radian frequency: The number of radians per second covered in circular or sinusoidal motion

random behavior: Action that never repeats itself and is inherently unpredictable

rarefaction: A decrease in density

recurrent laryngeal nerves: The paired branches of the vagus nerve that supply all of the intrinsic muscles of the larynx except for the cricothyroid muscles. The recurrent laryngeal nerves also carry sensory fibers (feeling) to the mucosa below the level of the vocal folds

reflux: (*See* **Gastroesophageal Reflux** and **Laryngopharyngeal Reflux**)

reflux laryngitis: Inflammation of the larynx due to irritation from gastric juice

refractive eye surgery: Surgery to correct visual acuity

registers: Weakly defined term for vocal qualities; often, register refers to a series of adjacent tones on the scale that sound similar and seem to be generated by the same type of vocal fold vibrations and vocal tract adjustments. Examples of register are vocal fry, modal, and falsetto; but numerous other terms are also used

regulation: The events by which a protein is produced or destroyed, and the balance between these two conditions

Reinke's space: The superficial layer of the lamina propria

relative average perturbation (RAP): A relative evaluation of short-term (cycle-to-cycle) variation of the pitch periods expressed in percent

relative voice rest: Restricted, cautious voice use

resonance: Peak occurring at certain frequencies (resonance frequencies) in the vibration amplitude in a system that possesses compliance, inertia, and reflection; resonance occurs when the input and the reflected energy vibrate in phase; the resonances in the vocal tract are called *formants*

resonator: With regard to the voice, refers primarily to the supraglottic vocal tract, which is responsible for timbre and projection

restoring force: A force that brings an object back to a stable equilibrium position

return map: Similar to phase plane plot, but analyzed data must be digital. This graphic technique represents the relationship between a point and any subsequent point in a time series

rhinorrhea: Nasal discharge; runny nose

rhotic: A vowel sound produced with r-coloring.

rima glottitis: The space between the vocal folds. Also known as the glottis

roll-off: Characteristics of filters specifying their ability to shut off frequencies outside the pass band; for example, if a low pass filter is set to 2 kHz and has a roll-off of 24 dB/octave, it will alternate a 4 kHz tone by 24 dB and a 8 kHz tone by 48 dB

rostral: Toward the mouth (beak)

sagittal: An anatomic plane that divides the body into left and right sides

sarcoplasmic reticulum: Connective tissue enveloping groups of muscle fibers

scalar: A quantity that scales, or adjusts size; a single number

second passaggio: "The second passage"; the second register change perceived in a voice

semicircular canal: Inner ear organ of balance

semi-vowel: A consonant that has vowel-like resonance

sensory: Having to do with the feeling or detection of other nonmotor input. For example, nerves responsible for touch, proprioception (position in space), hearing, and so on

sharp singing: Singing at a pitch (frequency) higher than the desirable target pitch

shimmer: Cycle-to-cycle variability in amplitude

shimmer percent: Is the same as shimmer dB but expressed in percent instead of dB. Both are relative evaluations of the same type of amplitude perturbation but they use different measures for this result: either percent or dB

simple harmonic motion: Sinusoidal motion; the smoothest back and forth motion possible

simple tone: (*See* **Pure Tone**)

singer's formant: A high spectrum peak occurring between about 2.3 and 3.5 kHz in voiced sounds in Western opera and concert singing. This acoustic phenomenon is associated with "ring" in a voice, and with the voices ability to project over background noise such as a choir or an orchestra. A similar phenomenon may be seen in speaking voices, especially in actors. It is known as the *speaker's formant*

singing teacher: Professional who teaches singing technique (as opposed to Voice Coach).

singing voice specialist: A singing teacher with additional training, and specialization in working with injured voices, in conjunction with a medical voice team

sinus of Morgagni: Often confused with ventricle of Morgagni. Actually, the sinus of Morgagni is not in the larynx. It is formed by the superior fibers of the superior pharyngeal constrictor as they curve below the levator veli palatini and the eustachian tube. The space between the upper border of the muscle and the base of the skull is known as the sinus of Morgagni, and is closed by the pharyngeal aponeurosis

sinusitis: Infection of the paranasal sinus cavities

sinusoid: A graph representing the sine or cosine of a constantly increasing angle; in mechanics, the smoothest and simplest back-and-forth movement, characterized by a single frequency, an amplitude, and a phase; tone arising from sinusoidal sound pressure variations

sinusoidal motion: The projection of circular motion (in a plane) at constant speed onto one axis in the plane

skeleton: The bony or cartilaginous framework to which muscle and other soft tissues are attached

smoothed amplitude perturbation quotient (sAPQ): A relative evaluation of long-term variation of the peak-to-peak amplitude within the analyzed voice sample, expressed in percent

smoothed pitch perturbation quotient (sPPQ): A relative evaluation of long-term variation of the pitch period within the analyzed voice sample expressed in percent

soft glottal attack: Gentle glottal approximation, often obtained using an imaginary /h/

soft phonation index (SPI): A measure of the ratio of lower frequency harmonic energy to higher frequency harmonic energy. If the SPI is low, then the spectral analysis will show well-defined higher formants

solid: A substance that maintains its shape, independent of the shape of its container

soprano acuto: High soprano

soprano assoluto: A soprano who is able to sing all soprano roles and classifications

sound level: Logarithmic, comparative measure of the intensity of a signal; the unit is dB

sound pressure level (SPL): Measure of the intensity of a sound, ordinarily in dB relative to 0.0002 microbar (millionths of 1 atmosphere pressure)

sound propagation: The process of imparting a pressure or density disturbance to adjacent parts of a continuous medium, creating new disturbances at points farther away from the initial disturbance

source-filter theory: A theory that assumes the time-varying glottal airflow to be the primary sound source and the vocal tract to be an acoustic filter of the glottal source

source spectrum: Spectrum of the voice source

spasmodic dysphonia: A focal dystonia involving the larynx. May be of adductor, abductor, or mixed type. Adductor spasmodic dysphonia is characterized by strain-strangled interruptions in phonation. Abductor spasmodic dysphonia is characterized by breathy interruptions

speaker's formant: (*See* **Singer's formant**)

special sensory nerves: Nerves responsible for hearing, vision, taste, and smell

spectrogram: Three-dimensional graphic representation of sound with time on the x axis, frequency on the y axis, and amplitude displayed as intensity of color

spectrograph: The equipment that produces a spectrogram

spectrum: Ensemble of simultaneously sounding sinusoidal partials constituting a complex tone; a display of relative magnitudes or phases of the component frequencies of a waveform

spectrum analysis: Analysis of a signal showing its partials

speech-language pathologist: A trained, medically affiliated professional who may be skilled in remediation of problems of the speaking voice, swallowing, articulation, language development, and other conditions

speed: The rate of change of distance with time; the magnitude of velocity

spinto: Literally means *pushed* or *thrust*. Usually applies to tenors or sopranos with lighter voice than dramatic singers, but with aspects of particular dramatic excitement in their vocal quality. Enrico Caruso was an example

spirometer: A device for measuring airflow

stable equilibrium: A unique state to which a system with a restoring force will return after it has been displaced from rest

staccato: Each note accented and separated

standard deviation: The square root of the variance

standing wave: A wave that appears to be standing still; it occurs when waves with the same frequency (and wavelength) moving in opposite directions interfere with each other

state space: In abstract mathematics, the area in which a behavior occurs

stent: A device used for shape, support, and maintenance of patency during healing after surgery or injury

steroid: Steroids are potent substances produced by the body. They may also be consumed as medications. (*See* **Anabolic steroids, Corticosteroids**)

stochastic: Random from a statistical, mathematical point of view

stop band: A band of frequencies rejected by a filter; it is the low region in a filter spectrum

strain: Deformation relative to a rest dimension, including direction (eg, elongation per unit length)

strain rate: The rate of change of strain with respect to time

stress: Force per unit area, including the direction in which the force is applied to the area

striking zone: The middle third of the musculomembranous portion of the vocal fold; the point of maximum contact force during phonatory vocal adduction

stroboscopy: A technique that uses interrupted light to simulate slow motion. (*See* also **Strobovideolaryngoscopy**)

strobovideolaryngoscopy: Evaluation of the vocal folds utilizing simulated slow motion for detailed evaluation of vocal fold motion

Strohbass (German): "Straw bass"; another term for *pulse register* or *vocal fry*

subglottal: Below the glottis

subglottal pressure: Air pressure in the airway immediately below the level of the vocal folds. The unit most commonly used is centimeters of water. That distance in centimeters that a given pressure would raise a column of water in a tube

subglottic: The region immediately below the level of the vocal folds

subharmonic: A frequency obtained by *dividing* a fundamental frequency by an integer greater than 0

subjective assessment: Evaluation that depends on perception and opinion, rather than independently reproducible quantifiable measures, as opposed to objective assessment

sulcus vocalis: A longitudinal groove, usually on the medial surface of the vocal fold

superior: above

superior laryngeal nerves: Paired branches of the vagus nerve that supply the cricothyroid muscle and supply sensation from the level of the vocal folds superiorly

support: Commonly used to refer to the power source of the voice. It includes the mechanism responsible for creating a vector force that results in efficient subglottic pressure. This includes the muscles of the abdomen and back, as well as the thorax and lungs; primarily the expiratory system

supraglottal: Above the glottis, or level of the vocal folds

supraglottic: (1) Above the level of the vocal folds. This region includes the resonance system of the vocal tract, including the pharynx, oral cavity, nose, and related structures. (2) Posterior commissure. A misnomer. Used to describe the posterior aspect of the larynx (interarytenoid area), which is opposite the anterior commissure. However, there is actually no commissure on the posterior aspect of the larynx

suprahyoid muscle group: One of the two extrinsic muscle groups. Includes the stylohyoid muscle, anterior and posterior bellies of the digastric muscle, geniohyoid, hyoglossus, and mylohyoid muscles

temporal gap transition: The transition from a continuous sound to a series of pulses in the perception of vocal registers

temporomandibular joint: The jaw joint; a synovial joint between the mandibular condyle and skull anterior to the ear canal

tenor: Highest of the male voices, except countertenors. Must be able to sing to C_5. Singer's formant is around 2800 Hz

tenore serio: Dramatic tenor

testosterone: The hormone responsible for development of male sexual characteristics, including laryngeal growth

thin voice: A term used by singers to describe vocal weakness associated with lack of harmonic richness. The voice often also has increased breathiness, noise, and weakness and is commonly also described as "thready"

thoracic: Pertaining to the chest

thorax: The part of the body between the neck and abdomen

thready voice: (*See* **Thin voice**)

thyroarytenoid muscle: An intrinsic laryngeal muscle that comprises the bulk of the vocal fold (paired). The medial belly constitutes the body of the vocal fold

thyroid cartilage: The largest laryngeal cartilage. It is open posteriorly and is made up of two plates (thyroid laminae) joined anteriorly at the midline. In males, there is a prominence superiorly known as the "Adam's apple"

tidal volume: The amount of air breathed in and out during respiration (measured in liters)

timbre: The quality of a sound. Associated with complexity, or the number, nature, and interaction of overtones

tonsil: A mass of lymphoid tissue located near the junction of the oral cavity and pharynx (paired)

tonsillitis: Inflammation of the tonsil

tracheal stenosis: Narrowing in the trachea. May be congenital or acquired

tracheoesophageal fistula: A connection between the trachea and esophagus. May be congenital or acquired

trajectory: In chaos, the representation of the behavior of a system in state space over a finite, brief period of time. For example, one cycle on a phase plane plot

transcription: Converting the message in DNA to messenger RNA

transfection: Infection by naked viral nucleic acid

transglottal flow: Air that is forced through the glottis by a transglottal pressure

transition: With regard to the vocal fold, the intermediate and deep layers of lamina propria (vocal ligament)

translation: Using messenger RNA to make proteins

transverse: Refers to an anatomic plane that divides the body across. Also used to refer to a direction perpendicular to a given structure or phenomenon such as a muscle fiber or airflow

tremolo: An aesthetically displeasing, excessively wide vibrato (*See* **Wobble**). The term is also used in music to refer to an ornament used by composers and performers

tremor: A modulation in activity

trill: In early music (Renaissance) where it referred to an ornament that involved repetition of the same note. That ornament is now referred to as a *trillo*

trillo: Originally a trill, but in recent pedagogy a rapid repetition of the same note, which usually includes repeated voice onset and offset

triphthong: Three consecutive vowels that make up the same syllable

tumor: A mass or growth

turbulence: Irregular movement of air, fluid, or other substance, which causes a hissing sound. White water is a typical example of turbulence

turbulent airflow: Irregular airflow containing eddies and rotating patterns

tympanic membrane: Eardrum

unilateral vocal fold paralysis: Immobility of one vocal fold, due to neurological dysfunction

unstable equilibrium: The state in which a disturbance of a mechanical system will cause a drift away from a rest position

unvoiced: A sound made without phonation, and devoid of pitch; voiceless

upregulation: Increased gene expression, compared with baseline

variability: The amount of change, or ability to change

variance: The mean squared difference from the average value in a data set

vector: A quantity made up of two or more independent items of information, always grouped together

velar: Relating to the velum or palate

velocity: The rate of change of displacement with respect to time (measured in meters per second, with the appropriate direction)

velopharyngeal insufficiency: Escape of air, liquid or food from the oropharynx into the nasopharynx or nose at times when the nasopharynx should be closed by approximation of the soft palate and pharyngeal tissues

velum: The area of the soft palate and adjacent nasopharynx.

ventral: Toward the belly

ventricle of Morgagni: Also known as *laryngeal sinus*, and *ventriculus laryngis*. The ventricle is a fusiform pouch bounded by the margin of the vocal folds, the edge of the free crescentic margin of the false vocal fold (ventricular fold), and the mucous membrane between them that forms the pouch. Anteriorly, a narrowing opening leads from the ventricle to the appendix of the ventricle of Morgagni

ventricular folds: The "false vocal folds," situated above the true vocal folds

ventricular ligament: A narrow band of fibrous tissue that extends from the angle of the thyroid cartilage below the epiglottis to the arytenoid cartilage just above the vocal process. It is contained within the false vocal fold. The caudal border of the ventricular ligament forms a free crescentic margin, which constitutes the upper border of the ventricle of Morgagni

ventricular phonation: (*See* **Dysphonia plica ventricularis**)

vertical phase difference: With reference to the vocal folds, refers to the asynchrony between the lower and upper surfaces of the vibratory margin of the vocal fold during phonation

vertigo: Sensation of rotary motion. A form of dizziness

vibrato: In classical singing, vibrato is a periodic modulation of the frequency of phonation. Its regularity increases with training. The rate of vibrato (number of modulations per second) is usually in the range of 5–6 per second. Vibrato rates over 7–8 per second are aesthetically displeasing to most people, and sound "nervous." The extent of vibrato (amount of variation above and below the center frequency) is usually one or two semitones. Vibrato extending less than ±0.5 semitone are rarely seen in singers although they are encountered in wind instrument playing. Vibrato rates greater than two semitones are usually aesthetically unacceptable, and are typical of elderly singers in poor artistic vocal condition, in whom the excessively wide vibrato extent is often combined with excessively slow rate

viscera: The internal organs of the body, particularly the contents of the abdomen

visceral pleura: The innermost of two membranes surrounding the lungs

viscoelastic material: A material that exhibits characteristics of both elastic solids and viscous liquids. The vocal fold is an example

viscosity: Property of a liquid associated with its resistance to deformation. Associated with the "thickness" of a liquid

vital capacity: The maximum volume of air that can be exchanged by the lungs with the outside; it includes the expiratory reserve volume, tidal volume, and inspiratory reserve volume (measured in liters)

vocal cord: Old term for vocal fold

vocal fold (or cord) stripping: A surgical technique, no longer considered acceptable practice under most circumstances, in which the vocal fold is grasped with a forceps, and the surface layers are ripped off

vocal fold stiffness: The ratio of the effective restoring force (in the medial-lateral direction) to the displacement (in the same direction)

vocal folds: A paired system of tissue layers in the larynx that can oscillate to produce sound

vocal fry: A register with perceived temporal gaps; also known as *pulse register* and Strohbass. (*See* **Pulse register**)

vocal ligament: Intermediate and deep layers of the lamina propria. Also forms the superior end of the conus elasticus

vocal tract: Resonator system constituted by the larynx, the pharynx and the mouth cavity

vocalis muscle: The medial belly of the thyroarytenoid muscle

vocalise: A vocal exercise involving sung sounds, commonly vowels on scales of various complexity

voce coperta: "Covered registration"

voce mista: Mixed voice (also voix mixed)

voce di petto: Chest voice

voce sgangherata: "White" voice. Literally means immoderate or unattractive. Lacks strength in the lower partials

voce di testa: Head voice

voce piena: Full voice

voice abuse: Use of the voice in specific activities that are deleterious to vocal health, such as screaming

voice box: (*See* **Larynx**)

voice coach: (1) In singing, a professional who works with singers, teaching repertoire, language pronunciation, and other artistic components of performance (as opposed to a singing teacher, who teaches technique); (2) The term voice coach is also used by acting-voice teachers who specialize in vocal, bodily, and interpretive techniques to enhance dramatic performance

voice misuse: Habitual phonation using phonatory techniques that are not optimal and then result in vocal strain. For example, speaking with inadequate support, excessive neck muscle tension, and suboptimal resonance. Muscular tension dysphonia is a form of voice misuse

voice range profile: (*See* **Phonetogram**)

voice rest: (*See* **Absolute voice rest, relative voice rest**)

voice source: Sound generated by the pulsating transglottal airflow; the sound is generated when the vocal fold vibrations chop the airstream into a pulsating airflow

voice turbulence index (VTI): A measure of the relative energy level of high frequency noise

voiced: A language sound made with phonation, and possessing pitch.

voiceless: (*See* **Unvoiced**)

volume: "Amount of sound," best measured in terms of acoustic power or intensity

vortex theory: Holds that eddys, or areas of organized turbulence, are produced as air flows through the larynx and vocal tract

Vowel color: refers to vowel quality, or timbre, and is associated with harmonic content

Waldeyer's ring: An aggregation of lymphoid tissue in the pharynx, including the tonsils and adenoids

waveform: A plot of any variable (eg, pressure, flow, or displacement) changing as time progresses along the horizontal axis; also known as a time-series

wavefront: The initial disturbance in a propagating wave

wavelength: The linear distance between any point on one vibratory cycle and a corresponding point of the next vibratory cycle

whisper: Sound created by turbulent glottal airflow in the absence of vocal fold vibration

whistle register: The highest of all registers (in pitch). It is observed only in females, extending the pitch range beyond F_6

wobble: Undesirable vibrato, usually with vibrato rate of 2 to 4 Hz, and extent greater than ± 0.5 semitone (*See also* **Tremolo**)

xerostomia: Dry mouth

Young's modulus: The ratio between magnitudes of stress and strain

Index